Handbook of Headache

Handbook of Headache

Randolph W. Evans, M.D.
Chief of Neurology
Park Plaza Hospital

Clinical Associate Professor
Department of Neurology
University of Texas Medical School at Houston

Clinical Associate Professor
Department of Family and Community Medicine
Baylor College of Medicine
Houston, Texas

Ninan T. Mathew, M.D., F.R.C.P. (C).
Director
Houston Headache Clinic

Clinical Associate Professor
Department of Neurology
University of Texas Medical School
Houston, Texas

Former President
American Headache Society

Immediate Past President
International Headache Society

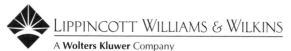

LIPPINCOTT WILLIAMS & WILKINS
A **Wolters Kluwer** Company
Philadelphia · Baltimore · New York · London
Buenos Aires · Hong Kong · Sydney · Tokyo

Acquisitions Editor: Anne M. Syd...
Developmental Editor: Sonya L. Seigafu...
Production Editor: Aureliano Vázquez...
Manufacturing Manager: Kevin Watt
Cover Designer: Kevin Kall
Compositor: Lippincott Williams & Wilkins Desktop Division
Printer: R.R. Donnelley-Crawfordsville

© 2000 by LIPPINCOTT WILLIAMS & WILKINS
530 Walnut Street
Philadelphia, PA 19106 USA
LWW.com

Printed in the USA

Library of Congress Cataloging-in-Publication Data
Handbook of headache / edited by Randolph W. Evans, Ninan T. Mathew.
   p. ; cm.
   Includes bibliographical references and index.
   ISBN 0-7817-1877-5
   1. Headache—Handbooks, manuals, etc.   I. Evans, Randolph W.
II. Mathew, Ninan T.
   [DNLM: 1. Headache—diagnosis—Handbooks. 2. Headache—therapy—Handbooks. WL 39 H2355 1999]
RB128.H346 1999
616.8′491—dc21   99-054157

10 9 8 7 6 5 4 3 2 1

Contents

Preface

Ninety percent of men and 95% of women have unprovoked headaches annually. Twenty-three million people in the United States have severe migraine headaches. The incidence of post-traumatic headaches is over 1 million persons per year. Furthermore, 9% of adults see physicians annually for headaches, making headaches one of the most common complaints of patients seeing primary care physicians.

Unfortunately, headache education during medical school and residency is frequently inadequate, and many physicians are less than enthusiastic about this topic. After reading this succinct volume, however, the primary care physician will be able to successfully diagnose and manage the great majority of headache patients. This book may also be of interest to neurologists since many uncommon topics are also examined.

The book begins with a general diagnostic approach to headaches. Then migraine, tension-type, chronic daily, cluster, first or worst, and posttraumatic headaches are reviewed. Chapters follow on headaches affecting various demographic groups including children and adolescents, women, and persons over the age of 50. Subsequent chapters cover short lasting head pains, vascular disorders, neoplasms, high and low pressure, HEENT disorders, other secondary headaches, and associated disorders. The final chapters feature interactive cases in "What's my Headache," and question and answer reviews in "The Headache Quiz." The book concludes with patient resources, educational materials, and a summary of alternative treatments.

With new diagnostic approaches and treatments becoming available, this is an exciting time for physicians and headache sufferers. We hope that, after you complete this book, you will be more confident and even enthusiastic in the evaluation and management of your patients with headaches.

We thank our editor at Lippincott Williams & Wilkins, Anne M. Sydor, Ph.D., for her encouragement and advice and the production team for their excellent work. Dr. Evans is indebted to his mentors in headache and neurology, K.M.A. Welch and Stanley H. Appel. He also appreciates the love and support of his wife, Marilyn, and children, Elliott, Rochelle, and Jonathan. Dr. Mathew appreciates the loving understanding of his wife, Sushila, whose support and encouragement have sustained him throughout his professional career. Dr. Mathew also appreciates the hard work of his transcriptionist, Ofelia F. Phillips, his office manager, Debbie Kennedy, and his study coordinator, Paula Gentry.

Randolph W. Evans, M.D.
Ninan T. Mathew, M.D.

About the Authors

Randolph W. Evans, M.D., is chief of Neurology at Park Plaza Hospital, and Clinical Associate Professor in both the Department of Neurology, University of Texas Medical School at Houston and the Department of Family and Community Medicine, Baylor College of Medicine. After receiving his B.A. from Rice University in 1974 and M.D. from Baylor College in 1978, Dr. Evans completed his internship and residency in Neurology at Baylor College of Medicine in 1982. He is board certified in Neurology and a fellow of the American Academy of Neurology and the American Headache Society. Dr. Evans is the co-editor of *Prognosis of Neurological Disorders*, first and second editions (1992 and 2000, respectively); editor of *Neurology and Trauma* (1996); and *Diagnostic Testing in Neurology* (1999); and associate editor of *Neurobase*. Dr. Evans is also the editor of four issues of "Neurologic Clinics," an issue of "Seminars in Neurology," and the author of numerous journal articles.

Ninan T. Mathew, M.D., is Director of the Houston Headache Clinic and Clinical Associate Professor in the Department of Neurology, University of Texas Medical School at Houston. He is immediate past-president of the International Headache Society, and immediate past-chairman of the Headache and Pain Section of the American Academy of Neurology. He is also the former president of the American Headache Society. He is on the editorial board of "Headache" and "Cephalalgia," and a regular reviewer for "Neurology," "Archives of Neurology," "Cephalalgia," and "Headache." Dr. Mathew has published more than 150 peer-reviewed articles and edited two volumes of "Neurologic Clinics" on headache and a monograph on cluster headaches.

Handbook of Headache

1

Diagnosis of Headaches

Randolph W. Evans

Headaches are a nearly universal experience, with a 1-year period prevalence of 90% and a lifetime prevalence of 99%. Twenty-three million Americans have migraines. Worldwide, an estimated 240 million persons suffer 1.4 billion migraine headaches yearly. Five percent of women and 2.8% of men have headaches 180 days or more per year. It is not surprising that headaches are one of the most common complaints seen by primary-care physicians. During a 1-year period in the United States, 9% of adults see physicians for headaches and 83% self-medicate. Television advertisements touting headache treatment with triptans, Tylenol, Motrin, and Excedrin Migraine are common.

The differential diagnosis of headaches is one of the longest in medicine, with more than 300 different types and causes (Table 1-1). The physician must diagnose headaches as precisely as possible.[1] Although most headaches are of benign and still poorly understood origin, some secondary headaches can have serious and sometimes life-threatening causes. As more specific medications become available, such as selective serotonin (5-HT$_1$) receptor agonists for migraine and cluster headaches or valproic acid for prophylaxis of migraine, accurate diagnosis is needed to choose the proper pharmacologic treatment.

For many of the headaches described in this book, the criteria of the 1988 International Headache Society (IHS) will be presented.[2] Since their introduction, the IHS criteria have become the worldwide standard for classification. Primary headaches, where there is no other underlying cause, include migraine, tension type, cluster, and miscellaneous headaches (such as benign exertional headaches). There are a large number of secondary headaches (Table 1-1), and the headaches are classified based upon their causes. A careful history, examination, and, in some cases, diagnostic testing usually permits headaches to be diagnosed correctly. However, sometimes a precise diagnosis may be impossible. For example, some benign headaches have both migraine- and tension-type features. Patients with chronic daily headaches may be difficult to classify.

PAIN-SENSITIVE STRUCTURES

Similar headaches can have different causes because there are a limited number of pain-sensitive structures (Table 1-2). Paradoxically, although all pain is felt in the brain, the brain parenchyma itself is not pain sensitive. The arachnoid, ependyma, and dura (except portions near vessels) are also not sensitive to pain. However, cranial nerves V, VII, IX, and X; the circle of Willis and proximal continuations; meningeal arteries; large veins in the brain and dura; and structures external to the skull (including scalp and neck muscles, cutaneous nerves and

Table 1-1.   Major categories of headache disorders

Migraine

Tension-type headache

Cluster headache and chronic paroxysmal hemicrania

Miscellaneous headaches unassociated with structural lesion
 Idiopathic stabbing, external compression, cold stimulus, benign
   cough, benign exertional, associated with sexual activity

Headache associated with head trauma

Headache associated with vascular disorders
 Acute ischemic cerebrovascular disorder, intracranial hematoma,
   subarachnoid hemorrhage, unruptured vascular malformation,
   arteritis, carotid or vertebral artery pain, venous thrombosis,
   arterial hypertension, associated with other vascular disorder

Headache associated with nonvascular intracranial disorder
 High and low cerebrospinal fluid pressure, intracranial infection,
   intracranial sarcoidosis and other noninfectious inflammatory
   disease, related to intrathecal injections, intracranial
   neoplasm, associated with other intracranial disorder

Headache associated with substances or their withdrawal
 Acute and chronic substance use or exposure, withdrawal after
   acute and chronic use, associated with substances with
   uncertain mechanism

Headache associated with noncephalic infection
 Viral infection, bacterial infection, other infection

Headache associated with metabolic disorder
 Hypoxia, hypercapnia, mixed hypoxia and hypercapnia,
   hypoglycemia, dialysis, other metabolic abnormality

Headache or facial pain associated with disorder of cranium, neck,
   eyes, ears, nose, sinuses, teeth, mouth, or other facial or cranial
   structures

Cranial neuralgias, nerve trunk pain, and deafferentation pain
 Persistent pain of cranial nerve origin, trigeminal neuralgia,
   glossopharyngeal neuralgia, nervus intermedius neuralgia,
   superior laryngeal neuralgia, occipital neuralgia, central
   causes of head and facial pain other than tic douloureux

Excerpted from Headache Classification Committee of the International
Headache Society. Classification and diagnostic criteria for headache disorders, cranial neuralgia, and facial pain. *Cephalalgia* 1988;8[Suppl 7]:1–96.

skin, the mucosa of paranasal sinuses, teeth, cervical nerves and
roots, and the external carotid arteries and branches) are sensitive to pain.

 In some cases, the location and source of the pain may be the
same (e.g., cheek or forehead pain from maxillary or frontal
sinusitis). However, because of referral patterns, the location of
the pain may not be the same as the source. For example, supratentorial structures are innervated by the ophthalmic division of
the trigeminal nerve, and the infratentorial or posterior fossa
structures are supplied by C_2 and C_3. Thus a cerebellar hemi-

**Table 1-2.   Pain-sensitive
structures that can cause headaches**

NOT the brain parenchyma

Transmitted through the trigeminal nerve and upper cervical
   segments

Intracranial structures
   Dura near vessels
   Cranial nerves V, VII, IX, X
   Circle of Willis and proximal continuations
   Meningeal arteries
   Large veins in the brain and dura

External to the skull
   Scalp and neck muscles
   Cervical nerves and roots
   Cutaneous nerves and skin
   Mucosa of the paranasal sinuses
   Teeth
   External carotid arteries and branches

sphere lesion generally refers pain posteriorly and an occipital
lobe lesion refers pain anteriorly.

   In addition, the caudal nucleus of the trigeminal nerve,
which is located from the midpons to the third cervical segment, also receives painful messages from the upper cervical
roots as well as the trigeminal nerve. Thus pain from the upper
cervical spine or posterior fossa can also be referred to the front
of the head.

THE HEADACHE HISTORY

   Most of the time, the headache history is essential to estab-
lishing the diagnosis.[3,4,4a] In the absence of an adequate headache history, unnecessary scans of the brain may be obtained or,
alternatively, a necessary scan may not be obtained. The key elements of the headache history are the following: temporal profile, headache features, associated symptoms and signs, aggravating or precipitating factors, relieving factors, evaluation and
treatment history, psychosocial history, family history, and a
complete medical and surgical history (Table 1-3). Table 1-4
gives examples of questions to ask to gather the key elements.

   Unfortunately for the busy clinician, some patients have more
than one type of headache. The presence of more than one type
may not be apparent at first. Both open-ended ("What are your
headaches like?") and close-ended ("Do you have nausea with the
headache?") approaches are necessary. Without specific prod-
ding, some patients will not remember to tell you about their
"sinus" or perimenstrual headaches or those they had when they
were younger that required bedrest. Other patients will need to
be told that the term *headache* includes any type and quality of
head and facial pain. A detailed account of each type is important. In some cases, it is helpful to ask about a history of mild
headaches and bad headaches. Some patients cannot clearly
remember or articulate features of the headache and will say

Table 1-3. Elements of the headache history

Temporal profile
  Age of onset
  Time to maximum intensity
  Frequency
  Time of day
  Duration
  Recurrence
Headache features
  Location
  Quality of pain
  Severity of pain
Associated symptoms and signs
  Before headache
  During headache
  After headache
Aggravating or precipitating factors
  Trauma
  Medical conditions
  Triggers
  Trigger zones
  Activity
  Pharmacologic
Relieving factors
  Nonpharmacologic
  Pharmacologic
Evaluation and treatment history
  Physicians and other health care providers
Psychosocial history
  Substance use
  Occupational and personal life
  Psychologic history
  Sleep history
  Impact of headache
Patient's own diagnosis
Family history
Complete medical and surgical history

something like, "It's just a headache, doc." When the patient has chronic headaches, sometimes it is necessary to provide a headache diary or have them record features of the headache(s) and then return for a later appointment. Examples follow of how the elements help you diagnose the headache.

Temporal Profile

Age of Onset

  Migraines usually begin before the age of 40; it is uncommon for them to start after the age of 50. In contrast, temporal arteritis typically begins after age 50 and is rare earlier.

Table 1-4. Helpful questions to ask for the headache history

Do you have different types of headaches or just one?

Where does the headache hurt?

When did you first start having these headaches?

What were you doing when the headache started?

How long before the headache is of maximal intensity?

How long does the headache last?

Does the headache recur?

How often do they occur?

What is the pain like? Is it a pressure, throbbing, pounding, aching, or stabbing?

Is the pain mild, moderate, or severe?

On a scale of 1 to 10, with 10 the worst and 1 the least, how would you rate the headache?

Do you have trouble with your vision before or during the headache?

Do you have other symptoms (e.g., nausea, vomiting, light sensitivity, noise sensitivity, discomfort with eye movement) with the headache?

Are signs (e.g., fever, ptosis, miosis) present?

Do you have triggers (e.g., menses, stress, foods, beverages, lack of sleep, oversleeping, strong odors, trigger zones) of your headaches?

Do activities (e.g., coughing, bending over, physical activity) make the headaches worse?

What (e.g., sleep, lying down in a quite room) makes the headache better?

Do your headaches have any impact on your life?

Do you take over-the-counter medications, vitamins, or herbs for your headaches? If so, how much and how often? Do you drink caffeinated beverages and, if so, what types and how many?

What prescription drugs have you tried and with what effect?

What doctors have you seen in the past for your headaches?

What other treatments (e.g., acupuncture, chiropractic, biofeedback, stress management, massage) have you tried and with what success?

Have you been under much stress lately?

Have you been depressed?

Do you have any parents or siblings with a history of migraines or bad headaches?

Time to Maximum Intensity

Thunderclap headaches, a severe headache with maximum intensity within 1 minute, can be caused by subarachnoid hemorrhage, carotid artery dissection, and migraine. Severe headaches can also have a gradual onset, such as migraine or viral meningitis.

Frequency

Primary headaches have widely variable frequency, ranging from a few migraines in a lifetime to cluster headaches that occur up to eight times each day.

Time of Day

Cluster headaches often occur during certain times of the day and may awaken the sufferer from sleep about the same time nightly. Although headaches that awaken people from sleep are usually benign (such as migraine, cluster, and hypnic), headaches can also result from brain tumors, meningitis, and subarachnoid hemorrhage. Tension-type headaches often occur in the afternoon.

Duration

Typical attack durations for primary headaches are as follows: migraine, 4 to 72 hours in adults; cluster headaches, 15 to 180 minutes; and tension-type headaches, 30 minutes to days. Trigeminal neuralgia is characterized by volleys of pain lasting a few seconds to less than 2 minutes.

Recurrence

About 30% of the time after using a triptan for migraine, the headache recurs.

Headache Features

Location

Cluster headaches are always unilateral, whereas about 60% of migraines are unilateral. Trigeminal neuralgia typically occurs unilaterally and is found more often in the second or third trigeminal distributions than in the first. Headaches from brain tumors or subdural hematomas can be bilateral or unilateral.

Quality of Pain

In about 50% of cases, migraine pain is throbbing, pounding, or pulsatile. Tension-type headaches consist of a sensation of pressure, aching, tightness, or squeezing. Cluster headaches are described as boring or burning. Trigeminal neuralgia is often an electrical or stabbing pain. Headaches due to brain tumors can produce a variety of pains, ranging from a dull, steady ache to throbbing.

Severity of Pain

When asking patients about severity, it is very helpful to use a scale of 1 (minimal) to 10 (the worst), even though the ranking may be subjective. For example, a similar headache rated a 7 by a stoic person may be rated a 12 by dramatic patients who want to emphasize the inadequacy of the 10-point scale to express their distress. Migraine pain can vary from mild to severe, and it can change from attack to attack. Severity of pain does not equate with the presence of life-threatening causes. The vast majority of severe headaches are due to migraine or cluster types. However, the new onset of severe headache should be taken very seriously. In contrast, some patients with headaches due to brain tumors or subdural hematomas may report a mild headache similar to a tension type that can be relieved by simple analgesics.

Associated Symptoms and Signs

Before the Headache

About 60% of migraineurs have a prodrome in the hours to days before the headache. Complaints may include changes in the mental state (e.g., irritability, depression, euphoria), neurologic symptoms (trouble with concentration; light, noise, and smell hypersensitivity), and general symptoms (diarrhea or constipation, thirst, sluggish feeling, food cravings, or neck stiffness). About 20% of migraines are those with an aura that generally develops over 5 to 20 minutes and lasts less than 60 minutes. The headache can begin before, during, or after the aura. The most common auras in descending frequency are visual, sensory, motor symptoms, and speech and language abnormalities.

Complaints prior to the headache are also very important in diagnosing other causes of headache. For example, low-grade fever and upper respiratory symptoms or diarrhea followed by headache are frequently present in viral meningitis.

During the Headache

Migraine is accompanied by nausea in 90%, vomiting in 30%, and light and noise sensitivity in 80%. These same symptoms are often present in headaches due to subarachnoid hemorrhage or meningitis. Ipsilateral conjunctival injection, tearing, and nasal congestion or drainage typically occur during cluster headaches. Ipsilateral ptosis and miosis are present in about 30% of cases.

After

After the headache resolves, many migraineurs complain of feeling tired and drained, with decreased mental acuity ("mashed potato brain"). Depression or euphoria is sometimes reported. In some systemic disorders, high fever and headache may be followed by other symptoms or signs.

Aggravating or Precipitating Factors

Trauma

Head and neck trauma are frequently followed by headaches. Headaches beginning after mild head injury are usually benign but raise concerns about a subdural or epidural hematoma present in up to 2%. Paradoxically, about 20% of those with milder degrees of head injuries or whiplash neck injuries may report headaches for months or years after the event, whereas those with more severe injuries may not have persistent headaches.

Medical Conditions

Other medical conditions may be associated with headaches. For example, although migraines often occur postpartum, preeclampsia and cortical venous thrombosis should be considered. During the second and third trimesters of pregnancy, migraines usually decrease in frequency. In 90% of cases, pseudotumor cerebri occurs in obese women. Paroxysmal hypertension with headaches suggests pheochromocytoma. New-onset headaches in someone who is HIV positive could be due to various causes such as cryptococcal meningitis. Headache in a person with a history of cancer (especially lung, breast, melanoma, colorectal, and hypernephroma) raises concern about metastatic disease. Persons with polycystic kidney disease have a 10% risk of having an intracranial saccular aneurysm.

Triggers

Eighty-five percent of migraineurs have one or more triggers. Various triggers include menstruation; stress or periods after stress; alcoholic beverages, especially red wine; foods such as chocolate, aged cheese, those containing monosodium glutamate, nitrates, and aspartame; environmental factors such as glare or flickering lights, loud noise, high altitude, heat and humidity, smoky rooms, and strong odors such as perfumes or cigarette smoke; and a missed meal or hunger. During periods of cluster headaches, alcohol can be a trigger. Tension-type headaches can be triggered by stress.

TRIGGER ZONES. Stimulation of certain areas of the face or mucous membranes of the mouth may trigger pain in trigeminal neuralgia. Washing the face, shaving, eating, speaking, feeling a breeze or cold air, and brushing the teeth may cause an attack. Glossopharyngeal neuralgia may similarly be triggered by swallowing, chewing, talking, coughing, or yawning.

ACTIVITY AND POSTURE. A variety of physical activities may trigger benign exertional headaches that can last 5 minutes to 24 hours, and such activities can also cause migraine. Coughing, sneezing, weightlifting, bending, stooping, or straining with a bowel movement can all trigger a bilateral headache of sudden onset that lasts less than 1 minute. Although usually benign, pathology such as Chiari malformations and posterior fossa tumors should be excluded (see Chapter 13). When these activities trigger a first, or worst, severe headache (see Chapter 6) lasting hours, subarachnoid hemorrhage should be considered. Exertional headache or jaw pain can occasionally be the presentation of angina. Physical activity and coughing may exacerbate migraine, postlumbar puncture headaches, and those due to brain tumors with mass effect. A severe explosive headache occurring just before or during orgasm can be due to benign orgasmic cephalalgia or subarachnoid hemorrhage. Low-cerebrospinal-pressure headaches can be brought on with sitting or standing and can be relieved by assuming the supine position. Headaches due to raised intracranial pressure may be worse in the supine position. The pain of acute frontal, ethmoid, and sphenoid sinusitis is worse when lying supine and better with the head in the upright position. Pain due to acute maxillary sinusitis is less when supine and worse in the upright position.

PHARMACOLOGIC TRIGGERS. Frequent use of many prescription or over-the-counter drugs can cause rebound headaches in susceptible persons or cause preventive medications to be ineffective. A detailed history of the use of acetaminophen, aspirin, caffeine (in many prescription and over-the-counter medications and beverages), butalbital, narcotics, triptans, ergotamine, and benzodiazepines is important. Headaches can be triggered or their frequency increased by the use of numerous medications, including oral contraceptives.

Relieving Factors

Nonpharmacologic Factors

Migraine headaches may resolve with sleep or improve with lying down in a dark, quiet room. Tension-type headaches may improve with relaxation for some people and with exercise in others. Massage or application of ice or heat may improve some headaches.

Pharmacologic Factors

Responses to prescription and over-the-counter treatments, including dosages and side effects, should be obtained in detail. Unless specifically asked, some patients will not volunteer use of nonprescription medications. Also ask about the use of herbs such as feverfew and vitamins such as riboflavin.

Evaluation and Treatment History

Other Physicians and Health Care Providers

It is very important to obtain a history of prior evaluations and treatment by physicians and other health professionals, including psychologists, chiropractors, acupuncturists, and physical therapists. In some cases, obtaining the medical records is essential. This can prevent unnecessary repeat testing or not trying a medication previously taken at too low a dose or for an inadequate period of time. Some patients are reluctant or do not disclose this information for various reasons, including their wish to get an independent evaluation or to conceal a history of medication abuse.

Psychosocial History

Substance Use

Ask about use and quantities of tobacco, alcohol, caffeine, and illicit drugs. Rebound headaches commonly occur from drinking as little as two to three cups of coffee daily.

Occupational and Personal Life

A variety of stressors can trigger and contribute to migraine and tension-type headaches. Occupational exposure to toxins should also be considered. The auto mechanic you see in the winter complaining of a headband-pressure-type headache in the afternoon that occurs only at work may have a headache triggered by high levels of carbon monoxide. A school history should be obtained from students.

Psychologic History

The treatment of many headaches requires addressing underlying or contributing psychologic factors, such as depression, stress, and anxiety.

Sleep History

The obese patient who snores may have sleep apnea that causes headaches in the morning. Sleep deprivation due to restless legs syndrome may contribute to migraine and tension-type headaches. Patients with sleep disturbance and frequent headaches may benefit from sedating tricyclic antidepressants. Sleep difficulties may be due to depression or anxiety.

Impact of Headache

What effect do the headaches have on occupational and personal life? Is the patient missing a lot of work, school, or home activities? Are there many "not tonight, I have a headache" nights damaging a relationship?

Patient's Own Diagnosis

In many cases, patients come to see you with their own diagnosis. You may think you have done a great job of diagnosing migraine correctly. However, the patient or family members think they have a headache due to "sinus," an aneurysm, a brain tumor, or spinal misalignment because their headache education is based upon sinus medication commercials, an internet search, anecdotes such as their cousin who had an aneurysm or their aunt with a brain tumor causing headaches, and visits with chiropractors. Patients often go through their differential diagnoses by seeing the ear, nose, and throat physician; optometrist; and chiropractor first. After getting a septoplasty, a new refraction, and manipulation without improvement, they may finally see a neurologist and receive a diagnosis of migraine. Before giving your diagnosis, simply ask what the patient or family members think is the cause. Then explain the basis for your diagnosis and how theirs is unlikely. Inappropriate demands for magnetic resonance imaging (MRI) or computed tomography (CT) scans can be averted and the patient may not shop around for other opinions.

Family History

A history of migraine is also present in perhaps 80% of first-degree relatives. Since more than 60% of those with migraine are not aware of the diagnosis, you may need to ask about a history of bad or sick headaches or perimenstrual headaches in family members. I have diagnosed numerous parents who came for their child's consultation with previously undiagnosed migraine. Perhaps 10% of those with a history of first-degree relatives with intracranial saccular aneurysm(s) have the same disorder. A family history of neurofibromatosis should also raise concern.

Complete Medical and Surgical History

A complete medical and surgical history is crucial not only to consider systemic causes of headache but also to be aware of possible contraindications to medications such as bronchial asthma and nonsteroidal antiinflammatory drugs or beta-blockers or coronary artery disease and triptans. A history of medication allergies or sensitivities is mandatory. (You know that you are in trouble with some patients who have chronic headaches when their list of drug "allergies" is longer than the Manhattan telephone directory or they are allergic to all pain pills (except Percodan.) Ipsilateral frontotemporal headaches can begin 36 to 72 hours after carotid endarterectomy and can last for months. Postural headaches after a lumbar laminectomy can be due to a dural tear and a cerebrospinal fluid (CSF) leak. A complete review of systems is also important. Galactorrhea and amenorrhea may be present in a woman with a pituitary macroadenoma causing headaches. Progressive weight loss and headaches may be present in cases of metastatic cancer or AIDS. Syncope and headaches could be due to a colloid cyst of the third ventricle.

PHYSICAL EXAMINATION

Abnormal vital signs such as fever or significantly elevated blood pressure may indicate the cause of the headache. A focused general examination may be informative. An erythematous oropharynx and posterior cervical adenopathy in a teenager with new-onset headaches often indicates infectious mononucleosis as the cause. In cases of possible meningitis or subarachnoid hemorrhage, neck stiffness or meningeal signs should be checked for. Findings of cervical region or suboccipital trigger points can suggest a myofascial cause of headaches. Temporomandibular joint tenderness, clicking, or limitation of movement may be seen when the joint is the source of headaches. In headaches due to frontal or maxillary sinusitis, there is usually tenderness to palpation over the affected sinus and nasal drainage.

Examination of arteries may be helpful. In patients with new-onset headaches over the age of 50, the superficial temporal artery should be checked for the presence of induration or a reduced or absent pulse consistent with temporal arteritis. Examining the carotids for pulses and bruits is important in patients at risk for atherosclerotic disease. The carotid bulb may be tender in cases of carotidynia or carotid dissection.

Even the skin exam may be useful. The teenager with acne and papilledema may have pseudotumor cerebri caused by Accutane. The patient with progressive headache and multiple café au lait spots may have neurofibromatosis and an intracranial schwannoma or meningioma. A skin rash, headache, and fever may signify viral meningitis or meningococcal meningitis.

Every patient seen for headaches should have at the least a screening neurologic examination, which can be performed within a few minutes. Although the exam is usually normal, you do not want to diagnose a patient with tension-type headaches when you might have discovered evidence of papilledema, a mild lateral rectus paresis, unequal pupils, a mild hemiparesis, or a Babinski sign if you had only bothered to perform a brief exam.

A SUMMARY OF THE FEATURES OF HEADACHES

Table 1-5 summarizes the features of the three most common primary headaches; Table 1-6 lists those of some secondary headaches.

Table 1-5. Features of some primary headaches

Feature	Migraine	Episodic tension-type	Episodic cluster
Epidemiology	18% of women, 6% of men 4% of children before puberty	90% of adults 35% of children ages 3–11	0.4% for men 0.08% for women
Female/male	3/1 after puberty, 1/1 before	5/4	1/5
Family history	80% of first-degree relatives	Frequent	Rare
Typical age at onset (years)	92% before age 40, 2% after age 50	20–40	20–40
Visual aura	In 20%	No	No
Location	Unilateral, 60%; bilateral, 40%	Bilateral > unilateral	Unilateral Especially orbital, periorbital, frontotemporal
Quality	Pulsatile or throbbing in 50%	Pressure, aching, tight, squeezing	Boring, burning, or stabbing
Severity	Mild to severe	Mild to moderate	Severe

Onset to peak pain	Minutes to hours	Hours	Minutes
Duration	4–72 hours May be <1 hour in children	Hours to days	15–180 minutes
Frequency	Rare to frequent	Rare to frequent	1–8 per day during clusters
Periodicity	Menstrual migraine	No	Yes Average bouts 4–8 weeks Average 1 or 2 bouts yearly
Associated features	Nausea in 90%, vomiting in 30%, light and noise sensitivity in 80%	Occasional nausea	Ipsilateral conjunctival injection, tearing, and nasal congestion or drainage Ptosis and miosis in 30%
Triggers	Present in 85% Numerous	Stress, lack of sleep	Alcohol, nitrates
Behavior during headache	Still, quiet, tries to sleep	No change	Often paces
Awakens from sleep	Can occur	Rare	Frequently

Table 1-6. Features of some secondary headaches

Headache type	Epidemiology	Age of onset	Location	Quality and severity	Frequency	Associated features	Comments
Trigeminal neuralgia	4.3/100,000/ year ♀/♂ = 1.6/1	Usually over 40 If <40, consider multiple sclerosis	Unilateral 96% 2nd or 3rd > 1st trigeminal division	Stabbing Electrical bursts Burning Last few secs <2 minutes	Few to many/ day	Trigger zone present >90%	Usually due to vascular compression of V. Scan needed to exclude occasional tumor
Brain tumor	Persona/yr in US 24,000 primaries 170,000 with metastases	Any age	Often bifrontal Unilateral or bilateral Any location	Variable can be pressure or throbbing Mild–severe	Occasional to daily. Usually progressive	Papilledema in 40% At time of diagnosis, headache present in 30% to 70%	Primaries in adults: lung, 64%; breast, 14%; unknown, 8%; melanoma, 4%; colorectal, 3%; hypernephroma, 2%
Pseudotumor cerebri	1/100,000/yr 90% are female 90% are obese	Mean of 30	Often bifronto–temporal but can occur in other locations and unilaterally	Pulsatile Moderate to severe	Daily	Papilledema in 95% Transient visual obscurations in 70% Intracranial noises in 60%	MRI scan preferred to better exclude cortical venous thrombosis and posterior fossa lesions

						VI nerve palsy in 20%	
Subarachnoid hemorrhage	30,000/yr in US due to saccular aneurysm	Mean of 50	Usally bilateral Any location	Usually severe but can be mild and gradually increasing	Paroxysmal	Often with nausea, vomiting, stiff neck, focal findings, syncope. Stiff neck absent in 36%	CT scan abnormal on first day 95%, third, 74%; 1 week, 50%. Lumbar puncture may be essential to diagnose
Temporal arteritis	In age >50, annual incidence 18/100,000 ♀/♂ = 3/1	Rare before 50 Mean age of 70	Variable Unilateral or bilateral Often temporo-frontal	Often throbbing / May be sharp, dull, burning, or lancinating Mild–severe	Intermittent to continuous	50% have PMR Jaw claudication in 38% 50% have absent pulse or tender STA	ESR within normal limits (WNL) in up to 36% CRP usually elevated STA biopsy false negative up to 44%

continued

Table 1-6. *Continued.*

Headache type	Epidemiology	Age of onset	Location	Quality and severity	Frequency	Associated features	Comments
Acute paranasal sinusitis	More common in children (in whom frontal and sphenoid sinusitis are rare) than in adults	Any age	Frontal—forehead, maxillary—cheek, ethmoid—between eyes, sphenoid—variable	Dull, aching Can be severe	Acute defined as fasting from 1 day to 3 weeks	Fever in about 50%. Nasal congestion and purulent nasal drainage usually present (less often in sphenoid)	Well visualized on routine MRI but not on routine CT scan of head. CT scan of the sinuses is the best study.
Subdural hematoma	Occurs in 1% after mild head injury in chronic cases, up to 50% without history of head injury	Any age	Unilateral or bilateral	Mild—severe May be aching, dull, or throbbing	Paroxysmal to constant	50% with normal neurology exam Alteration in consciousness and local findings may be present	MRI may detect occasional isodense subdural, which can be missed on CT scan

DIAGNOSTIC TESTING

Indications

For the vast majority of headaches, the diagnosis can be correctly made based upon the detailed history and examination without any testing at all. The decision for testing should be made on a case-by-case basis with guidelines suggested in the next section.[5–8] Other reasons that physicians order tests include the following: the quest for diagnostic certainty, faulty cognitive reasoning, the medical decision rule that holds that it is better to impute disease than to risk overlooking it, busy practice conditions in which tests are ordered as a shortcut, patient expectations, financial incentives, professional peer pressure where recommendations for routine and esoteric tests are expected as a demonstration of competence, and medicolegal concerns. The attitudes and demands of patients and families and the practice of defensive medicine are especially important reasons. A baseball player batting 0.990 could be paid $50 million yearly. However, a physician who is paid $50 for an office visit but has a similar "diagnosis average" and uses diagnostic testing appropriately could end up as a case on the civil docket.

Indicated testing may not be obtained in some circumstances. Under some managed-care plans, physicians may not order appropriate testing because of factors such as at-risk capitation and fear of deselection. Even when they order tests, insurance company reviewers may inappropriately deny certification as "not reasonable and not necessary." For many patients, testing is not obtained because of underinsurance and lack of funds. (There are now 40 million Americans without health insurance.)

Neuroimaging

A CT scan will detect most headaches caused by pathology. (Table 1-7 shows causes of headaches that can be missed on a routine CT scan.) The use of intravenous contrast may also reveal neoplasms and vascular malformations. The risk of reactions to intravenous contrast is as follows: mild, 10%; moderate, 1%; severe, .01%; and death, .002%. CT scan is superior to MRI for the demonstration of bony pathology, after acute head injury, and acute subarachnoid hemorrhage. However, numerous types of pathology can be missed on a routine CT scan.

MRI is superior to CT scan for evaluating headaches. The costs of CT scan and MRI are often about the same. In addition to general MRI contraindications, such as a pacemaker, about 8% of patients are claustrophobic, with about 2% to the point where they cannot tolerate the study. The yield of MRI may vary, depending on the field strength of the magnet, the use of paramagnetic contrast, the selection of acquisition sequences, and the use of magnetic resonance angiography and venography.

A routine MRI will demonstrate pathology of the paranasal sinuses, pituitary, posterior fossa, cortical veins (such as superior sagittal sinus thrombosis), and cervicomedullary junction (such as a Chiari malformation). In addition, MRI may find evidence of intracranial aneurysms, carotid dissection, infarcts, white matter abnormalities, congenital abnormalities, and neoplasms not seen on CT scan. Spiral CT scan and MRI angiography and

**Table 1-7. Causes of headache that can
be missed on routine CT scan of the head**

Vascular disease
  Saccular aneurysms
  Arteriovenous malformations (especially posterior fossa)
  Subarachnoid hemorrhage
  Carotid or vertebral artery dissections
  Infarcts
  Cerebral venous thrombosis
  Vasculitis (white matter abnormalities)
  Subdural and epidural hematomas
Neoplastic disease
  Neoplasms (especially in the posterior fossa)
  Meningeal carcinomatosis
  Pituitary tumor and hemorrhage
Cervicomedullary lesions
  Chiari malformations
  Foramen magnum meningioma
Infections
  Paranasal sinusitis
  Meningoencephalitis
  Cerebritis and brain abscess

venography are almost as sensitive as conventional cerebral angiography in the detection of aneurysms, arteriovenous malformations, arterial dissection, and venous thrombosis.

The yield of CT scan or MRI in patients with any headache and a normal neurologic examination is about 2%. A report of the Quality Standards Subcommittee of the American Academy of Neurology (AAN) in 1994 stated, "At this time, there is insufficient evidence to define the role of CT and MRI in the evaluation of patient with headaches that are not consistent with migraine."[9] Table 1-8 provides reasons to consider neuroimaging for headaches. Table 1-9 gives reasons to consider neuroimaging for children with headaches.

Patients who meet IHS criteria for migraine rarely have abnormal neuroimaging findings to explain the headache. The same AAN report stated, "In adult patients with recurrent headaches defined as migraine, including those with visual aura, with no recent change in headache pattern, no history of seizures, and no other focal neurologic signs or symptoms, the routine use of neuroimaging is not warranted. In patients with atypical headache patterns, a history of seizures, or focal neurologic signs or symptoms, CT or MRI may be indicated."

Electroencephalography

In the pre-CT-scan era, a skull series and electroencephalography constituted the standard testing for evaluation of headaches. Now, of course, CT and MRI scans are far superior to exclude structural lesions. The report of the Quality Standards Subcommittee of the AAN suggests the following practice para-

Table 1-8.   Reasons to consider neuroimaging for headaches

Temporal and headache features
  1. The "first or worst" headache
  2. Subacute headaches with increasing frequency or severity
  3. A progressive or new daily, persistent headache
  4. Chronic daily headache
  5. Headaches always on the same side
  6. Headaches not responding to treatment

Demographics
  7. New-onset headaches in patients who have cancer or who test positive for HIV infection
  8. New-onset headaches after age 50
  9. Patients with headaches and seizures

Associated symptoms and signs
  10. Headaches associated with symptoms and signs such as fever, stiff neck, nausea, and vomiting
  11. Headaches other than migraine with aura associated with focal neurologic symptoms or signs
  12. Headaches associated with papilledema, cognitive impairment, or personality change

Reasons obtained
  Tables 1-7 and 1-8
  The quest for diagnostic certainty
  Faulty cognitive reasoning
  The medical decision rule
  A shortcut in a busy practice
  Patient and family pressure
  Financial incentives
  Professional peer pressure
  Medicolegal issues: defensive medicine

Reasons not obtained
  Physician's fear of deselection and at-risk capitation
  Patient and/or family does not agree with necessity
  Lack of funds and underinsurance
  Insurance company's certification inappropriately denied

---

meter: "The electroencephalogram (EEG) is not useful in the routine evaluation of patients with headache. This does not exclude the use of EEG to evaluate headache patients with associated symptoms suggesting a seizure disorder such as atypical migrainous aura or episodic loss of consciousness. Assuming head imaging capabilities are readily available, EEG is not recommended to exclude a structural cause for headache."[10]

Blood Tests

Blood tests are generally not helpful for the diagnosis of headaches. However, there are numerous indications such as the following: erythrocyte sedimentation rate or C-reactive protein, to consider the possibility of temporal arteritis; a mono spot in a teenager with headaches, sore throat, and cervical adenopathy; a complete blood count (CBC), liver function test, HIV test, or

Table 1-9. Reasons to consider neuroimaging for children with headaches

1. Persistent headaches of less than 6 months' duration that do not respond to medical treatment
2. Headache associated with abnormal neurologic findings, especially if accompanied by papilledema, nystagmus, or gait or motor abnormalities
3. Persistent headaches associated with an absent family history of migraine
4. Persistent headache associated with substantial episodes of confusion, disorientation, or emesis
5. Headaches that awaken a child repeatedly from sleep or occur immediately on awakening
6. Family history or medical history of disorders that may predispose one to central nervous system lesions and clinical or laboratory findings suggestive of central nervous system involvement

Data from Medina LS, Pinter JD, Zurakowski D, et al. Children with headache: clinical predictors of surgical space-occupying lesions and the role of neuroimaging. *Radiology* 1997;202:819–824.

Lyme antibody in some patients with a suspected infectious basis; an anticardiolipin antibody and lupus anticoagulant in a migraineur with extensive white matter abnormalities on MRI; a TSH (thyroid stimulating hormone) level, since headache may be a symptom in 14% of cases of hypothyroidism; a CBC, since headache may be a symptom when the hemoglobin concentration is reduced by one-half or more; BUN (blood, urea, nitrogen) and creatinine, to exclude renal failure, which can cause headache; serum calcium, since hypercalcemia can be associated with headaches; CBC and platelets, because thrombotic thrombocytopenic purpura can cause headaches; and endocrine studies in a patient with headaches and a pituitary tumor.

Additionally, blood tests may be indicated as a baseline and for monitoring certain medications such as valproic acid for migraine prophylaxis, carbamazepine for trigeminal neuralgia, and lithium for chronic cluster headaches.

Lumbar Puncture

MRI or CT scan is always performed before a lumbar puncture for the evaluation of headaches except in some cases where acute meningitis is suspected. Lumbar puncture can be diagnostic for meningitis or encephalitis, meningeal carcinomatosis or lymphomatosis, subarachnoid hemorrhage, and high (e.g., pseudotumor cerebri) or low CSF (Table 1-10). In cases of blood dyscrasias, the platelet count should be 50,000 or greater before safely performing the lumbar puncture. The CSF opening pressure should always be measured when investigating headaches. When measuring the opening pressure, it is important for the patient to relax and at least partially extend the head and legs to avoid recording a falsely elevated pressure.

**Table 1-10. Causes of headache that
can be diagnosed by lumbar puncture**

1. Infection (meningitis and encephalitis)
2. Neoplastic disease (meningeal carcinomatosis and lymphomatosis)
3. Subarachnoid hemorrhage
4. High and low cerebrospinal fluid pressure

After neuroimaging as discussed, examples where lumbar puncture is often indicated include the following: the first or worst headache; headache with fever or other symptoms or signs suggesting an infectious cause; a subacute or progressive headache (e.g., an HIV-positive patient or a person with carcinoma); and an atypical chronic headache (e.g., to rule out pseudotumor cerebri in an obese woman without papilledema).

REFERENCES

1. Evans RW. Diagnosis of headaches. *Drugs Today* 1997;33:79–93.
2. Headache Classification Committee of the International Headache Society. Classification and diagnostic criteria for headache disorders, cranial neuralgia, and facial pain. *Cephalalgia* 1988; 8[Suppl 7];1–96.
3. Lance JW, Goadsby PJ. *Mechanism and management of headache,* 6th ed. Oxford: Butterworth Heinemann, 1998.
4. Silberstein SD, Lipton RB, Goadsby PJ. *Headache in clinical practice.* Oxford: Isis, 1998.
4a. Olesen J, Tfelt-Hansen P, Welch KMA (eds). The Headaches, 2nd edition. Philadelphia: Lippincott Williams, & Wilkins, 2000.
5. Evans RW. Diagnostic testing for the evaluation of headaches. *Neurol Clin* 1996;14:1–26.
6. Standards of Care Committee. *Standards of care for headache diagnosis and treatment as established by the National Headache Foundation.* Chicago: National Headache Foundation, 1996:1–30.
7. Frishberg BM. Neuroimaging in presumed primary headache disorders. *Semin Neurol* 1997;17:373–382.
8. Evans RW. The evaluation of headaches. In: Evans RW, ed. *Diagnostic testing in neurology.* Philadelphia: WB Saunders, 1999: 1–18.
9. American Academy of Neurology. The utility of neuroimaging in the evaluation of headache in patients with normal neurologic examinations. *Neurology* 1994;44:1353–1354.
10. American Academy of Neurology. Practice parameter: the electroencephalogram in the evaluation of headache. *Neurology* 1995;45:1411–1413.

Migraine

Ninan T. Mathew

INTRODUCTION AND EPIDEMIOLOGY

The last 15 years have witnessed a great deal of advance in our understanding of the pathophysiology, pharmacology, epidemiology and genetics of migraine. The International Headache Society (IHS) classifies headaches into primary headache disorders and secondary headache disorders (Chapter 1).[1] Migraine with and without aura, tension-type headache (episodic and chronic), and cluster headache (episodic and chronic) form most primary headache disorders (Table 2-1). The IHS diagnostic criteria are given in Table 2-2.

Prevalence of Migraine

The migraine prevalence in the United States is 17.6% for females and 6% for males using the IHS criteria for migraine diagnosis.[2] Similar high incidence is found in the European countries and most parts of the world except in China, where the prevalence is lower.[3] In the United States, among the females, Caucasians have more migraine (20.4%) than African-Americans (16.2%), with the Asians having the least prevalence of migraine (9.2%).[3] This may indicate a genetic component. Migraine prevalence is highest in the peak productive years of life (between 25 and 55 years of age). Prevalence is greater in females than in males after 12 years of age, but sex ratio varies with age. In children, both males and females have a fairly equal prevalence of migraine before the age of puberty. Three studies suggest that migraine prevalence may be increasing in the United States.[4–6] An analysis of data from the Centers for Disease Control showed that prevalence increased 60% from 25.8 per 1,000 population in 1981 to 41 per 1,000 population in 1989.

Impact of Migraine

The impact of headache disorders on individuals and on society is large and provides an important target for public health intervention. Despite widespread disability produced by migraine, this disorder is still underrecognized and undertreated.[7]

The public health significance of migraine has been of interest in the recent years. The high prevalence of this disorder is one of the measures of the significance of migraine. According to the American Migraine Study, there are 23 million people in the United States with severe migraine headache.[8] Most migraineurs experience frequent attacks. Twenty-five percent of women experience four or more severe attacks per month, 35% experience one to three severe attacks per month, and 40% experience one or less than one severe attack per month. Similar frequency patterns of migraine were observed in men.[2,8]

Table 2-1. IHS classification of primary headaches

1. Migraine
   1.1 Migraine without aura
   1.2 Migraine with aura
      1.2.1 Migraine with typical aura
      1.2.2 Migraine with prolonged aura
      1.2.3 Familial hemiplegic migraine
      1.2.4 Basilar migraine
      1.2.5 Migraine aura without headache
      1.2.6 Migraine with acute-onset aura
   1.3 Ophthalmoplegic migraine
   1.4 Retinal migraine
   1.5 Childhood periodic syndromes that may be precursors to or
       associated with migraine
      1.5.1 Benign paroxysmal vertigo of childhood
      1.5.2 Alternating hemiplegia of childhood
   1.6 Complications of migraine
      1.6.1 Status migrainosus
      1.6.2 Migrainous infarction
   1.7 Migrainous disorder not fulfilling preceding criteria
2. Tension-type headache
   2.1 Episodic tension-type headache
      2.1.1 Episodic tension-type headache associated with disorder
            of pericranial muscles
      2.1.2 Episodic tension-type headache unassociated with
            disorder of pericranial muscles
   2.2 Chronic tension-type headache
      2.2.1 Chronic tension-type headache associated with disorder
            of pericranial muscles
      2.2.2 Chronic tension-type headache unassociated with
            disorder of pericranial muscles
   2.3 Headache of the tension type not fulfilling preceding criteria
3. Cluster headache and chronic paroxysmal hemicrania
   3.1 Cluster headache
      3.1.1 Cluster headache, periodicity undetermined
      3.1.2 Episodic cluster headache
      3.1.3 Chronic cluster headache
         3.1.3.1 Unremitting from onset
         3.1.3.2 Evolved from episodic
   3.2 Chronic paroxysmal hemicrania
   3.3 Cluster headache–like disorder not fulfilling preceding
       criteria

More than 85% of women and more than 82% of men with severe headache had some headache-related disability.[8] About one-third were severely disabled or needed bedrest during the attack. Many other studies have examined various aspects of headache-related disability. Migraine is not just an episodic disease; it is also a chronic disease with episodic exacerbations. Many migraineurs live in fear, knowing that an attack will disrupt their ability to work, to take care of their families, or to meet social obligations. Thus there is some disability between attacks as well as during

**Table 2-2.   Diagnostic criteria
for migraine without and with aura**

Migraine without aura

A.   At least five attacks fulfilling B–D

B.   Headache attacks lasting 4–72 h (untreated or unsuccessfully treated)

C.   Headache with at least two of the following characteristics:
   1.   Unilateral location
   2.   Pulsating quality
   3.   Moderate or severe intensity (inhibits or prohibits daily activities)
   4.   Aggravation by walking stairs or similar routine physical activity

D.   During headache at least one of the following:
   1.   Nausea and/or vomiting
   2.   Photophobia and phonophobia

E.   At least one of the following:
   1.   History and physical and neurologic examinations do not suggest one of the disorders listed in groups 5–11 (headaches secondary to organic or systemic metabolic disease).
   2.   History and/or physical and/or neurologic examinations do suggest such disorder, but it is ruled out by appropriate investigations.
   3.   Such disorder is present, but migraine attacks do not occur for the first time in close temporal relation to the disorder.

Migraine with aura

A.   At least two attacks fulfilling B

B.   At least three of the following four characteristics:
   1.   One or more fully reversible aura symptoms indicate focal cerebral cortical and/or brain stem dysfunction.
   2.   At least one aura symptom develops gradually over more than 4 minutes or two or more symptoms occur in succession.
   3.   No aura symptom lasts more than 60 minutes. If more than one aura symptom is present, accepted duration is proportionally increased.
   4.   Headache follows aura with a free interval or less than 60 minutes. (It may also begin before or simultaneously with the aura.)

C.   At least one of the following:
   1.   History and physical and neurologic examinations do not suggest one of the disorders listed in groups 5–11 (headaches secondary to organic or systemic metabolic disease).
   2.   History and/or physical and/or neurologic examinations do suggest such disorder, but it is ruled out by appropriate investigations.
   3.   Such disorder is present, but migraine attacks do not occur for the first time in close temporal relation to the disorder.

attacks. These more chronic disabling effects generally have not been well studied. The health-related quality-of-life measurements have shown that, compared with such other chronic illnesses as hypertension, diabetes, and coronary artery disease, migraine has lower scores in physical functioning, role functioning (physical), bodily pain, and other health aspects.[9] Patients with chronic daily headaches have even lower scores in physical functioning, role functioning, bodily pain, and general health as well as mental health measures using the short form 36 (SF 36) instrument.[10]

Through its effect on individuals, migraine has a serious impact on society. In Washington County, Maryland, 8% of males and 14% of females missed all or part of a day of work or school because of headaches in the 4-week period prior to the interview.[11] Annual costs of lost productivity resulting from migraine in the United States have been estimated to range from $1.2 billion to $17.2 billion.

Data from a population-based sample of about 2,000 migraineurs show that most disabled, 50% of migraine sufferers, account for more than 90% of all work loss due to migraine. Because work loss is the principal driver of cost of illness, these findings imply that health care intervention should be directed to this most disabled segment of the migraine population.[12]

The direct cost of migraine from use of health care facilities is also substantial. National ambulatory medical care survey conducted from 1976 to 1977 reported that more than 10 million office visits to physicians were for headache. Migraine also results in frequent use of emergency rooms and urgent-care facilities. Many prescription and over-the-counter medications are taken for headache disorders.

Genetics of Migraine

Approximately 70% of patients with migraine give a positive family history of migraine. Genetic influence is most striking in migraine with aura.

Recent advances in genetics of migraine indicate that familial hemiplegic migraine (FHM), a rare variety of migraine, is linked to chromosome 19P and to at least one other locus. Several-point mutations in a gene on chromosome 19P that codes for a calcium channel α_1-subunit have been linked to FHM families.[13,14] Hereditary paroxysmal cerebellar ataxias are also linked to the same region on chromosome 19, suggesting a possible role of a calcium channel in these disorders. The calcium channel is a P/Q type, and specific medications with specific P/Q channel antagonism, which hopefully will be developed in the future, may have more specific effects on this type of migraine and related disorders. So far, there have been no convincing studies to show the same type of defect in migraine with and without aura. Other studies have indicated that dopaminergic genes may be involved in migraine.[15] At present, from the various genetics studies, it can only be concluded that multiple genes are involved in the pathogenesis of migraine and its frequent comorbid conditions. Rare causes of migraine may be monogenic, as in the case of familial hemiplegic migraine. Combinations of multiple genes cause common forms of migraine. The environmental and psychologic factors also play a part in the clinical manifestations of migraine.

DIAGNOSIS

Physicians should appreciate the fact that primary headache disorders, such as migraine, tension-type headache (Chap. 3), and cluster headache (Chap. 4), are much more common (about 90% of all headaches) than secondary headache disorders (Chap. 11, 12, 13). Headache disorders can exist without any obvious structural or metabolic cause. It is also important to emphasize that recurrent episodic headaches are rarely due to structural lesions.

Table 2-2 gives the universally accepted IHS criteria for diagnosis of migraine with aura and migraine without aura.

Positive Diagnosis of Migraine

Migraine is a syndrome with a wide variety of neurologic and nonneurologic manifestations; it is not simply a headache. Diagnosis of migraine is not obtained solely by exclusion of other disorders: positive diagnosis is possible. This positive diagnosis should be based on information about the attack profile, on identification of probable triggers, and on understanding of the clinical spectrum, variability, and natural history of migraine. Positive diagnosis requires a good history of the disorder, including accompanying symptoms and triggers. Also essential are brief physical and neurologic examinations, which can afford the most relevant information. A history of previous recurrent episodes, which is often neglected by physicians, and investigation of any family history are useful. About 70% of migraineurs have a positive family history.

The four different phases of migraine to be recognized are prodrome, aura, headache (during which associated symptoms are experienced), and recovery phase (Fig. 2-1). However, in a given patient and individual attack, only some of these stages may be present. For example, patients may have aura without headache or headache without any other stages. There is still a false impression among some physicians that aura is necessary for diagnosis of migraine. The same person can have both types of migraine (migraine with and without aura) at different times.

Prodrome and Aura

Prodrome is not always present in migraine. It may be difficult to identify, but if patients are specifically asked about premonitory symptoms in the 24-hour period before the headache, they often describe symptoms, such as irritability, excitability, hyperactivity, or depression, that they would not otherwise mention and that are helpful in diagnosis. The aura is more easily recognized, and information may be volunteered by the patient, but the physician must ask about this phase. Visual auras are the most common. Photopsia (e.g., spots, specks of colors, and lines) forms almost 75% of these paresthesias (Fig. 2-2)—often starting in the hand, going up the arm, and involving the face, lips, and tongue—and is the second most common aura.

Headache Phase

About 60% of headaches in migraine are unilateral or predominantly unilateral. It is important to emphasize that the

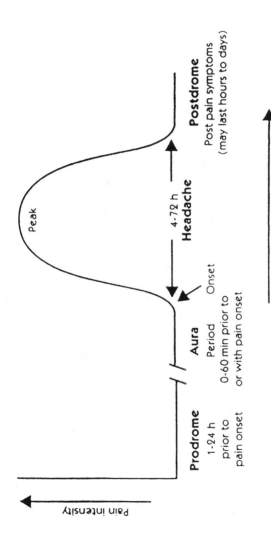

Figure 2-1. The four phases of a migraine attack.

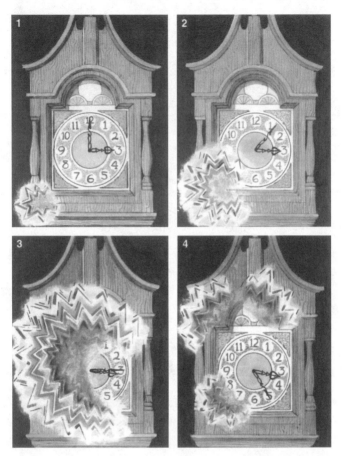

Figure 2-2. Scintillating, fortification scotoma of migraine appears in one portion of the visual field, typically enlarges to cover central fixation, and then "marches" toward the periphery and breaks apart. Entire phenomenon lasts 15–30 minutes. (Reprinted with permission from Hupp Sl, Kline LB, Corbett JJ. Visual disturbances of migraines. *Surv Ophthalmol* 1989;33:221–236.)

headache can switch sides: It can start on one side and go to the other side during the same attack, or it may be on different sides in different attacks. Although it is important to understand unilaterality and the ability of the headache to switch sides to reach a proper diagnosis, bilateral headache does not exclude the diagnosis of migraine.

A pulsating headache is not always diagnostic of migraine. For example, someone with a fever and vasodilatation may have a pulsating headache, as do some patients with brain tumors. Migraine headache is of moderate to severe intensity and is often aggravated by any activity or posture that increases intracranial pressure, such as coughing or sneezing, bending down, or climbing stairs.

The associated symptoms are also important. Nausea and/or vomiting often accompany headache and are helpful diagnostic features. They accompany any process that increases intracranial pressure or causes meningeal irritation. There may be heightened sensory perception, photophobia, phonophobia, and dislike of smells. There may also be orthostatic hypotension and dizziness. The behavior of patients during attacks may be altered: They may be irritable and seek to be left alone in a dark room, their verbal expression may be difficult, and their memory and concentration may be poor. This may be misdiagnosed as a psychologic condition. It is important to emphasize that such mental changes can occur during migraine attacks. Other features to support positive diagnosis of migraine are relief after sleep, relief after vomiting, exhaustion when the headache is over, and relief during pregnancy.

Trigger Factors for Migraine

Identification of a provocational trigger for a headache is evidence in support of the classification of the headache as benign: It is unusual for an organic disorder to show sensitivity to triggers. Physicians should be familiar with the common triggers for migraine listed in Table 2-3. It is important to emphasize that triggers vary between migraine attacks in any one patient, but identification of trigger factors is helpful in positive diagnosis of migraine.

A history of menstrual headaches or headache during ovulation almost certainly implies migraine, as does headache trig-

Table 2-3.   Common provocational triggers for migraine

Triggers for migraine	
Hormonal triggers	Menstruation, ovulation, oral contraceptive, hormonal replacement
Dietary triggers	Alcohol, nitrite-laden meat, monosodium glutamate, aspartame, chocolate, aged cheese, missing a meal
Psychologic triggers	Stress, period after stress (weekend or vacation), anxiety, worry, depression
Physical-environmental triggers	Glare, flashing lights, visual stimulation, fluorescent lighting, odors, weather changes, high altitude
Sleep-related triggers	Lack of sleep, excessive sleep
Miscellaneous triggers	Head trauma, physical exertion, fatigue
Drugs	Nitroglycerine, histamine, reserpine, hydralazine, ranitidine, estrogen

gered by alcohol, nitrite-laden food, and so on. Weekend headache or headache on the first day of vacation is common in migraine. For a person with a history of migraine, relatively minor head or neck trauma can trigger migrainelike episodes, which may respond to migraine treatments.

Provocative test for diagnosis with such agents as reserpine, histamine, or fenfluramine is not reliable and should not be used.[16] Nor are therapeutic tests useful.[16] In the past, doctors sometimes considered a positive response to ergotamine to be diagnostic of migraine. Now many physicians falsely believe that if a patient does not respond to sumatriptan, then he/she does not have migraine. Even with the new 5-HT$_1$ agonists, not all attacks respond to treatment, and response to drugs should never be a criterion for diagnosis.

Differential Diagnosis of Primary Headaches

It is important to make a differential diagnosis between migraine, tension-type headache (Chap. 3), and cluster headache (Chap. 4) because the optimal treatments may differ. Distinguishing characteristics are illustrated in Table 2-4, and all these features should be considered together to form the diagnosis. For example, 60% of migraines are predominantly unilateral, whereas all cluster headaches are unilateral, and tension-type headaches are bilateral. It is impossible to make a diagnosis of migraine from the location alone: It could be the back, front, or sides. The pain in tension-type headache is diffuse, whereas for cluster headache it is almost always periorbital or retroorbital.

The frequency of headaches varies greatly between patients. Tension-type headache might occur from once a month to 30 days a month. About 30% of migraineurs in the general population have more than four attacks a month, and clinic patients have even more. Cluster headaches are extremely severe, whereas tension-type headache is normally mild or moderate. The duration of attacks varies and it is important to emphasize that migraine may vary from the 4 to 72 hours specified in the International Headache Society (IHS) classification.[1] Children have shorter headaches, and some adults with chronic headaches may have prolonged migraine lasting for much longer than 72 hours. Cluster headache is of short duration and may be repeated many times a day.

The character of pain may be helpful in differential diagnosis: migraine headache is throbbing and pulsating; tension-type headache is dull; and cluster headache pain is described as sharp, boring, and not throbbing. Periodicity is important. Typically, cluster headache has a characteristic periodicity of 2 to 3 months of headache and remission for a year, whereas there are only rare examples of periodic migraine.

Aura preceding headache is invariably diagnostic of migraine and is not seen in the other primary headaches. Such autonomic features as watering from the eyes, redness of the eyes, and runny nose are diagnostic of cluster headache, but occasionally patients with migraine also have some autonomic features in and around the eyes. Vomiting, nausea, and photophobia are seen predominantly in migraine and are rare in other conditions. In migraine, movement often aggravates the headaches, whereas

Table 2-4. Differential diagnosis of primary headaches

Clinical features	Migraine	Tension-type headache	Cluster headache
Males: females	25:75	40:60	90:10
Lateralization	60% unilateral	Diffuse bilateral	100% unilateral
Location	Frontal, periorbital temporal, hemicranial	Diffuse	Periorbital
Frequency	1–4 per month	1–30 per month	1–3 per day for 3–12 months
Severity	Moderate/severe	Mild/moderate	Extremely severe
Duration	4–72 h	Variable	15 min–3 h
Pain character	Throbbing, pulsating	Dull	Sharp, boring
Periodicity	±	–	+++
Family history	+++	±	±
Associated symptoms			
Aura	+++	–	–
Autonomic features	±	–	+++
Nausea/vomiting	+++	–	±
Photo/phonophobia	+++	–	±
Exacerbation by movement	+++	–	–

cluster headache patients like to move around: Some run on the spot to get some relief from their pain.

Family history is important in diagnosis. It has been shown that, like migraine, chronic tension-type headache may be familial, whereas episodic tension-type headache is not.

Status migrainosus refers to a severe attack of migraine lasting for more than 72 hours. Patients are usually extremely sick with nausea, vomiting, and dehydration. This should be considered a medical emergency.

Complicated migraine with neurologic symptoms and signs, which is more often seen in the young, is described in Chapter 7.

Differentiation from Organic Disorders

Two particular diagnostic problems are organic conditions that mimic primary headache disorders and organic conditions that coexist with migraine because migraine is such a common disorder. For example, a patient may have a brain tumor or an aneurysm as well as migraine.

Normally, migraines begin gradually and take 3 to 4 hours to peak. Some patients have abrupt headaches that peak in seconds, called *crash migraine*[17] This type of abrupt-onset headache may resemble thunderclap headache (Chap. 5).[18] It is difficult to distinguish this from ruptured intracranial aneurysm. About 25% of thunderclap headaches arise from a rupturing aneurysm, whereas 75% are benign, migraine-like headaches. Sometimes carotid artery dissections cause an acute rapid-onset headache with facial pain, eye symptoms similar to an aura, partial Horner's syndrome, and severe unilateral head pain similar to migraine (Chapter 11). Diagnosis is facilitated somewhat because these conditions usually occur in a patient who has not had headaches before.

Table 2-5 lists particular warning signs that a physician should be aware of and investigate carefully (Chapter 1). So-called sudden-onset first headache and the "worst headache ever" should be investigated with neuroimaging. If that is negative, a lumbar puncture should be performed. There are case reports of negative computed tomography scan and lumbar punctures in patients with aneurysms,[18] so we recommend doing

Table 2-5. Headache alarms that should alert the physician to the need for further investigation

Sudden-onset "first" headache

"Worst headache ever"

Late-onset new headache

Headache with fever, rash, stiff neck

Progressively increasing headache

Headache with neurologic signs and symptoms other than aura

Headache with mental changes

Headache with papilledema

New-onset headache in a patient with cancer or HIV

at least a magnetic resonance angiography to explore subarachnoid hemorrhage and aneurysm.

Late-onset new headache refers to a person who has not had headaches before 55 years of age. Headache with fever, rash, and neck stiffness might arise from meningitis or other conditions. Headache with mental changes, especially in the elderly, might be caused by subdural hematoma. Headache with papilledema must be investigated for signs of intracranial pressure secondary to a brain tumor or idiopathic intracranial hypertension. New-onset headache in a person with cancer or HIV must also be investigated.

Treatment for sufferers of headaches would be greatly improved if doctors were more motivated and suitably educated to attempt differential diagnosis of the headache disorders. It should be recognized that secondary headache disorders are not common and usually can be excluded by a simple physical and neurologic examination coupled with a good history of previous headaches. The information obtained should then be used to diagnose the primary headache disorder and appropriate treatment programs should be applied. The benefits in avoiding unnecessary delay in adequate relief for the patient, reducing lost productivity, and negating the need for frequent follow-up visits should outweigh any additional time spent in the initial consultation.

Patients with migraine are more prone to tension-type headache in between their acute migraine attacks, leading to a mixed headache syndrome. The tension-type headaches in migraineurs are somewhat different from episodic tension-type headache. They are more frequent and more severe. They may be associated with nausea, photophobia, and phonophobia, unlike episodic tension-type headache. They may be triggered by the same factors that trigger their migraines. So these observations lead to the concept of a continuum in primary headache disorders. At one end of the spectrum is the typical migraine with aura and without aura; at the other end of the spectrum is the chronic tension-type headache. But in the middle of the spectrum, there are mixed forms of migraine and tension-type headache, which can sometimes become daily or nearly so in many patients.

Analgesic Rebound

One of the major factors that leads to transformation of episodic migraine into chronic daily headache (transformed migraine) with mixed features of migraine and tension-type headache is excessive use of analgesics.[19] This is referred to as *analgesic rebound headache.* The most commonly used medications, which lead to analgesic rebound, are over-the-counter pain medications, which contain caffeine. Some of the agents have caffeine up to 60 mg per tablet. It is not uncommon for chronic headache sufferers to take 8 to 10 tablets of analgesic per day. Prescription pain medications, particularly combination analgesics with barbiturates and caffeine, are also very high in the list that cause rebound headaches. Patients who have daily headache and take a large quantity of pain medications do not seem to respond to preventive medications used concomitantly.

The pain medications used daily make the headache process more resistant to treatment and very persistent. Detoxification from these medications will improve the headache frequency and will make the headache more responsive to preventive treatment.[20] Anybody with frequent headaches who is taking pain medications or over-the-counter prescriptions regularly should be evaluated for analgesic rebound and treated accordingly.

MANAGEMENT

Current Concepts in Acute Migraine Treatment

Doctors treating migraine face important decisions on how to optimize treatment for individual patients. Migraine patients would receive faster resolution of their pain and disability if physicians were more often able to identify successful therapies at the first consultation. This might be achieved by using assessment of the level of disability caused by migraine to assign patients to treatment groups rather than using the same sequence of treatment options for all patients. The development of strategies for optimizing therapy may also increase motivation to focus on, and communicate more widely about, headache-related disability.

A typical algorithm for treatment of primary headache disorders might be as follows:

1. Exclude secondary headache.
2. Diagnose the specific primary headache disorder.
3. Choose a treatment.

This simple algorithm is suboptimal for a number of reasons. First, primary headache disorders, such as migraine, are heterogeneous, and the nature, severity, and associated disability of attacks and the need for treatment vary among individuals.[27,28] Many people are able to control mild to moderate migraine with over-the-counter medications and do not require prescription drugs.[29] At the other end of the spectrum are those with frequent, severe, disabling attacks whose lives are completely disrupted. It is obvious that these two kinds of individuals differ in their treatment needs. The second reason that diagnosis does not give us enough information to optimize therapy is the enormous and expanding range of therapeutic options for migraine. Third, there are no systematic strategies for identifying individual patients for particular treatments or programs of care. Clinical trials are conducted by randomizing migraineurs diagnosed by the International Headache Society criteria,[1] and the results inform us that particular drugs are useful for migraine in general but they do not tell us which patients require which kinds of drugs.

Step Care

The mainstream approach to acute treatment of migraine in many countries might be termed *step care*. Patients are started at the bottom of the therapeutic pyramid, and if the treatments fail, the therapy is escalated. This is the approach recommended in some of the published treatment guidelines. The patient consults, migraine is diagnosed, and the patient starts at the bottom of the therapeutic pyramid. If patients are satisfied with the first-line treatment (usually simple analgesics), they continue it. If not, they may have a follow-up consultation and be prescribed treatment a second time (usually combination analgesics), or all too often they conclude that the doctor has nothing to offer and they lapse from care. If second-line treatment works, the patient is satisfied and continues on that treatment; if it does not work, either the patient lapses from care or, if the patient is highly motivated and the doctor allows it, the patient may receive a third-line treatment (specific antimigraine drugs). If this also fails, further options may be explored, such as an injectable rather than an oral triptan, or a different triptan therapy. Another option might be a complicated program to identify and avoid headache triggers. At some stage in this sequence of step-wise care there may be a referral from primary care to specialist tertiary care.

The fundamental assumption of step care is that all patients have the same treatment needs. This is a useful cost-effective methodology if the patient responds favorably to first-line therapy. The disadvantages of step-wise care are that successful treatment may be delayed, resources may be wasted on follow-up visits and failed prescriptions, patients and physicians may become discouraged, and patients may lapse from care.[30]

Stratified Care

Stratified care, on the other hand, stratifies attacks and patients according to their therapeutic need. Those with severe episodes, which are disabling, would then be assigned specific medications that have proven efficacy, and patients with mild or low disability, whose therapeutic needs are less, may be treated with simple analgesics. Patients and physicians should be flexible in using medications according to need. Patients and their attacks must be stratified. Patient education is highly essential in this respect.

Current Understanding of the Pathophysiology of Migraine

From various clinical and experimental data, it appears that the aura of migraine is a cortical phenomenon similar to cortical spreading depression.[21] On the other hand, pain of migraine may be due to activation of the trigeminal vascular system (the trigeminal nerve and the blood vessels it supplies, predominantly intracranial blood vessels, including dural vessels and major cerebral arteries). There are three components of migraine pain: (a) vasodilatation, predominantly of the intracranial blood vessels; (b) a rapid-onset neurogenic (sterile) inflammation in the perivascular area; (c) activation of the central trigeminal system—namely, the spinal tract of the trigeminal nerve (trigeminal nucleus caudalis) and its connections centrally.[22] One should also keep in mind that the trigeminal nucleus caudalis receives input from the upper cervical nerves and that neck pain becomes a part of migraine process.

Brain Stem Migraine Generator

Recent positron emission tomography studies suggest that the midbrain, periaqueductal dorsal raphe area is activated during migraine.[23] This activation is not reduced by sumatriptan, even though it reduces migraine pain. The preceding areas of the brain contain serotonin, norepinephrine, endorphin, and GABA systems. Perturbation in these areas of complex neurophysiologic interactions is thought to trigger a migraine attack.[24]

SEROTONIN AND MIGRAINE. Serotonin has been implicated in migraine pathophysiology for quite a long time. Intravenous serotonin may relieve a migraine attack; however, it is unpleasant for clinical use. Based on that observation, specific serotonin agonists were developed and sumatriptan was the first to be introduced in 1991.[25] Many of the drugs used in the acute treatment of migraine as well as prophylactic treatment of migraine have some link to serotonin metabolism.

Serotonin Receptors Among the various families of serotonin receptors in humans, $5\text{-}HT_1$, $5\text{-}HT_2$, and $5\text{-}HT_3$ are relevant to migraine. The $5\text{-}HT_1$ family of inhibitory receptors is subdivided into $5\text{-}HT_{1A}$, $5\text{-}HT_{1B}$, $5\text{-}HT_{1D}$, and $5\text{-}HT_{1F}$.[26] Most of the specific agents used in the treatment of acute migraine are $5\text{-}HT_{1B}/5\text{-}HT_{1D}$ agonists. Specific $5\text{-}HT_{1F}$ agonists are being tested at the present time. The $5\text{-}HT_{1B}$ postsynaptic receptor is on blood vessels. Intracranial blood vessels have a rich supply of these receptors. $5\text{-}HT_{1B}$ receptors are also found to a smaller degree in the coronary arteries; hence $5\text{-}HT_{1B}$ agonists would cause some degree of vasoconstriction of the coronary arteries.

The $5\text{-}HT_{1D}$ presynaptic receptor, on the other hand, is on trigeminal nerve endings. Stimulation of this receptor causes reduction in the release of vasoactive polypeptides, such as CGRP and substance P, and hence reduction in the degree of neurogenic inflammation.

$5\text{-}HT_2$ excitatory receptors are important, as many of the preventive medications that we use, such as methysergide and propranolol, are $5\text{-}HT_2$ antagonists.

The $5\text{-}HT_3$ family is also relevant to migraine pharmacotherapy. The nausea and vomiting associated with migraine may be partly due to stimulation of $5\text{-}HT_3$ receptors, which are found predominantly in the nausea, vomiting centers of the lower brain stem. $5\text{-}HT_3$ antagonists such as metoclopramide are useful in treating migraine-associated nausea.

Examples of Stratified Care

Tables 2-6 to 2-9 give treatment options according to the severity of migraine attack.

Mild migraine can very well be treated by simple analgesics, nonsteroidal antiinflammatory agents with or without metoclo-

Table 2-6.   Stratification according to severity of migraine—options

Mild:
   Simple analgesics
   NSAIDS
   Isometheptene
   (Metoclopramide may be added to reduce nausea and enhance
     absorption.)

Table 2-7. Stratification according to severity of migraine—options

Moderate:
  NSAIDS
  Isometheptene
  Ergotamine—oral, nasal
  Sumatriptan—oral, nasal
  Zolmitriptan—oral
  Naratriptan—oral
  Rizatriptan oral, MLT
  DHE—nasal
  (Metoclopramide may be added with oral agents)

Table 2-8. Stratification according to severity of migraine—options

Severe:
  Ergotamine–rectal
  +
  Antiemetic—rectal
  Sumatriptan–subcutaneous, nasal, oral
  Zolmitriptan–oral
  Naratriptan–oral
  Rizatriptan–oral, MLT
  DHE–intramuscularly, nasal

Table 2-9. Stratification according to severity of migraine–options

Extremely severe:
  Ketorelac–intramuscularly (60 mg)
  DHE IV
  +
  Metoclopramide
  Dopamine antagonists
  Opioids

pramide, and isometheptene. Moderate to severe headaches respond better to 5-HT$_{1D/1B}$ agonists, which will include ergotamine, dihydroergotamine (DHE), and triptans (see the following discussion). The choice of drug will depend on a number of factors, which will include the time to peak, associated symptoms (e.g., nausea and vomiting), and severity of the headache pain. For rapidly peaking headache, such as in cluster headache, crash migraine, and severe nocturnal migraine, subcutaneous sumatriptan is the drug of choice. Nasal sumatriptan is also very rapid in onset of action; therefore it may be considered under those circumstances. Oral medications in general take longer to work; however, oral sumatriptan, rizatriptan, and zolmitriptan have been shown to have a significant effect within an hour.

Some patients may need to have more than one drug available so that they can choose the one most suitable for the migraine attack in question.

Extremely severe headache, particularly in an emergency room, may be treated with intravenous dihydroergotamine with intravenous prochlorperazine or metoclopramide. The response to intravenous DHE is almost 80%. Those who cannot tolerate DHE or who have contraindications may be tried on a dopamine antagonist, such as intravenous chlorpromazine or perchlorperazine, droperidol, or intravenous diphenhydramine (Benadryl).

Therapeutic Options in the Treatment of Acute Migraine

Three classes of drugs, which have scientific validity in the treatment of migraine, include 5-HT$_1$ agonists, dopamine antagonists, and prostaglandin inhibitors.

5-HT$_1$ Agonists

PHARMACOLOGY. 5-HT$_1$ agonists can be divided into selective and nonselective (Table 2-10). All the triptans (sumatriptan, zolmitriptan, naratriptan, rizatriptan, eletriptan, almatriptan, and fravotriptan) are selective because of their specific affinity to 5-HT$_1$ group of receptors. Another group of drugs, which are specific 5-HT$_{1F}$ receptor agonists (SSOFRA), is currently under trial. On the other hand, the nonselective groups, which include ergotamine and dihydroergotamine, have a wider spectrum of receptor affinities outside the 5-HT$_1$ system. Dihydroergotamine and ergotamine also bind to dopaminergic receptors, which may account for the increased nausea associated with those medications.

PHARMACOKINETICS OF SELECTIVE 5-HT$_1$ AGONISTS (TRIPTANS). All triptans share a basic indole ring, with side chains being different. Because of the differences in the side chains, the pharmacokinetic properties also differ. Important pharmacokinetic parameters that determine efficacy are T-max, half-life (T$_{1/2}$), bioavailability, lipophilicity, CNS penetration, and other receptor affinities.[31] Table 2-11 lists the pharmacokinetics of triptans, and Table 2-12 shows the various triptan preparations used for migraine.

Sumatriptan, which is the gold standard of triptan therapy because of extensive experience worldwide with this drug, has a

Table 2-10.   Acute migraine–specific agents

5-HT$_1$ agonists
Selective
   Sumatriptan
   Zolmitriptan
   Naratriptan
   Rizatriptan
   Eletriptan
   Fravotriptan
   Almatriptan
Nonselective
   Ergotamine
   Dihydroergotamine

**Table 2-11. Pharmacokinetics of oral
5HT_{1B}/5HT_{1D} agonists**

Drug	T-max (hr)	T (1/2 hr)	Oral bioavailability (%)	Lipophilicity
Sumatriptan	2.5	2.5	15	-1.3
Zolmitriptan	2	2.5–3	40–48	-0.7
Rizatriptan	1.3	2	45	-0.7
Naratriptan	1.5–3	5–6.3	63 (men)	-0.2
			74 (women)	
Eletriptan	1–2	3.6–5.5	50	+0.5
Almotriptan	1.4–3.8	3.2–3.7	80	-0.35

T-max of 2 hours. Two agents which have been shown to have
lesser T-max are rizatriptan and eletriptan (1 to 1.5 hours).
Sumatriptan has a half-life of 2 hours and receptor binding is
reversible, resulting in relatively short-lasting biologic effects.
On the other hand, naratriptan has the highest half-life among
the currently available triptans, nearly 6 hours. Because of
longer half-life, the effect of naratriptan in relieving headache
symptoms persists for up to 24 hours, and the recurrence rate of
the headache is lower than that with sumatriptan.

Oral bioavailability is an important factor and may account
for consistency of response with repeated use. Sumatriptan
tablets have a low oral bioavailability (14%); all the second-gen-
eration triptans have better oral bioavailability. Naratriptan has
close to 70% bioavailability. The bioavailability of rizatriptan is
in the range of 40% to 45%, as is that of zolmitriptan

Lipophilicity determines whether the medications cross the
blood-brain barrier. All the new-generation triptans—namely,
zolmitriptan, naratriptan, rizatriptan, and eletriptan—cross the
blood-brain barrier, as does DHE. On the other hand, sumatriptan has not been shown to cross the blood-brain barrier when the
blood-brain barrier is intact. It is possible that during a migraine
attack, there is disruption of the blood-brain barrier and hence
that sumatriptan may get into the central nervous system.
Whether central effects of triptans have any clinical relevance to
efficacy is still not determined.

Most published reports of double-blind placebo controlled
studies are not head-to-head comparisons with sumatriptan.
Metaanalysis of published data from the literature of all the
triptans reveals that the efficacy range is not extremely different when appropriate doses are compared.[32] A few head-to-head
comparisons have been done, with rizatriptan and eletriptan
claiming better efficacy than 100-mg sumatriptan tablets.

CLINICAL USE OF TRIPTANS. **Sumatriptan (Imitrex).** Sumatriptan,
the first triptan to be introduced, is available in three forms:
tablet (25 mg, 50 mg, [100 mg in Europe]), nasal spray (5 mg, 20
mg), and 6 mg subcutaneously. Subcutaneous sumatriptan with a
96% bioavailability is the most efficacious of all triptans, with an

Table 2-12. Triptans

Generic name	Trade name	Company	Initial dose (mg)	Max dose in 24 h (mg)	Non-oral preparations (mg)
Sumatriptan	Imitrex	Glaxo-Wellcome	50 mg	200	Nasal spray: 20—maximum 40 mg/day Subcutaneous injection: 6—maximum 12 mg/day
Zolmitriptan	Zomig	Zeneca	2.5–5	10	
Naratriptan	Amerge	Glaxo-Wellcome	2.5	5	
Rizatriptan	Maxalt	Merck	10	30	
	Maxalt MLT		10	30	
Eletriptan	Relpax	Pfizer	40–80	80	

82% efficacy at 2 hours. The onset of action is extremely rapid, within 10 minutes, and is most appropriate for patients with a rapidly peaking headache condition, such as cluster headache and nocturnal severe crash migraine. Subcutaneous sumatriptan may be associated with more triptan symptoms, which include chest discomfort, heaviness of the chest and throat, paresthesias involving the head and neck and extremities, anxious feeling, and mild difficulty breathing. Fewer of these symptoms occur with the use of sumatriptan tablets and sumatriptan nasal spray. Sumatriptan is generally not associated with central nervous system symptoms, unlike the newer triptans, which cause such symptoms as somnolence, asthenia, and dizziness. Fifty milligrams of sumatriptan is the recommended starting dose. Up to four tablets are allowed in 24 hours. Tablets have a slower onset of action than subcutaneous sumatriptan. The time of onset of action is around 30 minutes, which is comparable to agents like rizatriptan. A 2-hour response is about 56% to 58%.

The recommended dose of sumatriptan nasal spray is 20 mg for adults. The efficacy of sumatriptan nasal spray is intermediate compared with the tablet or subcutaneous injection. The time of onset of action after sumatriptan nasal spray is about 15 to 20 minutes. Here again, if rapidity of onset of action is important, sumatriptan nasal spray is a good option.

Recurrence of headache is a problem with all the triptans. Recurrence rates vary anywhere from 20% to 45% reported from various studies. Recurrence can be treated with a second dose in most patients; however, some patients have multiple recurrences, overuse medications, and finally end up with a rebound phenomenon. If that happens, the patients will have to be switched to a long-acting triptan, such as naratriptan, and be started on preventive medications.

Sumatriptan has also been shown to be effective in special subgroups of migraine patients, such as women with menstrual migraine, migraineurs with asthma, those with early-morning migraine, and children. In children appropriate smaller doses are used.

Zolmitriptan. Zolmitriptan (Zomig) is available in 2.5-mg and 5-mg tablets and has been shown to have both central and peripheral action in the trigeminal system. From an efficacy point of view, 5 mg zolmitriptan may have a slightly higher 2-hour response rate. However, head-to-head comparison with 100 mg sumatriptan did not show any statistically significant difference in efficacy. One of the clinically helpful features of zolmitriptan is its consistency. The recurrence rate is somewhat similar to that of sumatriptan. It has been shown that a second dose of zolmitriptan is useful for recurrence and for patients who obtained partial relief after the first dose.

Naratriptan. Naratriptan (Amerge) is somewhat distinct from the other triptans because of its longer half-life and very good oral bioavailability. These features are translated into longer duration of action (up to 24 hours) and lower recurrence of headache.[33] However, the 2-hour efficacy rate of naratriptan is not as good as that of sumatriptan, zolmitriptan, rizatriptan, or eletriptan. Naratriptan may be most useful for patients with slow-onset prolonged migraine, such as in menstrual migraine and habitually prolonged nonmenstrual migraine episodes. Naratriptan has been shown to be more effective in moderate migraine attacks, whereas sumatriptan has better efficacy in severe attacks. Recurrence of the headache is lowest for naratriptan in comparison with other triptans. The tolerability of naratriptan is excellent. Many of the studies showed that adverse events were similar to that of placebo. Naratriptan is useful in sumatriptan nonresponders and those with multiple recurrences from sumatriptan.

Rizatriptan. Because of the shorter half-life and fairly good bioavailability some studies have shown that oral rizatriptan (Maxalt) results in a larger percentage of patients with relief at 2 hours than is obtained with the other oral triptans currently available. The pain-free response at 2 hours is also higher with rizatriptan. Maxalt MLT is a convenient route of administration, over the tongue. The medication dissolves quickly in the saliva which is swallowed without the need for water. There is no evidence that the efficacy of Maxalt MLT is superior to that of Maxalt tablets. The recurrence rate is around 40%; however, a second dose is generally effective for recurrence. Central side effects include somnolence, dizziness, and asthenia, which are seen slightly more with 10 mg than with smaller doses. The incidence of chest and other triptan symptoms is relatively low with the newer triptans.

From a review of the literature combined with clinical experience, it appears that there are no major differences among sumatriptan, zolmitriptan, and rizatriptan tablets. Naratriptan, on the other hand, is different and has certain potential indications, such as prolonged migraine. There are individual differences in the response to triptans. The physician, in cooperation with the patient, can determine which of the triptan tablets to try.

CLINICAL USE OF NONSELECTIVE 5-HT$_1$ AGONISTS. **Ergotamine.** The oral and rectal absorption of ergotamine is erratic, displaying great interindividual variation. Bioavailability is less than 5% for the oral dosage form but is considerably higher after rectal dosing.[34] Peak plasma concentrations are reached about 1 hour after oral or rectal dosing, but plasma levels after rectal administration are as much as 20 times higher.[35,36] The biologic effects of the drug last much longer than the drug's short elimination half-life of 2 to 3 hours would suggest. This is probably explained by the actions of one or more of its metabolites. The elimination half-life of its metabolites (20 hours) conforms closely to the duration of peripheral vasoconstriction after ergotamine administration.

Powerful and selective constriction of the external carotid artery and its branches is produced by ergotamine. Only slight alphaadrenergic blockage occurs at doses used clinically, and the vasoconstrictor effect is mediated by a direct effect on arterial serotonin receptors.[37] Ergot alkaloids have been found to depress the firing rate of serotonergic neurons of the brain stem raphe,[38] so that stabilization of serotonergic neurotransmission may be the major action of ergotamine, as appears to be the case for the preventive antimigraine drugs.[39]

An adequate dose should be taken as soon as possible and should *not* be divided into half-hourly or hourly supplements; if the initial dose fails, subsequent doses usually fail also. A subnauseating dose, if possible, should be determined. A dose that provokes nausea—probably a centrally mediated side effect—is too high and may even intensify a migraine attack. The appropriate dosage of ergotamine is best arrived at by titrating the patient's capacity to tolerate ergotamine during a headache-free period. The average dose of the suppository is one-half (1 mg), so that if encountering a patient for the first time during a headache attack, it is common to give 1 mg immediately and, if there is no improvement within 45 minutes, another 1 mg. Rectal administration is more effective. Nausea and vomiting are limiting side effects. Ergotamine is also contraindicated in coronary and peripheral artery disease.

Dihydroergotamine. About 10 years after the introduction to clinical medicine of ergotamine, DHE was studied for its effectiveness in aborting attacks of migraine and was found to be as good as ergotamine, if not better.[40] It was further noted in early studies that despite the close similarities in chemical structure, unlike ergotamine, DHE had minimal to no effects on peripheral arterial constriction. Modern studies have affirmed that DHE has only modest arterial effects[41] but is a potent venoconstrictor, allowing for its usefulness in the treatment of orthostatic hypotension. Like ergotamine, idiosyncratic hypersensitivity to the drug occasionally occurs, and rare instances of severe peripheral arterial spasm and coronary spasm have been reported.

DHE is presently available as a parenteral preparation and as a nasal spray. A major advantage of DHE over ergotamine is that the former can be given intravenously with far less nausea, and thus can terminate an acute attack quickly even when the attack is at its peak and attended by profuse vomiting and prostration.[42] A further advantage is that it does not result in physical dependence.[43]

DHE for Acute Migraine. Following parenteral administration, peak plasma levels of DHE are rapidly achieved: 15 to 45 minutes after it is given subcutaneously, 30 minutes after intramuscular administration, and 2 to 11 minutes following intravenous dosing, minutes after nasal administration. Plasma levels obtained after subcutaneous dosing are 40% lower than those after intramuscular administration of 1 mg. Therefore intramuscular administration of 1 mg is preferable to subcutaneous administration. Patients can be taught to self-administer intramuscular injection. After DHE nasal spray administration, plasma levels are achieved in 30 to 60 minutes.

For attacks that have already climaxed, the accepted protocol includes prochlorperazine, 5 mg intravenously, followed immediately by 0.75 mg DHE given slowly, over 2 to 3 minutes. If the attack has not begun to subside in 30 minutes, another 0.5 mg DHE is given intravenously (without prochlorperazine). Using this protocol in a prospective controlled study with patients entering a hospital emergency department because of headache, 85% were treated successfully, without the need for narcotic analgesics.[42]

DHE in Intractable Migraine. Mathew et al. have documented that episodic migraine may become incessant and refractory to standard therapy.[19] For many of these patients, drug dependence cycles have become established; for others, disabling headaches continue unabated, seemingly indefinitely. The use of DHE 1/2 ml given intravenously every 8 hours has revolutionized the therapeutic approach to this segment of the patient population, 90% of whom become headache-free within 2 days of treatment.[43] Metoclopramide 5 mg is used adjunctly with DHE.

Dopamine Antagonist and Prokinetic Agents

There is some evidence to suggest that dopaminergic symptoms may be activated during the initial phases of migraine, such as the prodrome of migraine.[15] The nausea and vomiting associated with migraine may also be due to activation of the dopaminergic system. In addition, there is a relative gastroparesis during acute migraine attacks, resulting in poor absorption of medications. Prokinetic agents such as metoclopramide increase gastric motility and enhance absorption, in addition to being effective antinausea drugs.

Antidopaminergic agents used in acute migraine are intravenous (IV) chlorpromazine, IV prochlorperazine, metoclopramide, IV droperidol, and domperidone. In an emergency room setting, these medications are definite alternatives to 5-HT$_{1D/1B}$ agonists. Recent reports indicate that IV diphenhydramine is a useful agent in the emergency room.

Prostaglandin Inhibitors

Prostaglandin inhibitors, such as nonsteroidal antiinflammatory agents, are effective in mild to moderate migraine. It has been shown that nonsteroidal antiinflammatory agents like indomethacin reduce the neurogenic inflammation in the trigeminal vascular system in experimental animals. Many NSAIDs have been shown to be as effective as ergotamine or more so. One report indicated that aspirin/metoclopramide combination is only slightly less effective than oral sumatriptan.[44] Naproxen sodium 550 to 750 mg is a fairly effective agent in mild to moderate headache. Intramuscular ketorolac (60 mg) is useful in many acute attacks. The new Cox$_2$ inhibitors may give us a better option, as they lack gastrointestinal side effects.

Rational Copharmacy in Acute Migraine

Combination of antimigraine agents may be useful in the treatment of acute migraine; for example, nonsteroidal antiinflammatory agents can be combined with ergotamine and with triptans. Antinausea medications (metoclopramide, a 5-HT$_3$ and dopamine antagonist) may be combined with nonsteroidals, triptans, ergotamine, or DHE.

OPIOIDS IN MIGRAINE TREATMENT. Opioids have no place in the routine management of acute migraines. However, opioid may be used in a controlled fashion when specific 5-HT$_{1D/1B}$ agonists are totally ineffective or when they are contraindicated, as in cases with ischemic heart disease. Mixing opioids with DHE and triptans may nullify the effect of these agents.

Prophylaxis of Migraine

Goals of prophylaxis include reduction in the frequency and severity of migraine attacks, increased responsiveness of acute attacks to abortive therapy, and improved quality of life. Table 2-13 lists indications for prophylatic treatment.

Ample clinical evidence suggests that there is a central neuronal hyperexcitability in patients with migraine.[45-52] A number of biochemical and neurophysiologic observations suggest that mobilization of serotonin (5-HT) may precipitate a migraine

Table 2-13. Indications for prophylactic pharmacotherapy

Two or more attacks a month that produce disability that lasts 3 or more days

Contraindication to, or ineffectiveness of, symptomatic medications

The use of abortive medication more than twice a week, or

Special circumstances, such as hemiplegic migraine or rare headache attacks producing profound disruption or risk of permanent neurologic injury.

attack.[53–56] Most of the prophylactic medications have some influence on central serotonergic symptoms. Agents that reduce the frequency and severity of migraine may have central effects that reduce activation of "migraine generators," decrease central neuronal hyperexcitability, raise the threshold for cortical spreading depression, and enhance central antinociception. The central effects of prophylactic agents may involve one or many of the following mechanisms: $5-HT_2$ antagonism, regulation of voltage-gated ion channels, modulation of central and peripheral neurotransmitters, enhancement of GABAergic inhibition, and alteration of neuronal oxidative metabolism.

Factors that influence choice of drugs for prophylaxis will depend on the patient profile, consisting of frequency and severity of attacks, disability, impact on quality of life, comorbidity, efficacy of the drug, side effect profile of the drug, and the risk-to-benefit ratio.

Agents that interfere with effective prophylaxis include concomitant use of analgesics, particularly combination analgesics, excess ergotamine, excessive $5-HT_{1B/1D}$ agonist, oral contraceptives, and vasodilator drugs, such as nitroglycerine and nifedipine. Table 2-14 lists medications currently in use for migraine prophylaxis.

Table 2-14. Currently used medications for migraine prophylaxis

Beta-adrenergic blocking agents: propranolol, timolol, metaprolol, nadolol

Tricyclic antidepressants: amitriptyline, nortriptyline, doxepin, protriptyline, desipramine, imipramine, Selective serotonin reuptake inhibitors (SSRIs)*

Calcium channel blockers: verapamil, flunarizine, diltiazem

$5-HT_2$ antagonists: methysergide, cyproheptadine, and pizotifen

Nonsteroidal antiinflammatory agent (NSAIDS): naproxen sodium

Antiepileptic agents: valproate sodium, gabapentin

Magnesium replacement: miscellaneous agents such as: clonidine, papaverine, riboflavin

*SSRI's, even though often used as an adjunct in the treatment of patients with chronic headache, have not been shown to have any significant antimigraine effect alone.

Reasons for failure of prophylactic therapy include incorrect diagnosis, failure to recognize comorbidity, inadequate dosage of medications, inadequate time period, and unrealistic expectations.

Practical Considerations in Prophylactic Pharmacotherapy

The following are some practical considerations in prophylactic pharmacotherapy:

1. *Start small, go slow.* It is extremely important to start with small doses of prophylactic medications initially and to build up the dosage gradually because patients tolerate the medications better with this strategy. For initial therapy, choose the most effective agent with the fewest side effects. Large doses of any of the agents on the first day may cause significant side effects and the patient may hesitate to continue the medication. This is particularly true of medications such as amitriptyline. Migraineurs frequently require a lower dose of a preventive medicine than is needed for other conditions.
2. *Give an adequate trial with the optimum dose* for at least 3 months before the medication is pronounced ineffective.
3. *Withdraw the medications gradually.* This is particularly important in beta-blockers, calcium channel blockers, and selective serotonin reuptake inhibitors (SSRIs). If the headaches are well controlled, a drug holiday can be undertaken following a slow taper program. Many patients experience continued relief after discontinuing the medication or may not need the same dose. A dose reduction may provide a better risk-to-benefit ratio.
4. *Combinations (co-pharmacy) may be needed* in many patients. Drug interactions have to be considered when combining medications.

Steps before prophylactic therapy is initiated include recognition of comorbidity, such as depression, panic attacks, anxiety, and bipolar illness. Analgesic/ergotamine/5-HT$_{1D}$ agonist rebound must be recognized. Such patients must be detoxified from analgesic/narcotic/sedative medications.

Always combine pharmacotherapy with nonpharmacologic approaches, including dietary adjustments, reducing triggers, physical exercise, relaxation using any suitable technique, particularly biofeedback and behavioral counseling.

Adequate contraception for women with potential to become pregnant is extremely important.

Whenever possible, use one agent at a time. There is a place for rational copharmacy, which will be discussed later.

LENGTH OF TREATMENT. There are no set rules for the length of treatment. Generally, prophylactic treatment is given for at least 6 months. It is very important that the patient understand that prophylactic medications take a number of weeks to show the desired effects. In many, the medications may have to be resumed after a while, and many patients with chronic migraine need continuous prophylactic therapy.

TACHYPHYLAXIS TO PROPHYLACTIC THERAPY. Clinical experience has indicated that tachyphylaxis becomes a problem in long-term management with prophylactic agents. Even very effective medication such as methysergide may produce tachyphylaxis after a while. Therefore it is important to monitor the patient over a period of time and to change medications if necessary.

Overall, assessment of the success of prophylactic therapy may become difficult because of spontaneous improvement in migraine, unpredictable cycles of worsening in some patients, and high placebo response.

Betaadrenergic Blocking Agents

Table 2-15 lists the usual dosages of the commonly used beta-adrenergic blocking agents.

The biologic basis of the effect of beta-blockers in migraine may include 5-HT$_{2B}$ antagonism, reduction of the amplitude of contingent negative variation (CNV), and blockage of the nitric oxide activity. The clinical efficacy of beta-blockers has been shown to have no correlation to its ability to enter the central nervous system, membrane-stabilizing properties, 5-HT$_2$ blocking properties, or beta receptor selectivity. Beta-blockers are particularly effective for patients with migraine associated with stress and hypertension. The antianxiolytic property of beta-blockers helps in this respect. All beta-blockers can cause fatigue, depression, memory disturbance, male impotence, and orthostatic hypotension, and all are contraindicated in patients with asthma and congestive heart failure. Beta-blockers should not be used in patients with depression or low energy.

For comparison purposes, Tfelt-Hansen and Welch[57] developed a scheme of rating clinical efficacy, scientific proof of efficacy, and potential for side effects rated from a scale from + to ++++.[57] Table 2-16 gives the rating. Beta-blockers in general are rated high in their clinical efficacy.

Antidepressants

TRICYCLIC COMPOUND. Antidepressants, particularly tricyclic compounds, are widely used in the prophylaxis of migraine and tension-type headache. Amitriptyline (Elavil and others) in dosages ranging from 10 to 200 mg per day is probably the most commonly used antidepressant.[28] The biologic basis of its action includes modulation of 5-HT and norepinephrine. Amitriptyline

Table 2-15. Beta-adrenergic blocking agents

Medication	Dosage
Propranolol (Inderal)*	40–240 mg/day in divided doses
Propranolol long-acting (Inderal LA)*	60–160 mg once daily
Nadolol (Corgard)	40–160 mg once daily
Timolol (Blocadren)*	Up to 20 mg twice daily
Metoprolol (Lopressor)	50–100 mg/day
Pindolol (Visken)	10–30 mg/day
Atenolol (Tenormin)	50–100 mg/day

*Approved by the FDA for migraine prophylaxis.

Table 2-16. Clinical efficacy,* scientific proof of efficacy,† and potential for side effects* rated on a scale from + to ++++ for some drugs used in migraine prophylaxis

Drug	Clinical efficacy	Scientific proof for efficacy	Side effect potential	Examples of side effects (examples of contraindications)
Beta-Blockers Propranolol, metoprolol, atenolol, nadolol, timolol	++++	++++	++	Tiredness, cold extremities, vivid dreams, depression (asthma, brittle diabetes, A-V [Atrio-Ventricular] conduction defects)
Antiserotonin drugs				
Methysergide	++++	++	++++	Chronic use: fibrotic disorders (cardiovascular diseases)
Pizotifen	+++	++	+++	Weight gain, sedation (obesity)
Calcium antagonists				
Flunarizine	+++	++++	+++	Sedation, weight gain, depression (depression, parkinsonism)
Verapamil	+	+	+	Constipation (bradycardia, A-V conduction defects)
NSAIDs				
Naproxen	++	+++	++	Dyspepsia, peptic ulcers (active peptic ulcers)
Tolfenamic acid	++	+++	++	

Tricyclic antidepressants

Amitriptyline	++	++	Sedation, dry mouth, weight gain (glaucoma)
SSRIs	++	+	
GABAergic agents			
Valproate	++++	++	Nausea, asthenia (liver disease)
Gabapentin	+++	+	
Miscellaneous			
Clonidine	+	+	Dry mouth
Dihydroergotamine	+	++	Nausea, diarrhea (ischemic heart disease)

Modified from Tfelt-Hansen P, Welch KMA. Migraine: prioritizing prophylactic treatment. In Olesen J, Tfelt-Hansen P, Welch KMA, eds. *The headaches* 2nd edition. Philadelphia: Lippincott Williams & Wilkins, 2000, p. 500.
*The rating is based on a combination of the published literature and personal experience.
†There have been no clinical studies with cyproheptadine.

has been shown to inhibit trigeminal neuron activation experimentally. The antidepressant effect adds to the clinical benefit even though the antimigraine effect of amitriptyline has been shown to be independent of the antidepressant effect.[58]

Tricyclic antidepressants are particularly effective in patients with frequent migraine attacks, migraine with medication overuse, migraine with insomnia, migraine with interictal tension-type headache, chronic daily headache, and migraine with depression.

Table 2-16 lists the comparative ratings of tricyclic antidepressants. Combination therapy of tricyclic antidepressants, particularly amitriptyline, with beta-blockers is a very practical way of treating patients with frequent headache, particularly those associated with depression, stress, anxiety, and sleep problems.

SSRIS. In one trial, fluoxetine, an SSRI antidepressant, was not found to be more effective than a placebo for migraine prophylaxis.[59] The same study reported that fluoxetine is useful in treating chronic daily headache.[59] However, SSRIs are used extensively in patients with chronic migraine, particularly because of comorbid depression. In a recent study, S-fluoxetine was found to produce statistically significant improvement of attack frequency, headache days per month, and patients' global impression of its usefulness.[60]

Venlafaxine (Effexor), the first specific serotonin and norepinephrine reuptake inhibitor, may be effective in migraine prophylaxis, but no studies have been performed.

Nefazodone (Serzone), with its central 5-HT$_2$ antagonist property along with beneficial effects on depression and anxiety, may be worthwhile using as a migraine prophylactic. Studies are in progress.

GABAergic Medications

Normally, balance exists between GABAergic inhibition and amino acid–mediated excitation in the central nervous system. It is possible that there is disinhibition due to decreased GABAergic inhibition that results in central neuronal hyperexcitability in migraine patients. This situation is similar to what one might see in epilepsy. GABA is highly concentrated in the visual cortex and periaqueductal area of the brain stem. GABA receptor subunits are expressed in cerebral blood vessels.[61]

VALPROATE. There is a dual site of action of valproate that results in reduction of migraine frequency and severity. The central action in the brain includes an elevation of brain GABA levels, reduction of the firing rates of serotonergic cells in the dorsal raphae,[62] and reduction of C-Fos activation in the trigeminal nucleus caudalis.[63] The peripheral effects include reduction of experimental neurogenic inflammation in the trigeminal vascular system, an effect mediated through GABA$_A$ receptor agonisum.[64] In recent years, a number of randomized double-blind placebo-controlled clinical trials have been done on valproate and migraine that have proved efficacious.[65–67] Comparative study with propranolol has shown that the efficacy of valproate is more or less equal to that of propranolol, as far as the frequency reduction and reduction of headache days per month are concerned.[68] The most common initial side effect of divalproex is nausea and/or vomiting, but as the treatment continues, this side effect gradually lessens. Gradually increasing small doses over a period of 2 to 3 weeks is recommended. Most patients benefit at doses of 500 to 1,500 mg/day. Other adverse effects include tremor, weight gain, asthenia, and loss of hair, which make valproate less acceptable to many. The fear of hepatotoxicity is unfounded in healthy individuals. Hepatitis and other hepatic dysfunctions are contraindications. There is no correlation between the blood levels of valproate and its clinical effect; therefore estimation of blood levels is not absolutely necessary. However, it is recommended that blood count and liver enzymes be tested periodically, preferably once every 3 months, to monitor any change in the profile. Divalproex is definitely contraindicated during pregnancy because of the teratogenic effects, particularly the neural tube abnormalities. Interaction with barbiturates should be kept in mind, and it is better to avoid barbiturate-containing, immediate-relief medications in patients receiving valproate.

Divalproex sodium (Depakote) is the only approved drug for migraine without any direct cardiovascular effects. Valproate is now approved for three different indications—epilepsy, migraine, and mania. Although beta-blockers remain the first-line drug of choice, valproate may be considered a first-line drug under many circumstances. When beta-blockers are contraindicated in such conditions as asthma, congestive cardiac failure, low blood pressure, orthostatic hypotension, and cardiac conduction defects, valproate becomes the first-line drug. Beta-blockers are known to produce depression in some patients; therefore they can be replaced by valproate. Patients with migraine who are on immunotherapy for allergy treatment should not take beta-blockers concomitantly and therefore may be switched to valproate. Beta-blockers are known to reduce exercise tolerance in those who exercise regularly. Valproate has no effect on exercise tolerance. When there is comorbid epilepsy and migraine or epilepsy and bipolar illness, valproate may be considered a first-line drug.

GABAPENTIN. *Gabapentin* has been shown to be effective in a randomized double-blind placebo-controlled trial for prophylaxis of migraine.[69] Gabapentin increases the GABA levels in the brain, but its precise mechanism of action is unknown. Gabapentin is a fairly well-tolerated medication, and doses of up to 2,400 mg/day are being tried. An initial open study showed efficacy of gabapentin in migraine and transformed migraine.[70] Gabapentin has been shown to have a beneficial effect on neuropathic pain states, such as diabetic neuropathy,[71] postherpetic neuralgia, trigeminal neuralgia, and complex regional pain syndrome. It has also been shown to be as effective as propranolol in the treatment of essential tremor.[72] The low side effect profile of gabapentin is a distinct advantage over valproate.

5-HT₂ Antagonists

Methysergide still remains one of the most effective antimigraine prophylactic agent; however, as shown in Table 2-16, the potential side effects make its use less than attractive.

Methysergide may cause weight gain and peripheral edema. With more than 6 months of use, retroperitoneal, pleuropericardial, and subendocardial fibrosis may occur, a rare complication (1/2,500). It appears to be an idiosyncratic reaction, as the great majority of patients do not develop this complication. Major vessel constriction, mesenteric vascular fibrosis, and small bowel infarction have been reported rarely. Concurrent use with other ergot alkaloids, betaadrenergic blockers, dopamine, erythromycin, or troleandomycin may increase the risk of arterial spasm and occlusion. Methysergide should be reserved for refractory severe migraine. Many clinicians recommend an interval without the drug for 4 weeks every 6 months, but whether this practice decreases toxicity is unclear. If one were to use methysergide over the long term, periodic checkups for fibrotic reactions—including chest x-ray, echocardiogram, and CT of the abdomen—are recommended.

Cyproheptadine appears to be a very effective drug in the prophylaxis of migraine in children and may be the drug of choice, even though there are no controlled trials. It has no major side effects except increased appetite and slight drowsiness.

Calcium Channel Blockers

The most commonly used calcium channel blocker for prophylaxis of headache conditions in the United States is *verapamil*.[73] Verapamil, however, has poor clinical efficacy in migraine compared with flunarizine. It is a well-tolerated medication; therefore many physicians are comfortable using it on a long-term basis. Verapamil is the drug of choice in the prophylaxis of cluster headache. Patients with complicated migraine with prolonged neurologic symptoms (prolonged aura) may benefit from verapamil prophylactic therapy. However, there are no studies to support that clinical impression. Many physicians use verapamil to treat transient migraine accompaniments, described by Miller Fisher.[74] Verapamil is especially useful in patients with comorbid hypertension or with contraindications for beta-blockers, such as asthma or Raynaud's disease.

It is interesting to note that many of the prophylactic agents for migraine effect voltage-gated ion channels, particularly calcium channels. These include the calcium channel blockers, such as flunarizine and verapamil, valproate, and propranolol through its membrane-stabilizing effect. Development of specific antagonists that act on P/Q type calcium channel (based on recent data of chromosome 19 abnormality) may improve prophylactic therapy in migraine.[14]

Nonsteroidal Antiinflammatory Drugs

Naproxen and tolfenamic acid are the two agents that have been tried for migraine prophylaxis. The clinical efficacy of both is not as good as that of the beta-blockers valproate or methysergide. The gastric and renal side effect potential prevents them from being long-term drugs. However, for short-term prophylaxis, particularly around the menstrual time, agents like naproxen sodium may be very effective.

Nonsteroidal antiinflammatory drugs act in multiple ways, producing prostaglandin inhibition, reducing the neurogenic inflammation perivascularly, and influencing central serotonin neurotransmission. There is no correlation between the degree of platelet inhibition and the prophylactic effectiveness of nonsteroidal antiinflammatory agents.

Miscellaneous Agents

MAGNESIUM. Even though magnesium deficiency in the brain is implicated in the pathophysiology of migraine, there is still no proof that magnesium replacement is of any benefit in migraine prophylaxis. The only double-blind placebo-controlled study in patients with migraine without aura (69 patients) reported negative results,[75] even though a previous small study in menstrual migraine reported magnesium to be effective.[76] Mauskop et al.[77] emphasized the importance of serum ionized magnesium measurements in determining the magnesium state in migraine patients and have used intravenous magnesium in patients found to have low ionized magnesium level.[77] These observations have not been confirmed yet.

RIBOFLAVIN. Based on theoretical considerations of possible altered mitochondrial energy metabolism in migraine[78,79] and the striking link between mitochondrial encephalomyopathy, lactic acidosis, and strokelike episodes (MELAS) and migraine,[80,81] high-dose riboflavin was studied in a double-blind placebo-controlled trial.[82] Riboflavin was used in the dosage of 200 mg twice a day, which reduced the frequency of migraine significantly compared with placebo.

Riboflavin (vitamin B_2) is the precursor of flavin mononucleotide and flavin adenine dinucleotide, coenzymes required for the activity of flavoenzymes involved in the transfer of electrons in oxidation-reduction reactions. A beneficial clinical response to high-dose riboflavin has been observed in some patients with mitochondrial myopathies[83] or encephalomyopathies[84] associated with mutations of mitochondrial DNA. If deficient mitochondrial energy reserve is a causal factor in migraine, logically riboflavin might have some beneficial effect.

Stratification of Migraine Prophylaxis

Continuous daily treatment with prophylactic medications is necessary when migraines are frequent and when migraines are associated with interictal nondescript tension-type headache. Patients with severe menstrual migraine or those who get headaches when visiting high altitudes may require *medication for a limited time*. In menstrual migraine, it is usually given 2 or 3 days before the menstruation and through the period. *Episodic prophylaxis* may be instituted when there is a known trigger for headache. For example, exercise-induced headache can be partially prevented by using medications like beta-blockers or indomethacin. The same applies to headache induced by sexual activity where the patient may take a prophylactic agent prior to the event.

The Role of Comorbidity in Prophylactic Treatment of Migraine

Comorbidity may result in certain therapeutic opportunities. Table 2-17 shows therapeutic opportunities provided by comorbid conditions. On the other hand, comorbidity may impose ther-

Table 2.17.   Comorbidity and therapeutic opportunities

Disorders	Medication
Migraine + hypertension	Beta-blockers
Migraine + angina	Calcium channel blockers
Migraine + stress	Beta-blockers
Migraine + depression	Tricyclic antidepressant (TCA), Selective serotinin reuptake inhibitor (SSRI)
Migraine + insomnia	TCA
Migraine + underweight	TCA
Migraine + epilepsy	Divalproex
Migraine + mania	Divalproex

apeutic limitations in using certain medications. Table 2-18 lists the therapeutic limitations because of comorbidity. Therapeutic limitations due to side effects are also a problem. Table 2-19 shows the therapeutic limitations as a result of side effects.

Rational Copharmacy

A primary antimigraine prophylactic agent can be combined with compatible agents for treating comorbidity (depression, anxiety, panic disorder, hypertension, sleeplessness). As long as the antimigraine drug and the drug used for comorbidity do not interact with each other, it is certainly logical to use combinations. Table 2-20 shows certain examples of rational copharmacy in migraine.

Table 2-18.   Comorbidity and therapeutic limitations

Migraine + epilepsy	Tricyclic antidepressant (TCA)
Migraine + depression	Beta-blockers
Migraine + obesity	TCA

Table 2-19.   Therapeutic limitations due to side effects

Asthma	Beta-blockers
Elderly with cardiac disease	Tricyclic antidepressant (TCA)
	Calcium channel blockers
	Beta-blockers
Athlete	Beta-blockers
Professions requiring quick recall and sharp cognitive ability	Beta-blockers TCAs
Liver dysfunction	Valproate

Table 2-20. Rational copharmacy

Suggested	Antidepressants	Beta-blocker
		Calcium channel blocker
		Divalproex
		Methysergide
	Methysergide	Calcium channel blocker
	Selective serotinin reuptake inhibitor (SSRI)	Tricyclic antidepressants
Caution	Beta-blocker	Calcium channel blocker
		Methysergide
	Monoamine oxidase inhibitor (MAOI)	Amitriptyline or nortriptyline
Contraindications	MAOI	SSRI
		Most tricyclic antidepressants (except amitriptyline or nortriptyline)
		Carbamazepine

Drug combinations are commonly used for patients with refractory headache disorders. Some combinations, such as antidepressants and beta-blockers, are suggested; others, such as beta-blockers and calcium-channel blockers, should be used with caution; and some, such as Monoamine Oxidase Inhibitor (MAOI) and SSRI, are contraindicated because of potentially lethal interactions (Table 2-20). Many clinicians find that the combination of an antidepressant (such as a tricyclic antidepressant or SSRI) and a beta-blocker act synergistically. Lance has advocated combining methysergide with a vasodilator such as a calcium channel blocker to decrease side effects. Divalproex, used in combination with antidepressants, is a logical choice to treat refractory migraine that is complicated by depression or bipolar illness. Some clinicians cautiously use the combination of phenelzine and amitriptyline in refractory headache patients.

Use of Abortive Medications Along with Preventive Treatment

Even though preventive agents reduce the frequency and severity of migraine attacks, many patients have breakthrough migraine or tension-type headache while on them. Menstrual migraine is a good example of the breakthrough headache. In general, preventive medications make acute agents more effective.

While using the preventive medication, one should make sure that they are not overused. A limit of use two times a week is recommended to prevent secondary failure of preventive treatment.

Table 2-21 shows the potential drug interactions between abortive and preventive agents.

Table 2-21.   Caution and contraindications for combining abortive and prophylactic antimigraine therapy

Agent	Caution	Contraindicated
Methysergide	Ergotamine, Dihydroergotamine, $5\text{-}HT_1$ agonists	
Monoamine oxidase inhibitors	Oral sumatriptan Zolmitriptan	Meperidine
	Rizatriptan	
		Sympathomimetics (Midrin)
Divalproex	Overuse of short-acting barbiturates	
Propranolol	Rizatriptan	
	Zolmitriptan	
Erythromycin	Eletriptan	

REFERENCES

1. International Headache Society. Classification and diagnostic criteria for headache disorders, cranial neuralgias, and facial pain. *Cephalalgia* 1988;8[Suppl 7]:1–96.
2. Lipton RB, Stewart WF. Migraine in the United States: Epidemiology and health care use. *Neurology* 1993;43[Suppl 3]:6–10.
3. Stewart WF, Lipton RB, Liberman J. Variation in migraine prevalence by race. *Neurology* 1996;16:231–238.
4. MMWR. Prevalence of chronic migraine headaches—United States, 1980–1989. *Morb Mortal Wkly Rep* 1991;40:331–338.
5. Stang PE, Yanagihara T, Swanson JW, et al. Incidence of migraine headaches: a population-based study in Olmstead County, Minnesota. *Neurology* 1992;42:1657–1662.
6. Pryse-Phillips W, Findlay H, Tugwell P, et al. A Canadian population survey on the clinical epidemiologic and societal impact of migraine and tension-type headache. *Can J Neurol Sci* 1992;19:333–339.
7. Lipton RB, Stewart WF, Celentano DD, et al. Undiagnosed migraine: a comparison of symptom-based and self-reported physician diagnosis. *Arch Int Med* 1992;152:1273–1278.
8. Stewart WF, Lipton RB, Celentano DD, et al. Prevalence of migraine headache in the United States: relation to age, income, race and other sociodemographic factors. *JAMA* 1992;267:64–69.
9. Dahlof C. Assessment of health-related quality of life in migraine. *Cephalalgia* 1993;13:233–237.
10. Monzon MJ, Lainez MJA. Quality of life in migraine and chronic daily headache patients. *Cephalalgia* 1998;18:638–643.
11. Linet MS, Stewart WF. Migraine headache: epidemiologic perspectives. *Epidemiol Rev* 1984;6:107–139.
12. Stewart WF, Lipton RB. Work-related disability: results from the American Migraine Study. *Cephalalgia* 1996;16:231–238.

13. Joutel A, Bousser MG, Biousse V, et al. A gene for familial hemiplegia migraine maps to chromosome 19. *Nat Genet* 1993;5: 40–45.

14. Ophoff RA, Terwindt GM, Vergouwe MN, et al. Familial hemiplegic migraine and episodic ataxia type-2 are caused by mutations in the Ca2+ channel gene CACNL1A4. *Cell* 1996;87: 543–552.

15. Peroutka SJ, Wilhoit T, Jones K. Clinical susceptibility to migraine with aura is modified by dopamine D2 receptor (DRD2) NCOI alleles. *Neurology* 1997;49:201–206.

16. Raskin NH. *Headache,* 2nd ed. New York: Churchill Livingstone, 1988.

17. Fisher CM. Painful states: a neurological commentary. *Clin Neurosurg* 1984;31:32–53.

18. Day JW, Raskin NH. Thunderclap Headache: symptom of unruptured cerebral aneurysm. *Lancet* 1986;2:1247.

19. Mathew NT, Reuveni U, Perez F. Transformed or evolutive migraine. *Headache* 1987;27:102–106.

20. Mathew NT, Kurman R, Perez F. Drug induced refractory headache: clinical features and management. *Headache* 1990;30: 634–638.

21. Lauritzen M. Cortical spreading depression. In: Olesen J, Tfelt-Hansen P, Welch KMA, (eds). *The Headaches*, 2nd edition. Philadelphia: Lippincott Williams & Wilkins, 2000:189–194.

22. Moskowitz MA. Basic mechanisms in vascular headache. *Neurol Clin* 1990;8:801–815.

23. Weiller C, May A, Limmroth V, et al. Brain stem activation in spontaneous human migraine attacks. *Nat Med* 1995;1:658–660.

24. Raskin NH, Hosobuchi Y, Lamb S. Headache may arise from perturbation of brain. *Headache* 1987;27:416–419.

25. Humphrey PPA, Feniuk W. Mode of action of the anti-migraine drug sumatriptan. *Trends Pharmacol Sci* 1991;12:444–446.

26. Ferrari MD, Saxena PR. On serotonin and migraine: a clinical and pharmacological review. *Cephalalgia* 1993;13:151–165.

27. Stewart WF, Shechter A, Lipton RB. Migraine heterogenicity. *Neurology* 1994[Suppl 4]:24–39.

28. Lipton RB, Stewart WF, Von Korff M. The burden of migraine: societal costs and therapeutic opportunities. *Neurology* 1997 [Suppl 3]:S4–S9.

29. Peters BH, Fraim CJ, Masel BE. Comparison of 650 mg aspirin and 1000 mg acetaminophen with each other, and with placebo in moderately severe headache. *Am J Med* 1983[Suppl June 14]: 36–42.

30. Lipton RB, Stewart WF. Clinical applications of zolmitriptan. *Cephalalgia* 1997;17[Suppl 18]:53–59.

31. Goadsby PJ. A triptan too far? *J Neurol Neurosurg Psychiatry* 1998;64:143–147.

32. Ferrari MD. "The triptan war. Anno 1998." Presented at the annual meeting of the American Academy of Neurology April 1998.

33. Mathew NT, Asgharnejad M, Peykamian M, et al. On behalf of the naratriptan treatment of migraine: results of a double-blind, placebo controlled, crossover study. *Neurology* 1997;49:1485–1490.

34. Perrin VL. Clinical pharmacokinetics of ergotamine in migraine and cluster headache. *Clin Pharmacokinet* 1985;10:334–352.

35. Ibraheem JJ, Paalzow L, Tfelt-Hansen P. Low bioavailability of ergotamine tartrate after oral and rectal administration in migraine sufferers. *Br J Clin Pharmacol* 1983;16:695–699.

36. Sanders SW, Haering N, Mosberg H, et al. Pharmacokinetics of ergotamine in healthy volunteers following oral and rectal dosing. *Eur J Clin Pharmacol* 1986;30:331–334.

37. Muller-Schweinitzer E. Studies on the 5-HT receptor in vascular smooth muscle. *Res Clin Stud Headache* 1978;6:6–12.

38. Muller-Schweinitzer E. Pharmacological actions of the main metabolites of dihydroergotamine. *Eur J Clin Pharmacol* 1984; 26:699–705.

39. Aghajanian GK, Wang RY. Physiology and pharmacology of central serotonergic neurons. In: Lipton MA, Dimascio A, Kollan KF, eds. *Psychopharmacology: a generation of progress.* New York: Raven Press, 1978:171–183.

40. Horton BT, Peters GA, Blumenthal LS. A new product in the treatment of migraine: a preliminary report. *Mayo Clin Proc* 1945;20:241–248.

41. Aellig WH. Investigation of the venoconstrictor effect of 8'hydroxydihydroergotamine, the main metabolite of dihydroergotamine in man. *Eur J Clin Pharmacol* 1984;26:239–242.

42. Callaham M, Raskin NH. A controlled study of dihydroergotamine in the treatment of acute migraine headache. *Headache* 1986;26:168–171.

43. Raskin NH. Repetitive intravenous dihydroergotamine as treatment for intractable migraine. *Neurology* 1986;36:995–997.

44. Tfelt-Hansen P. Sumatriptan for the treatment of migraine attacks: a review of controlled clinical trials. *Cephalalgia* 1993; 13:238–244.

45. Golla FL, Winter AL. Analysis of cerebral responses to flicker in patients complaining of episodic headache. *Electroencephalogr Clin Neurophysiol* 1959;11:539–549.

46. Schoenen J, Maertens de Noordhout A. Contingent negative variation and efficacy of beta-blocking agents in migraine. *Cephalalgia* 1986;6:229–234.

47. Nyrke T, Kangasniemi P, Land AH. Difference of steady-state visual evoked potentials in classic and common migraine. *Electroencephalogr Clin Neurophysiol* 1989;73:285–294.

48. Blin O, Azulay J, Masson G, et al. Apomorphine-induced yawning in migraine patients: enhanced responsiveness. *Clin Neuropharmacol* 1991;14:91–95.

49. Welch KMA, D'Andrea G, Tepley N, et al. The concept of migraine as a state of central neuronal hyperexcitability. *Neurol Clin* 1990;8:817–828.

50. Aurora SK, Ahmad BK, Alsayed F, et al. Cortical stimulation silent period is shown in migraine with aura. *Neurology* 1998;50[Suppl 4]:351–352.

51. Mathew NT, Mullani N. Migraine with persistent visual aura and sustained metabolic activation in the medial occipital cortex measured by PET. *Abstract Neurol* 1998;50[Suppl 4]: A350–A351.

52. Ramadan NM, Halvorson H, Vande-Linde A, et al. Low brain magnesium in migraine. *Headache* 1989;29:416–419.

53. Curran DA, Hinterberger H, Lance JW. Total plasma serotonin, 5-hydroxyindoleacetic acid and p-hydroxy-m-methoxymandelic

acid excretion in normal and migrainous subjects. *Brain* 1965; 88:997–1010.

54. Anthony M, Hinterberger H, Lance JW. Plasma serotonin in migraine and stress. *Arch Neurol* 1967;16:544–552.

55. Kimball RW, Friedman AP, Vallejo E. Effect of serotonin in migraine patients. *Neurology* 1960;10:107–111.

56. Peatfield RC, Olesen J. Migraine: precipitating factors. In: Olesen J, Tfelt-Hansen P, Welch KMA, eds. *The headaches.* New York: Raven Press, 1993:243.

57. Tfelt-Hansen P, Welch KMA. Migraine: prioritizing prophylactic treatment. In: Olesen J, Tfelt-Hansen P, Welch KMA, eds. *The headaches,* 2nd edition. Philadelphia: Lippincott Williams & Wilkins, 2000:499–505.

58. Couch JR, Ziegler DK, Hassaneur R. Amitriptyline in the prophylaxis of migraine: effectiveness and relationship of antimigraine and antidepressant effects. *Neurology* 1976;26:121–127.

59. Saper JR, Silberstein SD, Lake AE, et al. Double-blind trials of fluoxetine: chronic daily headache and migraine. *Headache* 1994;34:497–502.

60. Steiner TJ, Ahmed F, Findley LJ, et al. S-fluoxetine in the prophylaxis of migraine: a phase II double-blind randomized placebo-controlled study. *Cephalalgia* 1998;18:283–286.

61. LimmrothV, Lee WS, Cutrer FM, et al. Meningeal GABA$_A$ receptors located outside the blood brain barrier mediate sodium valproate blockade of neurogenic and substance P-induced inflammation: possible mechanism in migraine. *Cephalalgia* 1995;15:102.

62. Nishikawa T, Scatton B. Inhibitory influence of GABA on central serotoninergic transmission: raphi nuclei as the neuroanatomical site of GABAergic inhibition of cerebral serotoninergic neurons. *Brain Res* 1985;341:331–391.

63. Cutrer FM, Limmroth V, Ayata G, et al. Valproate reduces C-Fos expression in trigeminal Nucleus caudalis (TNC) after noxious meningeal stimulation. *Cephalalgia* 1995;15[Suppl 14]:96.

64. Cutrer FM, Moskowitz MA. Actions of valproate and neurosteroids in a model of trigeminal pain. *Headache* 1996;36:285.

65. Hering R, Kuritzky A. Sodium valproate in the prophylactic treatment of migraine double-blind study versus placebo. *Cephalalgia* 1992;12:81–84.

66. Jensen R, Brinck T, Olesen J. Sodium valproate has a prophylactic effect on migraine without aura: a triple-blind, placebo-controlled crossover study. *Neurology* 1994;44:647–651.

67. Mathew NT, Saper JR, Silberstein SD, et al. Migraine prophylaxis with Divalproex. *Neurology* 1995;52:281–286.

68. Kaniecki RG. A comparative study of propranolol and divalproex sodium in the prophylaxis of migraine. *Arch Neurol* 1997;54: 1141–1144.

69. Magnus-Miller L, Podolnick P, Mathew NTM, et al. Efficacy and safety of gabapentin (Neurontin) in migraine prophylaxis. American Pain Society Annual Meeting, 1998(abst).

70. Mathew NT. Gabapentin in migraine prophylaxis. *Cephalalgia* 1996;16:367.

71. Gorson KG, Schott C, Rand WM, et al. Gabapentin in the treatment of painful diabetic neuropathy: a placebo controlled double-blind, crossover trial. *Neurology* 1998;50:A103.

72. Girowell A, Kulisevsky J, Barbanog M, et al. A double-blind

placebo controlled comparative trial of gabapentin and propranolol in patients with essential tremor. *Neurology* 1988;50: A71–A72.

73. Silberstein SD, Lipton RB. Overview of diagnosis and treatment of migraine. *Neurology* 1994;44:6–16.

74. Fisher CM. Late life migraine accompaniments, further experience. *Stroke* 1986;17:1033–1042.

75. Pfaffenrath V, Wessely P, Meyer C, et al. Magnesium in the prophylaxis of migraine: a double-blind placebo controlled study. *Cephalalgia* 1996;16:436–440.

76. Facchinetti F, Sances G, Borella P, et al. Magnesium prophylaxis of menstrual effects on intracellular magnesium. *Headache* 1991;31:298–310.

77. Mauskop A, Altura BT, Cracco RQ, et al. Intravenous magnesium sulfate relieves migraine attacks in patients with low serum ionized magnesium levels: a pilot study. *Clin Sci* 1995;89:633–636.

78. Barbiroli B, Montagna P, Cortelli P, et al. Abnormal brain and muscle energy metabolism shown by 31P magnetic resonance spectroscopy in patients affected by migraine with aura. *Neurology* 1992;42:1209–1214.

79. Welch KMA, Levine SR, D'Andrea G, et al. Preliminary observations on brain energy metabolism in migraine studied by in vivo 31-phosphorus NNMR spectroscopy. *Neurology* 1989;39:538–541.

80. Dvorkin GS, Aderman F, Carpenter S. Classical migraine, intractable epilepsy and multiple strokes: a syndrome related to mitochondrial encephalomyopathy. Quoted in ref. 7.

81. Mosewich RK, Donat JR, DiMauro S, et al. The syndrome of mitochondrial encephalomyopathy, lactic acidosis, and stroke-like episodes presenting without stroke. *Arch Neurol* 1993; 50:275–278. In: Anderman F, Lugaresi E, eds. *Migraine and epilepsy.* Boston: Butterworths, 1987:203–232.

82. Schoenen J, Jacquy J, Lenaerts M. Effectiveness of high dose riboflavin in migraine prophylaxis: a randomized controlled trial. *Neurology* 1998;50:466–469.

83. Arts WFM, Scholte HR, Boggard JM, et al. NADH-CoQ reductase deficient myopathy: successful treatment with riboflavin. *Lancet* 1983;2:581–582.

84. Penn AMW, Lee JWK, Thuillier P, et al. MELAS syndrome with mitochondrial tRNA[Leu(UUR)] mutation: correlation of clinical state, nerve conduction, and muscle[31P] magnetic resonance spectroscopy during treatment with nicotinamide and riboflavin. *Neurology* 1992; 42:2147–52.

Tension-Type and Chronic Daily Headache

Ninan T. Mathew

CLASSIFICATION

Episodic tension-type headache (ETTH) is defined by the International Headache Society (IHS) as recurrent episodes of headaches. Older terms that are still sometimes used interchangeably include muscle contraction headache, tension headache, stress headache, and ordinary headache. ETTH is distinguished from chronic tension-type headache (CTTH) by the frequency of headaches.

CTTH and chronic daily headache (CDH) should not be used as synonyms. Although chronic daily headache is not yet a recognized IHS diagnosis, this chapter will point out the need for a modified classification to include CDH. Subtypes, which are discussed in this chapter, include chronic tension-type headache, transformed migraine, new daily persistent headache, and analgesic rebound headache, which can be associated with the other types (Table 3-1).

New data on epidemiology of frequent headaches[1-4] and the nature of "tension-type" headache in migraineurs[5-11] will add compelling arguments to consider chronic tension-type headache and tension-type headache in migraineurs a part of the migraine spectrum.

Limitations of the IHS Headache Classification of Chronic Headaches

Although the IHS headache classification has greatly enhanced the precision of diagnosis of migraine and cluster headache, its application in chronic headaches has been less than satisfactory. The main deficiencies of the IHS classification in this regard are as follows:

1. It is based purely on individual attacks of headaches and does not consider the natural history and evolution of primary headache disorders over a period of time.
2. The significant clinical relationship between migraine and tension-type headache is inadequately appreciated and totally ignored in the classification.
3. Even though tension-type headache and cluster headache are classified as episodic and chronic varieties, no mention is made of chronic varieties of migraine.
4. Mixed forms of headaches are not included.

Classification of Chronic Daily Headache

There is ample evidence to indicate that patients with chronic daily headache (CDH) are a heterogeneous group that can be subdivided into various categories. Approximately 20% of CDHs are primary (daily from the onset), whereas 80% are trans-

Table 3-1. Classification of chronic daily headache (CDH)

Chronic tension-type headache (CTTH)

Transformed migraine (TM)

New persistent daily headache (NPDH)

(All of the preceding categories can be associated with analgesic overuse.)

formed from intermittent headache. Table 3-1 shows an attempted broad classification of chronic daily headache (CDH).

Other forms of chronic headaches, such as chronic cluster headache, hemicrania continua, and chronic paroxysmal hemicrania, are described elsewhere in this book.

Chronic Daily Headache in Headache Clinic Population

Approximately 35% to 40% of patients who seek treatment at the headache centers suffer from daily or near-daily headache.[12] All those patients have headaches for more than 15 days a month or 180 days a year, which puts them in the category of chronic tension-type headache (CTTH) according to the IHS criteria.[1] Are they all chronic tension-type headache sufferers? Using the IHS criteria, Sanin et al. classified 400 patients attending a headache clinic.[13] The majority required more than two, often three or four, diagnoses. Even though migraine was the most common diagnosis, only one-fourth of those with a migraine diagnosis had it as the only diagnosis. Seventy-five percent of migraine patients had coexistent chronic tension-type headache (CTTH), drug-induced headache, or both. Ninety-six percent of patients diagnosed as having migraine with aura also suffered from migraine without aura. More than one-third of patients (37.7%) attending the clinic suffered from CDH (chronic cluster headache excluded), which is not included as a separate entity in the IHS classification. Pure CTTH formed only a small minority of CDH, whereas 86.6% of CDH had migraine as one of the diagnoses. Drug-induced headache was a prominent or second or third diagnosis.

Table 3-2 gives the relative incidence of subtypes of chronic daily headache clinic population.

Most patients seeking treatment in headache clinics have transformed migraine (TM), because their headaches are more severe and more disabling, as seen in the epidemiologic study of frequent headaches.[2]

EPIDEMIOLOGY

Although ETTH is common, the prevalence varies in different studies. In a telephone interview study of 13,345 subjects performed in Baltimore County, Maryland, the one-year prevalence of ETTH for adults was 38.3%, with 36% of males and 42% of females (for a female:male ratio of 1.16). Prevalence peaked in the fourth decade.[1] In a clinical interview and examination study of 740 subjects in Denmark, the one-year prevalence was 74%, including 63% of males and 86% of females.[13a] The lifetime prevalence of ETTH was 78%, with 69% males and 88% females.

Recent reports by Scher et al.[2] indicate an overall prevalence of frequent headaches (more than 15 days/month) to be 4.2% in

Table 3-2. Relative incidence of subtypes of chronic daily headache in headache clinic population

Authors	Total cases	Sex		Chronic tension-type	Migraine tension-type headache complex	
		Male	Female		Transformed migraine	Evolved from tension-type
Mathew et al. 1987 (ref. 2)	630	26%	74%	84 (14%)	487 (77%)	57 (9%)
Manzoni et al. 1987 (ref. 14)	250	24%	76%	57 (22.8%)	178 (71.2%)	8 (3.2%)
Manzoni et al. 1991 (ref. 15)	58	11%	89%	4 (7%)	44 (75%)	9 (15.5%)
Solomon et al. 1992* (ref. 16)	100	28%	72%	66 (66%)†	34 (34%)‡	-

*Reported that the majority evolved from migraine; pointed out the need for separate classification for chronic daily headache.
†Met International Headache Society (IHS) criteria for chronic tension-type headache.
‡Met IHS criteria for migraine.

the population. In that survey, CTTH was found to be 1.7 times more common than TM (CTTH 53%, TM 31%). Sixteen percent of those with frequent headache could not be classified as either CTTH or TM. Scher et al. found that TM is characterized by more severe pain and higher levels of disability than CTTH. This fact accounts for the higher percentage of patients with TM seen in the headache centers. Epidemiology of TM is similar to that of migraine because the gender ratio is 2.4 females:1 male and because there is an inverse relation with low educational level.

Epidemiology of CTTH has features in common with migraine and episodic tension-type headache (ETTH).[2] The gender ratio is intermediate. The relationship with educational level resembles that of migraine, not ETTH. CTTH patients reported severe pain twice as frequently as those with ETTH and missed work five times more often than those with ETTH. The disability profile of CTTH is similar to that of patients with migraine. Recent surveys have shown significantly increased familial risk of CTTH[3] patients; siblings and children of CTTH patients have 2.1- to 3.9-fold greater risk of CTTH than the general population,[3] again resembling migraine.

Castillo et al.[4] reported that in Spain the prevalence of CDH in the general population is 4.7%, of which 2.3% have CTTH and 2.4% have TM. Medication overuse was found to be prevalent in 41% of TM patients and 18% of the CTTH, indicating that TM patients have more severe pain, which requires more medication.

DIAGNOSIS

Episodic Tension-Type Headache

As defined by the IHS criteria, ETTH occurs with a history of at least 10 previous headache episodes. The number of days with such headache are less than 180/year (less than 15/month). The headache duration is from 30 minutes to 7 days. There is no aura or prodrome. The pain is usually dull and is described as aching, tightness, heaviness, pressure, soreness, band-like, or cap-like. Occasionally, the pain may be described as periodically pulsating. The pain is usually of mild or moderate intensity. The pain is typically bilateral with a bandlike distribution. Any region of the head alone or in combination may be involved. The frontal and temporal locations are more common than the occipital. In perhaps 10% of cases, the pain is unilateral, especially in the presence of oromandibular dysfunction, trigger points, or occipital neuralgia. The pain is not aggravated by physical activity and is not associated with nausea and vomiting. In fewer than 10% of cases, mild light or noise sensitivity may be present but not both (which suggests the diagnosis of migraine). ETTH may occur without precipitant or can be triggered by or associated with lack of sleep, psychosocial stress, emotional conflict, anxiety, and depression. Although ETTH may be associated with excessive contraction of pericranial muscles, in many cases there may be an underlying hypersensitivity of neurons in the trigeminal nucleus caudalis as a result of supraspinal facilitation.

Chronic Tension-Type Headache

Chronic tension-type headache is defined in the IHS classification, and the criteria for its diagnosis include (Table 3-3) an

Table 3-3.   IHS criteria for various forms of tension-type headache

Tension-type headache

At least two of the following pain characteristics:
1. Pressing/tightening (nonpulsating) quality
2. Mild or moderate intensity (may inhibit but does not prohibit activities)
3. Bilateral location
4. No aggravation by walking stairs or similar routine physical activity

Both of the following:
1. No nausea or vomiting (anorexia may occur)
2. Photophobia and phonophobia are absent, or one but not the other is present

At least one of the following:
1. History and physical and neurologic examinations do not suggest one of the disorders listed in groups 5–11 (headaches secondary to organic or systemic metabolic disease).
2. History and/or physical and/or neurologic examinations do suggest such disorder, but it is ruled out by appropriate investigations
3. Such disorder is present, but tension-type headache does not occur for the first time in close temporal relation to the disorder.

Episodic tension-type headache

Diagnostic criteria:
A. At least 10 previous headache episodes. Number of days with such headache <180/y (<15/mo)
B. Headache lasting from 30 min to 7 d

Chronic tension-type headache

Diagnostic criteria:
A. Average headache frequency 15 days/month (180 days/year) for 6 months

Tension-type headache associated with disorder of pericranial muscles

At least one of the following:
1. Increased tenderness of pericranial muscles demonstrated by manual palpation or pressure algometer
2. Increased electromyographic level of pericranial muscles at rest or during physiologic tests

Tension-type headache unassociated with disorder of pericranial muscles

No increased tenderness of pericranial muscles. If studied, electromyography of pericranial muscles shows normal levels of activity.

average headache frequency of at least 15 days per month (180 days per year) for 6 months and the ruling out of any organic or structural cause for headache. The headache has a pressing or tightening quality, is usually of mild or moderate severity (may inhibit but does not prohibit activities), has a bilateral location, and is not aggravated by physical activity. At least two of these pain characteristics must be met. There is no vomiting. Nausea, photophobia, or phonophobia may be present.

Two clinical types of chronic tension-type headache may be recognized: those associated with pericranial muscle tenderness, increased EMG level, or a combination of both factors; and those not associated with pericranial muscle tenderness with a normal EMG level. Patients with muscle tenderness show tenderness in the cervical muscles as well as in the pericranial muscles.

Episodic tension-type headache sometimes transforms into the chronic variety, whereas many other headaches are chronic from the onset, with no subsequent change in character. The essential difference between this type of headache and transformed migraine is the absence of a history of episodic migraine and the absence of clear-cut exacerbations with migrainous features.

Tension-Type Headache in Migraineurs

A great deal of evidence now suggests that tension-type headache in migraineurs and chronic tension-type headache may be different from episodic tension-type headaches. Tension-type headaches in migraineurs are frequent, severe, and of longer duration than those in nonmigraineurs.[5] They are associated with more photophobia, phonophobia, and nausea than tension-type headaches in nonmigraineurs.[6] Only migraineurs have episodes of tension-type headaches precipitated by alcohol, aged cheese, chocolate, and physical activity.[7] Tension-type headaches in migraineurs respond to agents such as sumatriptan.[8,9] Sumatriptan has a significant effect in chronic tension-type headache.[10] On the other hand, it has no clinically relevant effect in the treatment of episodic tension-type headache.[11]

The preceding observation plus the epidemiologic data on CTTH make a strong argument to consider tension-type headache in migraineurs and chronic tension-type headache, with many features in common with migraine, as different from episodic tension-type headache.

Transformed Migraine

The term *transformed migraine* was first introduced in 1987 by Mathew et al. to describe a common, daily, or near-daily headache condition that constituted 77% of CDH patients seen at the Houston Headache Clinic.[12] In two separate series, Manzoni et al. reported that 71% and 75%, respectively, of their patients transformed their headaches into a chronic daily pattern from a distinct episodic pattern.[14,15] Solomon et al. also recognized chronic daily headaches and mentioned that the majority of their 100 cases transformed from episodic migraine, even though actual percentages were not given.[16]

Probable factors aiding in the development of chronic daily headache from episodic headache include analgesic or ergotamine overuse, abnormal personality profile, stress, traumatic life events, hypertension, and medications. Analgesic or ergotamine overuse appears to be one of the most common factors that lead to chronic daily headache. Baldrati et al. reported analgesic or ergotamine overuse in 82% of their 50 patients who developed chronic migraine from an episodic pattern.[17] Typically, the patient describes a history of distinct attacks of migraine with or without aura starting in the teens or early twenties that eventually become more frequent.[18] In addition, the patient develops interparoxysmal tension-type headache, which also becomes more frequent, eventually leading to a daily or near-daily headache. Women in this group may show definite exacerbations of their migraine perimenstrually. Many of the headaches retain certain characteristics of migraine, whereas others are indistinguishable from CTH. Patients may suffer from a migraine one day and a tension-type headache the next. Periods of prolonged, persistent, and continuous headache lasting for many weeks may occur in many.[19]

Manzoni et al. analyzed the evolutionary pattern of transformed migraine (Table 3-4).[14,15] The majority maintained migraine attacks in addition to developing tension-type headache daily or nearly daily. Others lost the temporal profile of migraine but developed continuous headache with many migrainous features. It has been suggested transformed migraine should be subdivided into (a) migraine with interparoxysmal headache and (b) chronic migraine to accommodate these two presentations.[20] In general, the transformed migraine group showed higher incidence of family history of headache, more neurologic and gastrointestinal symptoms, aggravation

Table 3-4. Natural history of transformed migraine

Manzoni et al., 1987 (n = 178, ref. 14)	118/178	Maintained migraine attacks and developed interparoxysmal tension-type headache
		Frequency of migraine was more than 1/week in only 35 patients
	60/178	Lost the distinct migraine attacks and developed either a "steady" or a "fluctuating" pattern
Manzoni et al., 1991 (n = 44, ref. 15)	28/44	Maintained migraine attacks and developed interparoxysmal tension-type headache
		Lost the distinct migraine attacks and developed a continuous headache that exhibited most of the features of migraine, except the temporal profile

Table 3-5. Comparison of clinical characteristics of transformed migraine and chronic tension-type headache

Transformed migraine	Chronic tension-type
Headache >15 days/month >180 days/year	Headache >15/month >180/year
Previous history of distinct migraine attacks	No history of distinct migraine attacks
Increased incidence of headache in the family	Positive family history less prominent
Retains migrainous characters to a significant degree, intermittently or continuously	Migrainous features absent or very insignificant
Increased neurologic and gastrointestinal symptoms	Neurologic and gastrointestinal symptoms minimal
Menstrual aggravation	No particular aggravation during menstruation
More relief during pregnancy	Less relief during pregnancy
Excessive intake of analgesics	Excessive intake of analgesics
Responds to antimigraine therapy	Response to antimigraine therapy occurs, but less striking
Behavioral and psychologic factors prominent	Behavioral and psychological factors prominent

during menstruation, and relief during pregnancy, compared with other forms of chronic daily headaches, particularly CTH. Table 3-5 compares the clinical characteristics of transformed migraine and CTH.

Migraine, Chronic Tension-Type Headache Complex Evolved from Episodic Tension-Type Headache

A relatively small percentage of patients with CDH in the migraine-CTH headache complex, describe a history of evolution of the chronic headache from episodic tension-type headache (ETH) (Table 3-2). The figures varied from 3% to 15%. The frequency of headaches with migrainous features is significantly less in this group than that made up of patients with transformed migraine. Manzoni et al.[15] also found a subset of patients who developed CDH from the onset, without a history of previous migraine or tension-type headache. This is the primary variety of CDH, as opposed to the transformed variety. New persistent daily headache, mentioned later, is such a primary variety.

Transformational Factors and Types of Transformation

In approximately 80% of cases, the transformation from episodic headache to CDH is gradual, whereas it is sudden in about 20%. Factors aiding sudden transformation include trauma to the head and neck, flulike illness, aseptic meningitis, surgical interventions, myelography, and medical illnesses. In many cases the aiding factors are unknown.

The probable factors that influence gradual transformation of episodic headaches to the chronic daily form are listed earlier. Analgesic or ergotamine overuse and comorbidity (e.g., depression, anxiety, abnormal personality profile, and stress in family life and at work) appear to top the list. Drug-induced and non–drug-induced varieties are clearly identifiable.[21] There is a group of patients whose pain evolves spontaneously (without a history of analgesic overuse) into a chronic daily headache, as a course in the natural history of the disease. Manzoni et al. reported that in 22% of patients no apparent transformational factors could be found.[14]

Proposed Diagnostic Criteria for Transformed Migraine

Silberstein et al. field-tested the proposed 1994 criteria for classification of daily or near-daily headache and produced a new proposal for transformed migraine diagnostic criteria[21] (Table 3-6).

Table 3-6. Proposal for New Transformed Migraine Diagnostic Criteria

A. Daily or almost daily (more than 15 days/month) head pain for more than 1 month

B. Average duration of more than 4 hours/day

C. History of episodic migraine meeting any IHS criteria 1.1 to 1.6

D. At some time current headache meets IHS criteria for migraine 1.1 to 1.6 other than duration

E. At least one of the following:

  1. There is no suggestion of any organic (structural, infectious, or metabolic) causes.

  2. Such a disorder is suggested but is ruled out by appropriate investigations.

  3. Such a disorder is present, but first migraine attacks do not occur in close temporal relation to the disorder.

New Daily Persistent Headache

It is not uncommon to see patients who give a history of a fairly rapid onset of a persistent headache that continues on a daily basis.[22] This is a primary variety of CDH. These patients do not have a history of previous migraine or tension-type headache, nor do they give a history of trauma or psychologic stress. The patients may distinctly remember the "onset event" or the day or time when the headache started. Epstein-Barr virus–induced immune changes have been implicated as an etiologic factor.[23] However, this hypothesis has not been confirmed. The disease is usually self-limiting, but it is not uncommon to see patients continuing to have daily headache for a long period of time. In these patients, follow-up observations have not been adequate to produce any reliable data as to the ultimate prognosis.

Analgesic Rebound Headache

Excessive and daily use of immediate relief medications is seen in patients with CDH. Medication misuse headache has been variously referred to as *analgesic rebound headache, ergotamine rebound headache*, and *drug-induced headache. Rebound headache* is a term that is often used to characterize the headache-perpetuating tendency when immediate-relief medications are used very frequently.

There appears to be some confusion between the terms *recurrence* and *rebound. Recurrence* may be defined as the recurrence of the same headache, which was significantly relieved by an abortive antimigraine agent. Recurrence should happen within the natural duration of that migraine attack. Recurrence of the same headache may arise when $5-HT_1$ agonists are used in acute migraine.

Rebound headache, on the other hand, can be defined as perpetuation of head pain in chronic headache sufferers, caused by frequent and excessive use of immediate relief medication. It can also be defined as "a self-sustaining, rhythmic, headache-medication cycle characterized by daily or near daily headache and irresistible and predictable use of immediate relief medications as the only means of relieving headache attacks."[24]

Evidence for Rebound

The most convincing evidence for analgesic-ergotamine rebound is the fact that mere discontinuation of these medications results in significant improvement. Ample data in the literature support the existence of analgesic/ergotamine rebound headache.[25–30] Silverman et al.[31] reported that moderate or severe headache occurred in 52% of patients on caffeine withdrawal based on a double-blind cessation of caffeine consumption. In a recent survey of physicians engaged in the treatment of headache, more than 40% of the respondents (174) indicated that analgesic rebound is present in at least 20% of their patients with headache.[32] Table 3-7 lists the commonly used immediate-relief medication in a group of 200 patients with CDH.[27]

Agents commonly associated with rebound in decreasing order include butalbital/caffeine/aspirin/acetaminophen combinations, caffeine-containing analgesic combinations, opioids, and ergota-

Table 3-7. Daily symptomatic or immediate-relief medications*

Medications	Average no. of tablets per week	Range of no. of tablets per week	No. of patients	% of patients
Butalbital/aspirin/acetaminophen/caffeine with or without codeine	30	14–86	84	42%
Natural or synthetic codeine-containing preparations	28	10–84	80	40%
Aspirin or acetaminophen with caffeine	42	14–108	50	25%
Ergotamine with or without phenobarbital	15 mg.	6–42 mg	44	22%
Acetaminophen	52	15–105	34	17%
Propoxyphene	26	14–56	32	16%
Nasal decongestants and antihistamines	14	6–30	24	12%
Aspirin	28	10–64	8	4%

Reproduced from Mathew NT, Kurman R, Perez F. Drug induced refractory headache: clinical features and management. *Headache* 1990;30:634–638.

mine. Triptans have been reported to cause multiple recurrences and rebound, but the incidence is extremely low.

Clinical Features of Analgesic Rebound Headache

A number of clinical characteristics help us in identifying the occurrence of analgesic rebound headache in patients with primary headache disorders.[27] The following are the clinical features of analgesic rebound:

1. The headaches are refractory, daily, or nearly daily.
2. The headaches occur in a patient with primary headache disorder who uses immediate-relief medications very frequently, often in excessive quantities.
3. The headache itself varies in severity, type, and location from time to time.
4. The slightest physical or intellectual effort will bring on headaches. In other words, the threshold for head pain appears to be low.
5. Headaches are accompanied by asthenia, nausea, and other gastrointestinal symptoms; restlessness; anxiety; irritability; memory problems; and difficulty in intellectual concentration and depression. Those consuming large quantities of ergot derivatives may experience cold extremities, tachycardia, paresthesias, diminished pulse, hypertension, lightheadedness, muscle pain of the extremities, weakness of the legs, and depression.
6. Headaches exhibit a drug-dependent rhythmicity. Predictable early-morning (2:00 A.M. to 5:00 A.M.) headaches are frequent, particularly in patients who use large quantities of analgesic, sedative, caffeine. or ergotamine combinations. Barbiturate-containing analgesics such as Fiorinal and Esgic suppress rapid eye movement (REM) sleep; this results in REM rebound and severe headache on awakening.
7. There is evidence of tolerance to analgesics over a period of time, so that patients need to increase doses as time goes by.
8. Withdrawal symptoms are observed when the patients are taken off pain medications abruptly.
9. Spontaneous improvement of headache occurs on discontinuing the medications.
10. Concomitant prophylactic medications are relatively ineffective while the patients are consuming large excess amounts of immediate-relief medications.

Patterns of Medication Consumption in Patients with Analgesic Rebound

Many patients consume analgesics in anticipation of headache. Fear of pain drives them to take medication even before the headache develops. There is a predictable and irresistible pattern of use in many patients. Multiple medications are used concomitantly, both prescription and nonprescription (Table 3-8). Ferrari and Sternieri[33] analyzed the reasons for daily analgesic consumption in chronic headache disorders. The reasons given by the patient were as follows: consumption under medical advice to take the analgesic at the moment of need (57%); inability to cope with pain (67%); apprehension about headache devel-

Table 3-8. Pattern of consumption of symptomatic medications

Number of preparations of symptomatic medications consumed concomitantly	No. of patients ($n = 200$)	Patients (%)
1	70	35
2	86	43
≥ 3	44	22

Reproduced from Mathew NT, Kurman R, Perez F. Drug induced refractory headache: clinical features and management. *Headache* 1990;30:634–638.

oping if drug is not taken (62%); recurrence of pain soon after previous consumption (30%); the notion that there is no other cure (61%); the analgesic makes headache more bearable and enables the patient to function at work (62%); reduction of tension and anxiety (41%); and a means of inducing sleep (18%). It should be noted that many patients gave more than one of the preceding reasons for daily analgesic consumption.

The behavioral aspects of the analgesic consumption are important. Relief of pain gives a negative reinforcement and changes in the mood produced by some of the agents containing barbiturates or stimulants such as caffeine may give a positive reinforcement for the behavior that results in excessive use of immediate-relief medications. It is very rare for these patients to use habit-forming doses of barbiturates, which are usually above 600 to 800 mg/day. Therefore addiction does not appear to be a problem in most patients, although there are exceptions, with drug-seeking behavior.

Analgesic use does not usually interfere with the execution of normal social and/or occupational roles, as happens when the abuse substance is a narcotic or alcohol. On the contrary, the analgesic represents a kind of necessary crutch for everyday functioning.

Development of tolerance is evidenced by escalating consumption with no apparent adverse consequences. Withdrawal symptoms on discontinuation can be very prominent and include restlessness, sleeplessness, increased headache, diarrhea, and occasional seizures, especially in those who consume large amounts of butalbital-containing analgesics. Increased headache pain with decreased analgesic efficacy occurs over time.

Consequence of Rebound

Clinical evidence from various centers around the world points to the fact that rebound phenomenon alters the natural history of migraine.

Analogous Phenomena to Rebound Headache

There are few analogous phenomena to rebound headache in medicine. These include worsening of nasal congestion by frequent use of decongestants, insomnia aggravated by sleeping pills, chronic constipation because of frequent laxative use, and idiopathic edema caused by diuretics.

Mechanisms of Analgesic Rebound

Analgesic rebound phenomenon is actually a paradoxical response. Those taking most medications experience most pain. The question then arises, "Is a high level of pain experience the cause of high analgesic consumption, or is the overuse of analgesics due to certain psychologic predispositions?" That leads to the question, "Is analgesic rebound headache due to addictive behavior?"

There is no evidence of addictive personality in these patients.[28] Sensation-seeking behaviors are not high in these patients with chronic headache.[34]

Relapses of migraine occur in migraineurs who have been placed on analgesics for other ailments.[35] The association between analgesic overuse and headache has been studied in conditions other than primary headache disorders. Chronic overuse of analgesics does not cause increased headache in nonmigraineurs. For example, studying a group of arthritis patients who were consuming fairly large amounts of analgesics regularly for arthritis did not show increased incidence of headache.[36] There is no major difference between various types of analgesics used in the treatment of chronic headache in producing analgesic rebound headache.[37] The conclusion from various clinical observations and studies is that analgesic rebound headache may be restricted to those who are already headache sufferers.

Pathogenesis of analgesic-induced headache is not clearly understood, although evidence suggests involvement of 5-hydroxy tryptamine (5-HT) in the process.[38-40] Hering et al.[38] reported reduction in whole-blood 5-HT in patients with analgesic rebound headache that was normalized on discontinuing the analgesics. This rise in 5-HT level in the whole blood paralleled the improvement in headache frequency. Patients with analgesic-induced headaches have lower basal content of platelet 5-HT, reduced 5-HT uptake ability when incubated with excess of the amine, and a greater density of $5-HT_2$ receptors on platelet membrane than migrainous patients without analgesic-induced headache.[39,40] These observations suggest that chronic analgesic overuse interferes with the intrinsic pain modulatory system by depletion of 5-HT and consequently upregulation of its postsynaptic receptors. Therefore it is likely that analgesic-induced headache is at least partly due to defective mechanisms of 5-HT uptake caused by analgesic use.

Alteration in the central pain modulation mechanism may account for perpetuation of headache.

Sicuteri postulated central opioid receptor impairment as an underlying mechanism for chronic headaches.[41-43] Natural opioids play a vital role in regulating pain. Sicuteri pointed out the neurochemical and other similarities between chronic headaches and morphine abstinence syndrome.[42,43] Both involve central serotonin and dopamine systems. Their prominent symptoms include headache, anhedonia, autonomic symptoms, and hypernociception. Intrinsic opioids act on the central nervous system to limit pain. Impairment of the opioid system would lower the pain threshold in

Table 3-9. The possible neurophysiologic mechanisms of CDH

Long-term plasticity/central sensitization/central functional reorganization

Kindling

Activation of nociceptive facilitatory systems, such as "on cells" in the ventral medial medulla

Lack of inhibitory modulation

---

patients with chronic headache. Prolonged use of analgesics may lead to suppression of antinociceptive opioids, thus resulting in heightened pain sensitivity, if the drug use were to be discontinued.

Table 3-9 lists possible neurophysiologic mechanisms of chronic daily headache.

Lance et al. postulated that further suppression or down-regulation of an already partly suppressed or abnormal antinociceptive system due to excessive symptomatic medications is a possible explanation for analgesic rebound headache in migraineurs.[36] Alterations in the density and function of postsynaptic neuronal receptors as a result of chronic medication use may be another explanation for the refractory headache these patients develop (central sensitization and long-term plasticity).

A phenomenon akin to "kindling" seen in epilepsy may be operating in chronic headaches also.

Activation of facilitatory nociceptive "on cells" in the ventral medulla as a result of excessive analgesic/narcotic use may be another explanation. "On cells" in the ventromedial medulla facilitate nociceptive reflex response such as tail flick response and show increased firing during naloxone-induced morphine withdrawal.[44] Mechanisms such as this, even though not adequately understood, may give a physiologic basis for analgesic-induced headache.

COMORBIDITY

Behavioral and Psychiatric Comorbidity

A number of recent publications have dealt with behavioral and psychiatric comorbidity of migraine.[45–50] Those observations are highly relevant to chronic daily headache, as most severe chronic daily headaches are transformed migraine. Breslau et al.[47] found that the estimated risk for major depression associated with prior migraine, adjusted for sex and education, was 3.2. The risk for migraine associated with prior depression was 3.1. The bidirectional influences, with each disorder increasing the risk of onset of the other, were shown by the preceding study.[47] A "shared etiology" between migraine and depression is implicated. A history of migraine is also associated with increased lifetime rates of anxiety disorders, illicit drug use disorders, nicotine dependence, and suicide attempts.[45,46] Those with a history of migraine were more likely to report job absenteeism, assess their general health as fair or poor, and use mental health services.[45,46] Breslau and Andreski[48] reported that migraine was associated with increased

Table 3-10. Behavioral scales in chronic daily headache (CDH)

Type of CDH	Zung Depression Scale score	Beck Depression Scale	Type A behavior pattern
Chronic tension-type headache (n = 84)	53 ± 9.9*	11 ± 8.6*	42 ± 4.7
Transformed migraine (n = 489)	52 ± 10.8*	13 ± 10.3*	50 ± 9.2*
Control episodic migraine (n = 100)	34 ± 4.2	8 ± 2.4	42 ± 4.8

*$p < 0.05$, compared with controls (episodic migraine). Adapted with permission from Mathew NT, Reuveni U, Perez F. Transformed or evolutive migraine. *Headache* 1987;27:102–106.

incidence of "neuroticism," defined as a general emotional overactivity, which may lead to neurotic disorders under stress. Merikangas et al. also observed strong association between migraine and depression, bipolar illness, anxiety, and panic disorders.[49,50] The preceding epidemiologic studies confirm the association between migraine and primary psychiatric and behavioral disorders such as depression, anxiety, and neuroticism, which have been reported in the clinic-based population.

Table 3-10 shows the behavioral scales, including Zung Depression Scale,[51] Beck Depression Scale,[52] and Type A Behavioral Pattern[53] in a series of 573 patients with chronic daily headache (48 with chronic tension-type headache and 489 with transformed migraine).[12] When compared with episodic migraine patients, chronic daily headache patients show significant elevation of depression scales. In addition, transformed migraine patients show elevated Type A behavioral pattern scores.[12]

Minnesota Multiphasic Personality Inventory

In our series, based on the Minnesota Multiphasic Personality Inventory (MMPI), an abnormal personality profile was found in 61% of patients with CDH compared with 12.2% of patients in the episodic migraine group ($p < 0.01$). Of the CDH patients, 56% showed elevations of scales 1, 2, and 3 (i.e., hypochondriasis, depression, and hysteria), with most showing typical V configuration. Thus "neuroticism" was found to be significantly higher with patients with chronic daily headache. No statistical difference among the various types of CDH was found. Various combinations of elevated scales of 6, 7, 8, and 9 were seen in 21% of CDH patients, and those elevated scales were seen more frequently in the most persistent and intractable cases.

The psychiatric comorbidity in CDH was assessed by Sandrini et al. in a series of 98 patients.[54] DSM-III-R criteria were used to diagnose psychiatric conditions. Only 9.2% had no psychiatric diagnosis. Anxiety disorders were observed in 72.4%; mood disorders, in 55.1%; combined anxiety and mood disorders, in 46%; and somatoform disorders, in 3.1%. Of those with mood disorders, one-third suffered from major depression.

Neurologic Comorbidity

Coexistence of migraine and idiopathic intracranial hypertension without papilledema may result in refractory chronic daily headache.[55] A spinal tap to measure the cerebrospinal fluid (CSF) pressure is the only way to diagnose this condition. Headache characteristics of the two conditions may be very similar. In a refractory case of chronic daily headache with migrainous features, a spinal tap to rule out raised CSF pressure is in order.[55] Another comorbid neurologic condition associated with chronic daily headache is sleep apnea.[56]

Quality of Life in CDH Patients

Health-related quality of life (HQL) using short-form (SF to 36) questionnaire in 115 patients (62 migraine patients and 53 CDH patients) revealed that patterns of disability were similar in migraine and CDH patients, but CDH was marked by a lower level of health scales.[57] Patients with CDH had a significantly worse pain score in physical functioning, role functioning (physical), bodily pain, general health perceptions, and mental health than patients with migraine headache.

Disability in CDH

Assessment of disability in a series of 201 CDH patients using the migraine disability assessment score (MIDAS)[58] showed very high MIDAS.[59] The mean MIDAS was 70, with 21 being the upper limit of normal. Scores were significantly higher than those seen in patients with episodic migraine. The MIDAS in CDH showed a high correlation with the number of headache days (frequency).[59] MIDAS in CDH also correlated with the level of anxiety and depression, as measured by Beck anxiety and depression scales.

MANAGEMENT

ETTH is typically treated with aspirin and/or acetaminophen often combined with caffeine or alternatively with nonsteroidal antiinflammatory drugs (such as ibuprofen, napoxen sodium, or ketoprofen). Moderate intensity ETTH may respond to prescription drugs such as combinations containing butalbital or acetaminophen, isometheptene, and dichloroalphenazone (Midrin). To prevent habituation and rebound, the use of combination analgesics should usually be limited to 10 events or 24 tablets or capsules. Patients with frequent ETTH may benefit from prophylactic medication using tricyclic antidepressants such as amitriptyline, nortriptyline, or protriptyline or alternatively from SSRI drugs such as fluoxetine. Nonmedication approaches that benefit some patients include progressive relaxation training, biofeedback, hypnosis, acupuncture, and physical therapy modalities.

The two major factors that determine the prognosis of CDH are analgesic rebound and comorbidity. The first step in the management of CDH is to determine the presence or absence of rebound phenomenon. A person suffering from headache despite consuming analgesics and ergotamine on a daily basis could fall into the category of drug-induced headache or analgesic rebound headache. Concomitant use of prophylactic medications in this situation is usually ineffective.

Behavioral, psychologic, and disability aspects of CDH need to be considered when treating patients with this form of headache.

A multimodality approach is essential for satisfactory results, and a combination of pharmacologic and behavioral interventions is necessary.

It is important to make as comprehensive a diagnosis as possible and to attempt to recognize the subtype of CDH the patient is suffering from. Those with transformed migraine are significantly more responsive to treatment than those with CTH. In all subtypes, the analgesic rebound has to be looked for.

Essential principles are the following:

1. Discontinuation of the offending medications to detoxification.
2. Attempts to break the cycle of continuous headache by pharmacotherapeutic agents.
3. Initiation of prophylactic pharmacotherapy.
4. Management of breakthrough headaches by specific agents such as triptans.
5. Concomitant behavioral intervention, which includes biofeedback therapy, cognitive behavioral therapy, individual counseling, family therapy, physical exercise, and dietary instructions.
6. Adequate instructions about ill effects of medications, with special focus on analgesics.
7. Continuity of care.

The multimodality approach to treatment outlined earlier can be undertaken as either an outpatient or an inpatient.

Outpatient Treatment

Outpatient treatment is most suitable for highly motivated patients who are not very high consumers of opioids/butalbital/tranquilizers containing analgesics. Outpatient management consists of (a) gradual reduction of the overused medications; (b) substitution of naratriptan 2.5 mg BID or a nonsteroidal antiinflammatory agent (NSAIDs) including COX_2 inhabitants during the withdrawal period; (c) introduction of appropriate prophylactic pharmacotherapy; (d) treatment of breakthrough headache with specific antimigraine drugs such as a triptan; and (e) a combination of all the preceding with behavioral approaches and education.

Inpatient Treatment

Inpatient treatment is indicated in those who fail outpatient treatment, who consume very large quantities of opioids/butalbital/tranquilizers containing analgesics, with very significant psychologic and behavioral comorbidities as well as medical comorbidities.

Essential differences in the inpatient approach are a more aggressive supervised withdrawal of offending medications, use of agents to reduce the effect of abrupt withdrawal, intravenous administration of medication around the clock to break the cycle of headache, initiating prophylaxis that often includes a rational combination of medications to treat comorbidities and adjustment of the dosages. A hospital stay of 5 to 6 days is necessary in most cases, which may be extended to 10 or 15 days in more complicated cases.

Detoxification

Discontinuation of daily analgesics, narcotics, sedatives, caffeine, and ergotamine is the first step. A rare patient with triptan-induced rebound may also have to be taken off those medications, substituting with a triptan with a low recurrence rate such as naratriptan.

Abrupt withdrawal of analgesics and narcotics is possible; however, it should be done under close supervision. Detoxification from opioids can be aided by using clonidine. Clonidine reduces the clinical symptoms of opioid withdrawal. Two number 2 (0.2 mg) transdermal clonidine patches may be applied on the first day of withdrawal, to be changed after 1 week and discontinued after 2 weeks. Oral clonidine can be used after the first week.

Butalbital Withdrawal

The most commonly prescribed and overused medication for the treatment of chronic headaches and the most common cause of analgesic rebound is butalbital/caffeine/aspirin/acetaminophen combinations with or without codeine. Butalbital is a short-acting barbiturate. Barbiturate withdrawal symptoms may include apprehension, muscle weakness, tremors, postural faintness, amnesia, twitches, seizures, and psychosis or delirium. Seizures usually occur on the second or third day of withdrawal but can occur up to the eighth day. To avoid seizure and other withdrawal reactions, a long-acting barbiturate may be substituted. Phenobarbital 30 mg three times daily for the first 2 days and 30 mg daily for the next 2 days is recommended during the withdrawal period.[60]

Breaking the Cycle of Headache

To further aid the withdrawal of agents containing opioids/butalbital/caffeine and to help break the cycle of headache, any one of the following or an appropriate combination of these is recommended:

NSAIDs:
  Naproxen[61]
  Tolfenamic acid[62]
  Ketoprofen
  Diclofenac
Methylergonovine[63]
Sumatriptan SC injections[64]
Oral corticosteroids[65]
Naratriptan oral
Intravenous (IV) dihydroergotamine[66,67]
IV prochlorperazine[68]
IV chlorpromazine[69]
IV droperidol[70]
IV diphenhydramine[71]
IV valproate sodium[72]
IV dexamethasone[73]

Intravenous Dihydroergotamine

In most transformed migraine patients, the daily headache cycle can be broken by repetitive intravenous administration of dihydroergotamine (DHE).[66,67] A test dose of 0.33 ml of DHE with 5 mg of metoclopramide or 10 mg of prochlorperazine may be used, followed by 0.5 ml of DHE with one of the antinausea medications every 6 hours for 48 to 72 hours. Some patients may require the therapy for a few additional days. Approximately 70% to 80% of patients do respond to DHE. Diarrhea, leg cramps, and chest pain are seen as side effects in some patients. DHE is contraindicated in coronary and peripheral vascular disease.

Alternate Intravenous Medications

In those who cannot tolerate DHE or when it is contraindicated, alternative intravenous medications are possible. These include chlorpromazine or prochlorperazine.[68,69] In some patients, 12.5 mg of chlorpromazine given intravenously (piggy back) infused in 15 minutes every 6 hours for 2 days has been found to be effective. Orthostatic hypotension is a possible side effect, and precautions should be taken to prevent dizziness and syncope as a result of it.

Prochlorperazine at 5 to 10 mg given intravenously is also effective and can be repeated. Extrapyramidal dystonic reactions are possible side effects that can be counteracted by benztropine mesylate (Cogentin). Anecdotal reports also indicate the use of intravenous dexamethasone.[73] Although there are no controlled studies to prove its clinical efficacy, those who have prolonged migraine seem to respond to such therapy. It can be combined with DHE or prochlorperazine.

Intravenous Valproate Sodium

Recently, intravenous valproate sodium (Depacon) has been found to be useful for status migrainosus and can be given to break the cycle of CDH.[74] Five hundred milligrams of valproate sodium diluted in 50 ml of IV saline given as fast drip are recommended. This can be repeated every 8 hours for 2 days.

Triptans to Break the Cycle

Diener et al.[64] found that repeated subcutaneous injections of sumatriptan may be useful in breaking the cycle of CDH (transformed from migraine). Because of the excellent tolerability of naratriptan, prolonged effect, and very low recurrence rate, naratriptan tablets 2.5 mg BID are being used during the withdrawal period. Controlled studies are in progress.

Prophylactic Pharmacotherapy

Depending on the type of CDH, prophylactic pharmacotherapy can be planned. Those with transformed migraine may respond to antimigraine prophylactic agents effectively, provided detoxification from analgesic has been achieved already. The clinician may choose a prophylactic agent or a combination of prophylactic agents, depending on the clinical diagnosis and comorbid factors. There is a place for *rational copharmacy* in the prophylactic treatment of CDH. For example, one can combine a primary antimigraine prophylactic agent, such as a beta-blocker, methysergide, or divalproex sodium, with agents that act on the psychiatric comorbid conditions, such as depression or anxiety. A combination of antidepressants or antianxiety agents with antimigraine prophylactic agents is a rational way of approaching the treatment of persistent CDH. Prophylactic medications are dealt with extensively in the section on migraine.

Bonuccelli et al.[65] treated patients with analgesic rebound headache with dexamethasone (4 mg intramuscularly) for 2 weeks followed by amitriptyline (50 mg/day) for 6 months. Acute exacerbations were treated with sumatriptan. They reported good response with this combination treatment. In an open study, divalproex sodium used prophylactically reduced the frequency and severity of CDHs of a transformed migraine type.[74]

For chronic tension-type headache amitriptyline is the drug of choice.

Concomitant Behavioral Therapy

Concomitant behavioral intervention, including biofeedback therapy, individual cognitive behavioral therapy, family therapy, physical exercise, and dietary instructions, is imperative for successful management of patients with CDH. Details of these modes of treatment are beyond the scope of this chapter. Physical therapy (heat, massage, ultrasonography) to neck muscles may help partially. Selected application of trigger point injections may help as well.

Education

Adequate instruction about the nature of the patent's disorder and the ill effects of certain medications used in excessive and frequent quantities, particularly analgesics and narcotics, should be emphasized. Patients must understand that this disorder is biologic and that neurochemical and physiologic changes produce the headache. They should also realize that behavioral factors, such as anxiety, depression, inability to relax, and stress, influence this process a great deal, making headaches more frequent, more severe, and more difficult to manage. Every program that deals with CDH should include education.

Continuity of Care

CDH is usually a prolonged problem occupying years of a person's life, and none of the preventive medications are 100% effective. Adverse effects prevent prolonged use of many medications. Patients develop tachyphylaxis to many medications. Therefore continuity of care with frequent follow-up and adequate physician/patient communication is essential for the long term.

Psychiatric Referral

CDH is not a primary psychiatric disorder, although comorbidities are important. Referral to a psychiatrist should not be an "end-of-the-road" referral. If a psychiatrist is consulted, the consultation should be in conjunction with the medical treatment. The physician who takes care of these patients has full control of all aspects of treatment, and the psychiatric treatment should only be an adjunct in the overall management.

PROGNOSIS OF CDH

A long-term follow-up study has looked at the prognosis for CDH.[75] A group of 489 patients was followed for an average of 42 months (range, 18 to 72 months). Thirty-eight patients (8%) were lost to follow-up. Of the remaining 451 patients, 140 (31%) showed significant recurrence of headaches despite continuing efforts to use prophylactic medications, dietary control, behavioral treatment, and avoidance of analgesics, sedatives, and daily ergotamine. Most of these 140 patients continued to have periodic exacerbations of headache with episodes of status migrainosus and low-grade daily headache. They continued to need some symptomatic medications or showed a tendency to use prescribed substitute medications such as isometheptene in excessive quantities. They were frequent visitors to the headache clinic compared with patients who showed improvement. In some, repeated hospitalizations were necessary. Ninety-two patients (20%) were unable to work, and the rest were relatively unproductive in their work. Many had to change jobs frequently because of absenteeism.

Pini et al.[76] evaluated 102 patients with chronic daily headache with analgesic rebound attending a headache center in Italy. They divided the group into those who underwent day hospital treatment followed by prophylactic therapy and those who were given prophylactic therapy immediately. Both groups improved, with no difference with respect to hospital treatment or outpatient treatment. After 4 months of follow-up, 28% of patients reverted to daily analgesic use. These patients took barbiturate-containing mixtures in higher percentages than other drugs. More patients who were treated as outpatients relapsed compared with those who were treated in the day hospital.

Overall, from the experience of many centers treating chronic daily headache patients, approximately one-third of patients appear to show relapse of their daily headache and may have a tendency to return to taking pain medications regularly unless they are supervised very carefully. In patients with this persistent, intractable chronic daily headache, the behavioral, psychologic, and neuroendocrine features are strikingly different from those with CDH who show improvement (Table 3-11).[75] MMPI

Table 3-11. Behavioral, psychologic, and neuroendocrine features in intractable chronic daily headache (CDH)

	Intractable CDH (31%) ($n = 140$)		CDH improved group ($n = 311$) (69%)	
	No. of patients	%	No. of patients	%
Abnormal MMPI	140	100*	158	48
Alcoholism among parents	82	58*	51	17
Physical, emotional, sexual abuse	74	52*	26	8
Positive dexamethasone suppression test	42	30*	34	11

	Depression scores in intractable CDH	
	Intractable CDH ($n = 140$)	Improved group of CDH ($n = 311$)
Zung Depression Scale	62 ± 9.9*	51.2 ± 8.8*
Beck Depression Scale	16 ± 6.6*	12.2 ± 8.9

*$p < 0.01$

was abnormal in 100% of intractable cases. High scores and hypochondriasis, depression, and hysteria (scores 1, 2, and 3) were consistent, and combinations of high scores of 6, 7, 8, and 9 were seen in 56% of those with intractable CDH. Among the parents of patients with intractable CDH, a high incidence of alcoholism was found. A high incidence of physical, emotional, and sexual abuse was also discovered in this group when compared with those who were treated successfully. The Zung Depression Scale and the Beck Depression Inventory were also higher in the intractable group when compared with the improved group.

Therefore it appears that there is a group with very persistent intractable chronic daily headache that is resistant to all currently available forms of treatment. It may signify some permanent abnormalities in the pain control systems of the brain.

REFERENCES

1. Schwartz BS, Stewart WF, Simon D, et al. Epidemiology of tension-type headache. *JAMA* 1998;279:381–383.
2. Scher A, Stewart WF, Liberman J, et al. Prevalence of frequent headache in a population sample. *Headache* 1997;37:330.
3. Russell MB, Ostergaard S, Bendtsen L, et al. Familial occurrence of chronic tension-type headache. *Cephalalgia* 1999;19: 207–210.
4. Castillo J, Munoz P, Guitera V, et al. Epidemiology of chronic daily headache in the general population. *Headache* 1999;39: 190–196.
5. Rasmussen BK, Jensen R, Schroll M, et al. Interrelations between migraine and tension-type headache in general population. *Arch Neurol* 1992;49:914–918.
6. Iversen HK, Langemark M, Andersson PG, et al. Clinical characteristics of migraine and episodic tension-type headache in relation to old and new diagnostic criteria. *Headache* 1990;30: 514–519.
7. Ulrich V, Russell MB, Jensen R, et al. A comparison of tension-type headache in migraineurs and in non-migraineurs: a population-based study. *Pain* 1996;67:501–506.
8. Cady RK, Gutterman D, Saiers JA, et al. Responsiveness of non-IHS migraine and tension-type headache to sumatriptan. *Cephalalgia* 1997;17:588–90.
9. Lipton RB, Cady RK, O'Quinn S, et al. Effects of sumatriptan on the full spectrum of headaches in individuals with disabling IHS migraine. *Cephalalgia* 1999;19:370.
10. Brennum J, Kjeldsen M, Olesen J. The $5HT_1$-like agonist sumatriptan has a significant effect in chronic tension-type headache. *Cephalalgia* 1992;12:375–379.
11. Brennum J, Brinck T, Schriver L, et al. Sumatriptan has no clinically relevant effect in the treatment of episodic tension type headache. *Eur J Neurol* 1996;3:23–28.
12. Mathew NT, Reuveni U, Perez F. Transformed or evolutive migraine. *Headache* 1987;27:102–106.
13. Sanin LC, Mathew NT, Bellmeyer LR, et al. International Headache Society (IHS) Headache Classification as applied to a headache clinic population. *Cephalalgia* 1994;14:443–446.
13a. Rasmussen BK, Jensen R, Schroll M, et al. Epidemiology of headache in a general population—a prevalence study. *J Clin Epidemiol* 1991;44:1147–1157.

14. Manzoni GC, Micieli G, Granella F, et al. Daily chronic head-ache: classification and clinical features—observation on 250 patients. *Cephalalgia* 1987;7[Suppl 6]:169–170.
15. Manzoni GC, Sandrini, Zanferrari C, et al. Clinical features of daily chronic headache and its different subtypes. *Cephalalgia* 1991;11[Suppl 11]:292–293.
16. Solomon S, Lipton RB, Newman LC. Clinical features of chronic daily headache. *Headache* 1992;32:325–329.
17. Baldrati A, Bini L, D'Alessandro R, et al. Analysis of outcome predictors of migraine towards chronicity. *Cephalalgia* 1985;5 [Suppl 2]:195–199.
18. Giglio JA, Bruera OC, Leston JA. Influence of transformation factors on chronic daily headache. *Cephalalgia* 1995;15[Suppl 14]:165.
19. Mathew NT, Stubits E, Nigam MP. Transformation of episodic migraine into chronic daily headache: an analysis of factors. *Headache* 1982;22:66–68.
20. Manzoni GC, Granella F, Sandrin G, et al. Classification of chronic daily headache by International Headache Society criteria: limits and new proposals. *Cephalalgia* 1995;15:37–43.
21. Silberstein SD, Lipton RB. Classification of daily and near daily headache: field trial of revised IHIS criteria. *Neurology* 1996; 47:871–875.
22. Vanast WJ. New daily persistent headache: definition of a benign syndrome. *Headache* 1986;26:318–320.
23. Vanast WJ, Diaz-Mitoma F, Tyrrell DLJ. Hypothesis: chronic benign daily headache is an immune disorder with a viral trigger. *Headache* 1987;27:138–142.
24. Saper JR, Jones JM. Ergotamine dependency. *Clin Neuropharmacol* 1986;9:244.
25. Dichgans J, Diener HO, Gerber WD, et al. Analgetika-induzierter dauerkopfschmerz. *Dtsch Med Wochenschr* 1984;109:369.
26. Kudrow L. Paradoxical effects of frequent analgesic use. In: Critchley M, Friedman A, Gorini S, Sicuteri F, eds. *Advances in neurology*, vol. 33. New York: Raven Press, 1982:335.
27. Mathew NT, Kurman R, Perez F. Drug induced refractory headache: clinical features and management. *Headache* 1990;30: 634–638.
28. Michultka DM, Blanchard EB, Appelbaum KA, et al. The refractory headache patient II high medication consumption (analgesic rebound) headache. *Behav Res Ther* 1989;27:411–420.
29. Pini L, Bigarelli M, Vitale G, et al. Headaches associated with chronic use of analgesics: a therapeutic approach. *Headache* 1996;36:433–439.
30. Rapoport AM, Weeks RE, Sheftell FD, et al. Analgesic rebound headache: theoretical and practical implications. *Cephalalgia* 1985;5[Suppl 3]:448.
31. Silverman K, Evans SM, Strain EC, et al. Withdrawal syndrome after the double blind cessation of caffeine consumption. *N Engl J Med* 1992;327:1109–1114.
32. Rapoport AM, Stang P, Gutterman DL, et al. Analgesic rebound headache in clinical practice—data from a physician survey. *Headache* 1996;36:14–19.
33. Ferrari A, Sternieri E. Chronic headache and analgesic abuse. In: *Ten years of headache research in Italy*. De Marinis M, Granella F, eds. Rome: CIC Edizioni Internazionali, 1996:44–54.

34. Wang W, Timsit-Berthier M, Schoenen J. Negative correlation between sensation seeking behavior and intensity dependence of auditory evoked potentials in migraine. *Cephalalgia* 1995;15 [Suppl 14]:65.
35. Isler H. Migraine treatment as a cause of chronic migraine. In: Rose FC, ed. *Advances in migraine research and therapy.* New York: Raven Press, 1982:159.
36. Lance E, Parkes C, Wilkinson M. Does analgesic abuse cause headaches de novo? *Headache* 1988;28:61.
37. Bowlder I, Kikan J, Gansslen-Blumberg S, et al. The association between analgesic abuse and headache—coincidental or causal? *Headache* 1988;28:494.
38. Hering R, Glover V, Patichis K, et al. 5-HT in migraine patients with analgesic rebound headache. *Cephalalgia* 1993;13:410–412.
39. Srikiatkhachorn A, Govitrapong P, Limthavon C. Up-regulation of 5-HT$_2$ serotonin receptor: a possible mechanism of transformed migraine. *Headache* 1994;34:8–11.
40. Srikiatkhachorn A, Anthony M. Platelet 5-HT and 5-HT$_2$ receptors in patients with analgesic induced headache. *Cephalalgia* 1995;15[Suppl 14]:83.
41. Sicuteri F. Opioid receptor impairment: underlying mechanism in "pain diseases"? *Cephalalgia* 1981;1:77–82.
42. Sicuteri F. Natural opioids in migraine. In: Critchley M, ed. *Advances in neurology.* New York: Raven Press, 1982:523–533.
43. Sicuteri F. Is acute tolerance to 5-hydroxytryptamine opioid dependent? Its absence in migraine sufferers. *Cephalalgia* 1983; 3:187–190.
44. Fields HL, Heinricher MM. Brainstem modulation of nociceptor-driven withdrawal reflexes. *Ann NY Acad Sci* 1989;563:34–44.
45. Breslau N, Davis GC, Endreski P. Migraine, psychiatric disorders and suicide attempts: an epidemiological study of young adults. *Psychiatry Res* 1991;37:11–23.
46. Breslau N, Davis GC. Migraine, physical health and psychiatric disorder: a prospective epidemiologic study in young adults. *J Psychiatr Res* 1993;27:211–221.
47. Breslau N, Davis GC, Schultz LR. Migraine and major depression: a longitudinal study. *Headache* 1994;34:387–393.
48. Breslau N, Andreski P. Migraine, personality, and psychiatric comorbidity. *Headache* 1995;35:382–386.
49. Merikangas KR, Angst J, Isler H. Migraine and psychopathology: results of the Zurich cohort study of young adults. *Arch Gen Psychiatry* 1990;47:849–853.
50. Merikangas KR, Angst J. Headache syndromes and psychiatric disorders: association and familial transmission. *J Psychiatr Res* 1993;27:197–210.
51. Zung WWK. A self-rating depression scale. *Arch Gen Psychiatry* 1965;12:63–70.
52. Beck AT, Ward CM, Mendelsohn M, et al. An inventory for measuring depression. *Arch Gen Psychiatry* 1961;5:561–571.
53. Friedman M, Rosenman R. *Type A behavior and your heart.* New York: Knopf, 1974.
54. Sandrini G, Verri AP, Barbieri E, et al. Psychiatric comorbidity in chronic daily headache. *Cephalalgia* 1995;15[Suppl 14]:163.
55. Mathew NT, Ravishanker K, Sanin LC. Coexistence of migraine and idiopathic intracranial hypertension without papilledema. *Neurology* 1996;46:1226–1230.

56. Guilleminaut C, Dement WC. *Sleep apnea syndrome.* New York: Liss, 1978.
57. Monzon MJ, Lainez MJ. Quality of life in migraine and chronic daily headache patients. *Cephalalgia* 1998;18:638–643.
58. Stewart WF, Lipton RB, Kolodner K, et al. Reliability of the migraine disability assessment score in a population-based sample of headache sufferers. *Cephalalgia* 1999;19:107–114.
59. Villarreal SS, Mathew NT, Shahial N, et al. Disability in chronic daily headache: factors affecting MIDAS scores. *Headache* 1999; 39:384.
60. Sands GH. A protocol for butalbital, aspirin and caffeine (BAC) detoxification in headache patients. *Headache* 1990;30:491–496.
61. Mathew NT. Amelioration of ergotamine withdrawal symptoms with naproxen. *Headache* 1987;27:130–133.
62. Ala-Hurula V, Mylyla VV, Hokkanen E, et al. Tolfenamic acid and ergotamine abuse. *Headache* 1981;21:240–243.
63. Graff-Radford SB, Bittar CT. The use of methylergonovine (methergine) in the initial control of drug induced refractory headache. *Headache* 1993;33:390–393.
64. Diener HC, Haab J, Peters C, et al. Subcutaneous sumatriptan in the treatment of headache during withdrawal from drug-induced headache. *Headache* 1991;31:205–209.
65. Bonuccelli U, Nuti A, Lucetti C, et al. Amitriptyline and dexamethasone combined treatment in drug-induced headache. *Cephalalgia* 1996;6:197–200.
66. Raskin NH. Repetitive intravenous dihydroergotamine as therapy for intractable migraine. *Neurology* 1986;36:995–997.
67. Silberstein SD, Schulman EA, Hopkins MM. Repetitive intravenous DHE in the treatment of refractory headache. *Headache* 1990;30:334–339.
68. Coppola M, Yealy DM, Leibold RA. Randomized, placebo-controlled evaluation of prochlorperazine versus metoclopramide for emergency department treatment of migraine headache. *Ann Emerg Med* 1995;26:541–546.
69. Lane PL, Ross R. Intravenous chlorpromazine-preliminary results in acute migraine. *Headache* 1985;25:302–304.
70. Wang SJ, Silberstein SD, Young WB. Droperidol treatment of status migrainosus and refractory migraine. *Headache* 1997;37:377–382.
71. Swidan SZ, Hamel RL, Saper JR, et al. The efficacy of intravenously administered diphenhydramine versus dihydroergotamine, ketorolac, chlorpromazine, and droperidol in the treatment of refractory daily chronic headache. *Neurology* 1999;[Suppl 2]:A255.
72. Mathew NT, Kailasam J, Meadors L, et al. Intravenous valproate sodium (Depacon) aborts migraine rapidly: a preliminary report. *Cephalalgia* 1999;19:373.
73. Saadah HA. Abortive migraine therapy in the office with dexamethasone and prochlorperazine. *Headache* 1994;34:366–370.
74. Mathew NT, Ali S. Valproate in the treatment of persistent chronic daily headache: an open label study. *Headache* 1991;31:71–76.
75. Mathew NT, Kurman R, Perez F. Intractable chronic daily headache: a persistent neurobiobehavioral disorder. *Cephalalgia* 1989; 9[Suppl 10]:180–181.
76. Pini L, Bigarelli M, Vitale G, et al. Headaches associated with chronic use of analgesics: a therapeutic approach. *Headache* 1996; 36:433–439.

Cluster Headache

Ninan T. Mathew

Cluster headache (CH), one of the most severe forms of head pain, is a typical example of a periodic disease and is distinct from other forms of headache. The term *cluster headache* recognizes periodicity as a major clinical feature of the disorder.[1,2]

CLASSIFICATION AND CLINICAL TERMS

The Headache Classification Committee of the International Headache Society (IHS) recognizes three major forms of CH: episodic, chronic, and the variant, chronic paroxysmal hemicrania (CPH).[3] Table 4-1 shows the IHS classification. The terms used in describing CH include *attack,* meaning individual attacks of headache pain; *cluster period,* the period during which patients have repeated attacks; *remission,* a period of freedom from attacks; and *minibouts,* periods of attacks lasting less than 7 days.

Episodic CH is characterized by cluster periods of 7 days to 1 year, periods of remission of more than 14 days up to months or years, and occasional minibouts. Chronic CH is characterized by absence of remission for 1 year or short remissions of less than 14 days, increased frequency of attacks, and relative resistance to pharmacotherapy.

CLINICAL MANIFESTATIONS

CH, predominantly a disease of males (the male-to-female ratio is 9:1), has an approximate prevalence of 0.1% to 0.4% in the general population.[4] It usually begins between the ages of 20 and 40 years, although there are well-documented cases outside that range.

The unique head pain profile, periodicity, and autonomic features distinguish CH from other headache disorders.

Headache Pain Profile

The *head pain profile* consists of rapid onset of headache, reaching a peak intensity in 10 to 15 minutes and lasting 30 to

Table 4-1.   IHS classification: cluster headache and chronic paroxysmal hemicrania

3.1 Cluster headache (CH)
   3.1.1 CH periodicity undetermined
   3.1.2 Episodic CH
   3.1.3 Chronic CH
      3.1.3.1 Unremitting from onset
      3.1.3.2 Evolved from episodic
3.2 Chronic paroxysmal hemicrania
3.3 CH-like disorder not fulfilling preceding criteria

45 minutes. The pain may remain severe for an hour or more and then, after a period of fluctuating peaks of pain, rapidly subsides, leaving the sufferer exhausted. Headache is almost always unilateral, the most common sites of pain being orbital, retroorbital, temporal, supraorbital, and infraorbital, in order of decreasing frequency. Rare cases occur outside this trigeminal territory.[5] A few to several attacks usually occur with a frequency range of one a week to eight or more per day.

In any cluster period, the pain remains on the same side and may affect that side year after year. Occasionally, the pain may be contralateral in a subsequent cluster; even more rarely, it alternates from side to side, headache to headache. The pain is of terrible intensity and is usually described as boring or tearing, like a "hot poker in the eye," or as if "the eye is being pushed out." This is distinctly different from the dull throbbing of migraine.

Periodicity

There is a clocklike regularity in the timing of attacks,[6] a phenomenon thought to be due to dysfunction of hypothalamic biologic clock mechanisms. Onset shortly after falling asleep is common and, at least in some subjects, corresponds to the onset of rapid eye movement (REM) sleep.[7]

Nocturnal attacks also occur during non-REM periods.[7] Sleep apnea and resultant oxygen desaturation could act as triggers for CH attacks.[8] At times, three or four attacks per night rapidly lead to sleep deprivation, which in turn can result in frequent daytime naps, often with further painful attacks. Circannual periodicity also occurs.

Autonomic Symptoms

Parasympathetic overactivity resulting in ipsilateral lacrimation, injection of the conjunctiva, and nasal stiffness or rhinorrhea is regular. Partial sympathetic paralysis resulting in ptosis and miosis also occurs. Facial flushing or pallor, scalp and facial tenderness, tenderness of the ipsilateral carotid artery, and bradycardia are other common associated features.

Some of these features also occur in patients with CPH or other conditions, such as dissection of the carotid artery, but the temporal profile of CH is virtually specific.

Behavior During Attacks

During the attack, patients find it difficult to lie down, as it aggravates pain. Some patients pace the floor or sit up in a posture that gives maximum relief.[7] This is distinct from migraine, during which the patient retreats to a dark, quiet room. The CH patient may behave in irrational and bizarre ways, moaning, crying, or screaming, and may threaten suicide. Some patients find relief by physical exercise such as jogging in place. They may press on the eye or temple with the hand or with an ice pack or a hot washcloth. Many prefer to be alone or to go outside, even in cold weather. After an attack, the patient may be exhausted. Fear of a further attack with the onset of sleep can lead to prolonged attempts to remain awake. This futile behavior results in the rapid onset of REM activity when sleep eventually overcomes the subject, and a further attack often occurs within minutes of falling asleep.

Provocation of Attacks

Alcohol frequently triggers an attack while the patient is in an active cluster phase. In patients with periods of remission, alcohol rarely precipitates an attack during a pain-free period. Most subjects give up the use of alcohol as soon as they realize a cluster period has begun. Some patients who are receiving prophylactic treatment can consume alcohol without developing an attack. Some can imbibe without any effect on the attacks, regardless of the phase of the disorder, and a very small percentage actually use excessive quantities of alcohol to try to get to sleep without causing an attack to develop. Unlike migraine, CH may be precipitated by any type of alcoholic beverage—beer, spirits, and wine have the same effect. Whether alcohol acts simply as a vasodilator is uncertain.

Other vasodilators, such as nitroglycerin tablets[9] and histamine, also induce attacks of CH in susceptible subjects. Transient, mild hypoxemia occurs following the administration of nitroglycerin.[10] Kudrow and Kudrow reported that CH in patients in remission and nonheadache controls had no headache following nitroglycerin, despite transient oxygen desaturation.[11] In the active cluster group, low-grade oxygen desaturation persisted, never returning to baseline, and resulted in cluster attacks. Altitude hypoxemia and sleep apnea-induced hypoxemia also can induce DH attacks during the cluster period. Kudrow and Kudrow offered the hypothesis, based on these observations, that the carotid body chemoreceptors are involved in CH pathogenesis.[12]

Food items and food additives do not appear to be involved in the pathogenesis of CH, as in migraine. The frequency of smoking is greatly increased among CH patients, and some achieve remission after abstinence.

For patients in the episodic phase, the factors that determine the beginning and end of a cluster period or a period of remission are unknown. Stress, depression, and psychologic factors seem to have less importance in the pathogenesis of CH than in other headache types. The behavior of some patients during attacks that resembles a manic episode, the periodicity of CH, and beneficial effects of lithium in some patients suggest some resemblance to manic-depressive illness.

Course

Both the episodic form and the chronic form of CH continue to occur for many years. In the episodic form, remissions may last, but the subject remains at risk for a recurrence until old age. In a large series of patients followed by Krabbe,[13] only a small minority appeared to have lost the propensity to attacks with age. The chronic form may revert to the episodic form.[14]

PATHOPHYSIOLOGY

A comprehensive pathophysiologic explanation to account for various aspects of CH is still lacking. Four elements that need explanation are pain, vasodilation, autonomic features, and periodicity.

Pain and vasodilation are due to the activation of the trigemi-novascular system. A number of observations have indicated vasodilation of the ophthalmic artery during an attack of CH. These include tonometry, corneal indentation, pulse amplitude studies, and thermography showing focal hyperthermia. Doppler studies showing decreased velocities in the ophthalmic artery, conventional angiography showing dilation of the ophthalmic artery,[15] and, recently, magnetic resonance angiographic studies confirming the same.[16] Vasodilation has been shown to follow the onset of pain and is not the initial event.[17] In addition to the vasodilation, there is neurogenic inflammation. Calcitonin gene-related peptide (CGRP)[18] and vasoactive intestinal polypeptide (VIP) are increased in the ipsilateral external jugular vein, whereas substance P (SP) and neuropeptide Y are normal. These indicate activation of the trigeminovascular system and cranial parasympathetic pathways.

Somatostatin, a SP inhibitor, reduces the intensity and dura-tion of CH.[19] Sumatriptan and dihydroergotamine (DHE), which block perivascular neurogenic inflammation, are very effective agents in relieving CH. Activation of the trigeminovascular sys-tem with involvement of bipolar SP neurons and resultant axonal reflex may be a reasonable explanation for the neuro-genic inflammation in CH.

Autonomic involvement such as Horner's syndrome and parasympathetic activation needs to be explained along with the pain. It has been proposed that a lesion in the cavernous sinus, possibly venous vasculitis, is the underlying cause of CH. Lesions of the cavernous sinus, where the nociceptive fibers of the fifth nerve, the sympathetic and parasympathetic fibers, come together, are a reasonable explanation for the occurrence of pain and autonomic symptoms concomitantly.[20] Evidence for lesions such as venous vasculitis in the cavernous sinus consists of abnormal orbital phlebography during cluster periods[21]; increased gallium 67 uptake in the cavernous sinus, demon-strated during cluster periods; dilation of the ophthalmic artery during an attack;[16] reports of pericarotid tumors, such as pitu-itary adenoma, causing clusterlike headache; response to steroids; lack of propensity to shift sides; and rare propensity to have bilateral attacks. Some authors feel that there is a similar-ity between CH and Tolosa-Hunt syndrome.[22]

Even though an intracavernous sinus lesion may explain most symptoms of attack, one of the most distinguishing features of CH—the periodicity—is difficult to explain. Involvement of the hypophyseal branches of the carotid artery and veins draining to the cavernous sinus, with the resultant changes in the perfusion of the hypothalamus, is a possible explanation for periodicity.[20]

Role of Hypothalamus and Biologic Clock Mechanisms

Circadian periodicity of individual attacks and periodic occur-rence of cluster periods indicate a disordered biologic clock. Hor-monal studies in CH patients give further evidence of a disor-dered central pacemaker. Alterations of secretory circadian rhythms of melatonin, cortisol, testosterone, beta-endorphin, beta-lipoprotein, and prolactin have been shown during cluster periods. Most of these rhythms return to normal during remission.[23] The circadian pacemaker, believed to be located in the suprachiasmatic nuclei (SCN), has interconnections with the brain stem serotonergic centers and the nuclei of the trigeminal nerve. A disturbance in the central pacemaker mechanism may thus act as a trigger for the activation of the trigeminovascular system. There are data that demonstrate a relationship between the frequency of CH and changes in the number of daylight hours (photoperiods).[24]

Using positron emission tomography (May et al.[25]) showed activation of ipsilateral inferior hypothalamic gray matter during the acute pain stage of CH, indicating hypothalamus as the primary generator of CH.

EXAMINATION

The only abnormal physical sign that may be seen between attacks of CH, either permanently or for a few hours, is an ipsilateral partial Horner's syndrome with a minor degree of upper-lid ptosis and miosis. Pharmacologic testing of the pupillary response suggests the Horner's syndrome is a third-order neuron disorder.[26]

During an attack, an ipsilateral Horner's syndrome, conjunctival injection, tearing, and nasal obstruction are common. Flushing and ipsilateral facial sweating are relatively rare. An occasional patient will complain of swelling of the temple, cheek, palate, or gums ipsilateral to the pain. In most instances, swelling cannot be detected by an examiner, although occasionally there is apparent edema and soft-tissue swelling in the region described by the sufferer.

Results of neurogenic imaging studies, including computed tomography (CT) and magnetic resonance imaging (MRI) scans of the head and neck, are normal, and cerebral angiography, performed between attacks, is unremarkable. Arteriography or magnetic resonance angiography (MRA) during the attack has been performed only a few times.[15,16] In the best-documented cases, the carotid artery appeared to be in spasm or to be irregularly compressed in the region of the siphon, with dilated ophthalmic artery.[15,16]

DIAGNOSIS

The diagnosis of CH, which is primarily clinical, is based on the history of the attacks, a careful description of the pain, the temporal profile, the trigger factors, and the associated autonomic manifestations. The rapid escalation of the pain, the predominance of nocturnal attacks, and the limited duration of each headache are important details of the history. Despite the rarity of associated structural abnormalities, it is appropriate to obtain a neuroimage, preferably MRI of the brain or a contrast-enhanced CT.

Differential Diagnosis

CH is distinguished from *migraine* by the male predominance, strict unilaterality of pain, short-lived attacks (45 minutes to 1 hour), multiple attacks per day, associated autonomic features, restlessness and inability to lie down during the attack, and periodicity (clustering) of attacks. Migraines tend to occur pri-

Table 4-2.   Comparison of cluster headache and migraine

Clinical Feature	Cluster Headache	Migraine
Gender ratio (M:F)	90:10	25:75
Unilateral pain	-100%	-68%
Duration	15–180 minutes	4–72 hours
Associated with		
Nausea	+	+++
Photophobia, phonophobia	+	+++
Exacerbation by movement	-	+++
Family history	+	+++
Neurologic aura	-	+
Autonomic features, such as lacrimation, rhinorrhea, and ptosis	+++	±

marily in females. Attacks may be associated with prodrome or aura and may last a number of hours to days. Nausea, vomiting, and photophobia are prominent features in migraine; they are absent in CH (Table 4-2) Variants of CH are listed in Table 4-3. These will be discussed in detail in the chapter on short-lived headache.

Symptomatic Cluster Headache

Symptomatic CHs[27] are CH-like attacks that occur as a result of an underlying intracranial lesion. Parasellar meningioma, adenoma of the pituitary, calcified lesion in the region of the third ventricle, anterior carotid artery aneurysm, epidermoid tumor of the clivus expanding into the suprasellar cistern, vertebral artery aneurysms, nasopharyngeal carcinoma, ipsilateral large hemispheric arteriovenous malformation, and upper cervical meningioma have been reported to produce symptomatic CH,

Table 4-3.   Cluster headache variants

A. Those that differ in frequency, duration, or treatment response
    Paroxysmal hemicranias
        Episodic (EPH)
        Chronic (CPH)
    Hemicrania continua
    Short-lasting unilateral, neuralgiform headache with
        conjunctival injection and tearing (SUNCT)
    Hypnic headache

B. Those with mixed features of cluster headache and another
        primary headache disorder
    Cluster–migraine syndrome
    Cluster–tic syndrome

C. Those with an underlying organic pathologic process
    Symptomatic cluster headache

which should be suspected when clinical features are atypical. Atypical features include the following:

1. Absence of typical periodicity seen in episodic CH—in other words, the headaches behave more like chronic CH.
2. A certain degree of background headache that does not subside between attacks.
3. Inadequate or unsatisfactory response to treatments that are effective in idiopathic CH, such as oxygen inhalation or ergotamine,
4. Presence of neurologic signs other than miosis and ptosis.

A careful neurologic examination is essential. Diminished corneal reflex and other signs of involvement of the fifth nerve and signs of involvement of other cranial nerves have to be looked for. Most cases of symptomatic CH reported have had some parasellar abnormality, especially around the distal portions of the carotid artery in the cavernous sinus area, where nociceptive fibers of the trigeminal nerve and sympathetic and parasympathetic nerves come together.

Clusterlike headaches have been reported following head and facial trauma involving the trigeminal nerve territory.[28,29]

Differentiating from Trigeminal Neuralgia

Trigeminal neuralgia is a short-lived lancinating pain confined to the second and third divisions of the trigeminal nerve. The most common areas of pain are perioral, around the angle of the mouth, or periorbital, in the distribution of the second division of the trigeminal nerve. Presence of trigger zones of the face, stimulation of which brings on severe attacks, is characteristic of trigeminal neuralgia. The patient prefers not to touch the face, unlike the patient with CH, who may press on the areas to obtain some relief. Trigeminal neuralgia is more common above 50 years of age. Each attack lasts for only a few seconds.

MANAGEMENT OF CLUSTER HEADACHE

Treatment of Acute Attacks of Cluster Headache

Acute attacks are of sudden onset and of short duration. Therefore agents that give immediate relief are essential. Only agents that reach the site of action rapidly are effective in acute CH. Analgesics and oral ergotamine, which are effective in migraine, tend not to be useful in CH, as their rate of onset is slow relative to severe and short-lasting CH pain. The most effective agents are oxygen inhalation[30] and subcutaneous sumatriptan.[31,32] Nasal sumatriptan[33] and oral zolmitriptan[34] have been evaluated recently.

Oxygen

The recommended dose for oxygen inhalation by facemask is 7 liter per minute for 10 minutes at the onset of headache. Approximately 60% to 70% of patients respond to oxygen, the effect being evident in approximately 5 minutes. Oxygen may delay an attack rather than abort it completely in some patients. Oxygen has a significant cerebral vasoconstrictive property and reduces calcitonin gene-related peptide (CGRP) release during CH attacks.[35]

Sumatriptan

SUBCUTANEOUS SUMATRIPTAN. In a double-blind placebo-combined study, it was shown that 15 minutes after treatment 74% of active and 26% of placebo-treated patients had reported relief.[2]

With subcutaneous sumatriptan the headache relief is very rapid, commencing within 5 minutes. The recommended dose is 6 mg subcutaneously. Increasing the dose from 6 mg to 12 mg did not result in either more responders or quicker effect.[36] Long-term repeated use of sumatriptan for acute attacks of CH has been investigated.[37] In the first 3 months of 24-month European multicenter open study[37] to assess the safety and efficacy of subcutaneous sumatriptan (6 mg) in the long-term acute treatment of CH, 138 patients were treated for a maximum of two attacks daily with a single 6-mg injection. (The effect of oral sumatriptan is slower than that of subcutaneous injection; hence oral administration is not the ideal route for CH attacks.) A total of 6,353 attacks were treated.

Adverse events, reported in 28% of sumatriptan-treated attacks, were qualitatively similar to those seen in long-term trials for migraine. Their incidence did not increase with frequent use of sumatriptan. There were no clinically significant treatment effects on vital signs, electrocardiographic recordings, or laboratory parameters.

Headache relief (a reduction from very severe, severe, or moderate pain to mild or no pain) at 15 minutes was obtained for a median of 96% of attacks treated. There was no indication of tachyphylaxis or increased frequency of attacks with long-term treatment.

This study demonstrated that, in long-term use, 6 mg of subcutaneous sumatriptan is a well-tolerated and effective acute treatment for CH.

Preemptive treatment with oral sumatriptan in a regimen of 100 mg three times daily does not affect either the timing or the frequency of headache.[38] Sumatriptan is contraindicated in patients with ischemic heart disease or uncontrolled hypertension. Both oxygen and sumatriptan reduce CGRP in the external jugular vein during a CH attack, whereas opioids do not.[35]

INTRANASAL SUMATRIPTAN. In 26 patients, four consecutive attacks were treated alternately with nasal spray and subcutaneous injection.[34] Treatment was given within 5 minutes of onset of pain, and the time interval for the start and completeness of pain relief, provided these occurred within 15 minutes of administration, were recorded by the patient. After completion of the study, the patients were also asked to indicate which treatment they preferred, based on efficacy, side effects, and handling of the preparation. Forty-nine of the 52 treatments with injection resulted in complete relief of pain within 15 minutes, with a mean of 9.6 minutes. The remaining three attacks were reduced by a mean of 86.7% at 15 minutes. Only seven of the 52 treatments with nasal spray in the nostril ipsilateral to pain resulted in complete relief within this time period, with a mean of 13.0 minutes. In 18 of these treatments pain was reduced by a mean of 42.2% at 15 minutes, whereas no effect on pain was obtained at this time in the remaining 27 treatments. The effect was almost identical when the nasal spray was administered in the nostril on the nonpainful side. As an overall judgment, only two of the 26 patients preferred nasal spray to injection. Conclusion of the study indicates that sumatriptan nasal spray 20 mg/dose is less effective than subcutaneous injection in relieving pain in the great majority of CH sufferers.

Zolmitriptan

In a randomized, placebo-controlled, three-period, crossover study, adult patients with an established diagnosis of CH were given three oral doses (placebo, 5 mg and 10 mg zolmitriptan) for the acute treatment of three CHs.[34] Headache was rated on a five-point verbal scale of nil, mild, moderate, severe, very severe and patients were asked to treat attacks of moderate or greater severity. Headache response was an improvement of two or more points on this scale.

Zolmitriptan is the first orally administered triptan to demonstrate efficacy in the acute treatment of episodic CH. Zolmitriptan (10 mg and 5 mg) provided relief from CH at 30 minutes following treatment in patients with episodic CH and was well tolerated.

The intention to treat population consisted of 124 patients who took trial medication. Most (73%) had episodic CH; the rest (27%) had chronic CH. Of the 124, 102 treated three attacks, 13 treated two attacks, eight treated one attack, and one was lost to follow-up. Considering both episodic and chronic CH, response rates were 30% for placebo (PLB), 33% for zolmitriptan 5 mg (Z-5), and 41% for zolmitriptan 10 mg ($p = 0.11$; Z-10). A similar but significant dose response was seen for the subgroup of patients with episodic CH: 29% (PLB, $n = 83$), 40% (Z-5, $n = 83$; $p = 0.11$), and 47% ($p = 0.102$; Z-10, $n = 79$). There was no evidence for a headache response in chronic CH patients. For episodic patients, mild or no pain 30 minutes after treatment was observed in a higher proportion of patients who were treated with zolmitriptan compared with placebo, 42% (PLB), 57% (Z-5; $p = 0.01$), and 60% (Z-10; $p = 0.01$). Response rates for mild/no pain at 30 minutes in patients with chronic CH were not significantly better than placebo.

Dihydroergotamine

Dihydroergotamine (DHE), available in injectable and nasal form in the United States, is effective in the relief of acute attacks of CH. Intravenous injection gives rapid relief in less than 10 minutes, whereas intramuscular injection and nasal DHE take longer.

Ergotamine

Ergotamine, available only in tablet or suppository form, is not useful in acute management, as it takes longer to be effective and the attack may subside spontaneously before the medicine has a chance to work. However, some patients may respond fairly quickly to the suppository form of ergotamine. In general, oral or suppository ergotamine is not highly effective in the management of acute attacks of CH because of the delayed action.

Topical Local Anesthetics

Locally applied lidocaine nasal drops have been reported to be effective.[39] The use of 4% lidocaine nasal drops is recommended. Patients are told to lie supine with the head tilted backward toward the floor at 30 degrees and turned to the side of the headache. A medicine dropper may be used and the dose (1 ml of 4% lidocaine) may be repeated once, 15 minutes after the initial dose. The beneficial effect is purely from local anesthetic action that interferes with the nociceptive circuits involving the nasal mucosa and the sphenopalatine ganglion and, in turn, decreases the afferent activity in the trigeminal system. Many physicians, however, do not find lidocaine a reliable agent.

Analgesics and Narcotics

Analgesics and narcotics have little value in the treatment of acute attacks of CH. As the pain is of short duration and is self-limited, administration of oral medication is futile most of the time because these medications reach the bloodstream in adequate levels only after the headache is almost terminated. Repeated use may result in habit formation. In most patients, narcotics are not necessary. In patients with coronary artery disease, in whom $5HT_{1B/D}$ agonists are contraindicated, butorphanol nasal spray (Stadol) may be used to relieve pain.

Prophylactic Pharmacotherapy of Cluster Headache

Prophylactic pharmacotherapy is the mainstay in the management of CH. Medications are used daily during the cluster period for the episodic variety and continuously for the chronic variety.[40] The most effective agents include ergotamine, verapamil, lithium carbonate, corticosteroids, methysergide, and valproate. Indomethacin is specific for paroxysmal hemicrania. Beta-adrenergic blocking agents and tricyclic antidepressants are of no particular value.

Principles of prophylactic pharmacotherapy include starting medications early in the cluster period and using them daily until the patient is free of headache for at least 2 weeks, tapering the medications gradually rather than abruptly withdrawing them toward the end of the treatment period, and restarting them at the beginning of the next cluster period. The side effects of the medications must be explained to the patient in every case. A few attacks occur despite preventive medications, and in those situations, abortive agents such as oxygen or sumatriptan can be used.

The *criteria for selection of a particular medication* for prophylactic treatment depend on previous response to prophylactic medications, adverse reactions to medications, presence of contraindications for the use of a particular medication, type of CH (episodic versus chronic versus CPH), age of the patient, frequency of attacks, timing of attack (nocturnal versus diurnal), and expected length of cluster period. Combinations of two or more medications may be necessary for proper control in some patients.

If a patient is seen in the midst of a series of CHs and indicates that previous clusters have lasted a few weeks or a few months, he is probably still in the episodic phase of the disease. For such an individual, prophylactic therapy will probably be needed for only a limited time, and this permits the use of regimens that would not be suitable for long-term or continuous use.

Corticosteroids

Although there is little understanding of the beneficial mode of action, a short course of corticosteroids is one of the most effective means of providing quick protection against frequent attacks of CH. Several regimens have proven effective; each was an empiric choice, and other dosages might be equally effective. Provided that there are no known medical contraindications, a tapering course of oral prednisone can be given as follows: prednisone (60 mg) as a single morning dose for 3 days, followed by a 10-mg reduction every third day, thereby tapering the dose to zero over 18 days. The prednisone is given each morning to reduce interference with sleep; despite this, many subjects feel stimulated while on the higher doses.

For some patients, the corticosteroid taper is sufficient to give protection from the attacks, and by the time the course is over, the current cluster period has ended. It often happens that the headaches return as the dose is lowered. To prevent a return of the attacks when the corticosteroids are withdrawn, we initiate prophylactic therapy with oral ergotamine or verapamil, along with corticosteroid. (This allows time for verapamil and ergotamine to become effective when the effects of corticosteroid wane.) In some patients, repeat of the corticosteroid taper may be required, as the CH attacks return with full vigor. Repeat courses of corticosteroids should be avoided, whenever possible, as repeat courses might induce serious steroid side effects such as weight gain, fluid retention, gastric irritation, hyperglycemia or a more permanent side effect such as osteonecrosis. For these patients, an alternative form of prophylaxis is indicated.

Corticosteroids are also useful in chronic CH; however, when the medication is tapered, the headache tends to return. If steroids are going to be effective, they are usually effective after the first couple of doses, and certainly by the third day as a general guideline.

The mechanism of action of steroids in CH is speculative. Suppression of the inflammatory reaction, possibly in the cavernous sinus area (venous vasculitis), is a possible explanation. It is also possible that corticosteroids exert some control on serotonergic neurotransmission in the central nervous system (CNS). The side effects of steroids prevent long-term use. Necrosis of the joints and bones is of particular concern. In general, use of corticosteroids should be limited to short periods of time as an attempt to break the cycle of headache in the episodic variety and for extreme flare-ups in the chronic variety. Long-term use should be avoided.

Ergotamine

One milligram of ergotamine tartrate twice a day given prophylactically is very useful. There is no evidence that ergotamine causes rebound phenomenon in CH, as it does in migraine. Ergotamine is particularly useful in controlling nocturnal attacks when taken at bedtime. Ergotamine is contraindicated in peripheral and cardiovascular disease.

Verapamil

Verapamil is the prophylactic drug of choice in both episodic and chronic CH; doses typically range between 120 and 480 mg daily in divided doses, but doses up to 1200 mg daily have been used in chronic CH.[41] Constipation and water retention are the usual side effects. Verapamil can be combined with ergotamine, and this combination is the treatment of choice in episodic CH prophylaxis. Prior to initiating the calcium blocker, it is appropriate to perform an ECG to rule out any cryptic conduction defect. Hypotension, peripheral edema, and severe constipation are potential side effects.

Methysergide

Methysergide is useful as a prophylactic agent. It is best indicated in younger patients with CH. In older patients with potential atherosclerotic heart disease, this agent must be used with care. Methysergide has a number of side effects, including muscle cramps and muscle pain, water retention, and fibrotic reactions (retroperitoneal, pleural, pulmonary, and cardiac valvular). As the duration of episodic CH is usually less than four months, the use of methysergide is quite acceptable for that period of time. However, in chronic CH, methysergide must be used with caution, with provision for drug holidays between treatment periods. Six months of treatment with 2-month drug holidays is essential if the patient is to have repeated treatments with methysergide. Investigations, including periodic chest roentgenogram, echocardiogram, and intravenous pyelogram (IVP), are recommended to check for the development of any fibrotic reactions.

Intravenous Dihydroergotamine (DHE)

If different combinations of corticosteroid, ergotamine, verapamil, and methysergide do not result in a remission of the cluster period, a 3- to 4-day course of intravenous DHE (0.5 ml every 6 hours) is helpful in breaking the cycle.[42]

Lithium Carbonate

Lithium carbonate is used mostly in the prophylactic treatment of chronic CH, even though it is also helpful in the episodic variety.[43,44] Lithium is a mood-stabilizing agent. The mechanism of the beneficial action of lithium in CH is not fully understood. Lithium stabilizes and enhances serotonergic neurotransmission within the CNS. The usual dose of lithium is 600 to 900 mg per day in divided doses. Lithium levels should be obtained within the first week and periodically thereafter. The serum level required for therapeutic response is usually 0.4 to 0.8 meq/L, which is less than the standard recommended dose in cases of manic-depressive psychosis. Patients who respond to lithium experience dramatic relief in the first week. Chronic CH patients appear to be more responsive than those with episodic patterns. Approximately 20% of chronic CH may become episodic on lithium treatment, and many patients may require an additional agent such as ergotamine or verapamil with lithium.[45] As months go by, there is a tendency for the effect of lithium to wane, and some patients have become resistant to lithium after months of treatment.[45] Lithium dose does not appear to prevent alcohol-induced CH.

The side effects of lithium need to be carefully monitored. Neurotoxic effects such as tremor, lethargy, slurred speech, blurred vision, confusion, nystagmus, ataxia, extrapyramidal signs, and seizures may occur if toxic levels are reached. Concomitant use of sodium-depleting diuretics should be avoided, as sodium depletion will result in high lithium levels and neurotoxicity. Long-term effects such as hypothyroidism and renal complications must be monitored in chronic CH patients who use lithium for a long time. Polymorphonuclear leukocytosis is a common reaction to lithium often mistaken for occult infection.

Sodium Valproate

Sodium valproate, 600 to 2,000 mg per day in divided doses, has been reported to be an effective agent in reducing the frequency of CH attacks.[46] Valproate is fairly well tolerated. Lethargy, tremor, weight gain, and hair loss are some of the common side effects. The valproate level must be maintained between 50 and 100 µg/ml, and periodic estimations of blood count and liver enzymes are essential. Valproate should not be used in patients with hepatic disorders.

Intravenous sodium valproate, which has recently been shown to be effective in migraine, may be worthwhile in CH.[47]

Topical Capsaicin

It has been suggested that treatment of CH patients with topical capsaicin may desensitize sensory neurons by depleting the nerve terminals of substance P. In a double-blind placebo-controlled study using intranasal capsaicin (0.025% cream) applied via a cotton-tipped applicator 0.5 inch up the nostril, ipsilateral to the side of the headache twice daily for 7 days, patients who received the active drug had significantly less frequent and less severe attacks.[48] Application of capsaicin in the eye should be avoided. Local burning sensations in the nasal mucosa were an unpleasant side effect. Further experience is needed before this mode of therapy is recommended for routine use.

Transdermal Clonidine

Some clinical as well as pharmacologic indications suggest that a reduction of the noradrenergic tone occurs in CH, during both the active and remission periods. But sharp fluctuations of the sympathetic system may trigger the attacks. Clonidine, an alpha-2-adrenergic presynaptic agonist, regulates the sympathetic tone in the central nervous system. Therefore a continuous administration of low-dose clonidine could be beneficial in the active phase of CH by antagonizing the variations in noradrenergic tone. After a run-in week, transdermal clonidine (5 to 7.5 mg) was administered for 1 week to 13 patients suffering from CH, either episodic (eight cases) or chronic (five cases).[49] During clonidine treatment, the mean weekly frequency of attacks dropped from 17.7 ± 7.0 to 8.7 ± 6.6 ($p = 0.0005$); the pain intensity of attacks measured on the visual analog scale, from 98.0 ± 7.2 to 41.1 ± 36.1 mm ($p = 0.001$); and the duration, from

59.3 ± 21.9 to 34.3 ± 24.6 min (p = 0.02). This open pilot study strongly suggests that transdermal clonidine may be an effective drug in the preventive treatment of CH. Its efficacy may be due to its central sympathoinhibition, which reduces or prevents the occurrence of fluctuations of noradrenaline release that may induce the attacks.[49]

In another study, a 2-week course of transdermal clonidine (5 mg the first week, 7.5 mg the second week) preceded by a 5-day run-in period was administered to 16 patients with episodic CH in an active cluster period. In five patients, the painful attacks disappeared after the seventh day of treatment.[50] For the group as a whole, no significant variations in headache frequency, pain intensity, or attack duration were observed between the run-in period and the first and second weeks of treatment (ANOVA).[50] Further studies are necessary to clarify the effectiveness of transdermal clonidine in the prophylaxis of episodic CH.

Indomethacin

Indomethacin is particularly useful in the treatment of CPH. Benefit usually appears within 48 hours. Indomethacin is a powerful prostaglandin inhibitor and reduces cerebral blood flow. Other indomethacin-responsive headache syndromes include hemicrania continua, benign exertional headache, benign cough headache, idiopathic stabbing headache, and headache associated with sexual activity.[51]

Prioritization of Prophylactic Therapy

For episodic CH, ergotamine 1 mg twice a day is the first choice, followed by verapamil 360 to 480 mg a day. In more resistant cases a combination of ergotamine and verapamil is recommended. Methysergide 2 mg three to four times a day is an effective alternative, especially in younger patients. Methysergide should not be combined with ergotamine. Corticosteroids may be used for short periods to break the cycle of headache or to treat severe exacerbations.

For chronic CH, the preference is a combination of verapamil and lithium. In more resistant cases of chronic CH, triple therapy using ergotamine, verapamil, and lithium, or using methysergide, verapamil, and lithium may be considered. There is very little experience with valproate for CH; therefore it is considered a low priority. Careful monitoring of blood levels of lithium and valproate is essential.

Nerve Blocks and Injections

OCCIPITAL NERVE STEROID INJECTION. Injections of 120 mg of methylprednisolone with lidocaine into the greater occipital nerve ipsilateral to the site of attack have been reported to have resulted in remissions lasting from 5 to 73 days.[52] This procedure is a reasonably effective temporary measure to give the patient freedom from pain for a short period of time. Decrease in the afferent input to the trigeminal vascular system via C2 and the spinal tract and nucleus of the trigeminal nerve may be the mechanism by which occipital nerve injections help CH control.

BLOCKADE OF SPHENOPALATINE GANGLION. Blockade of the sphenopalatine ganglion using cocaine or lidocaine is a useful temporary measure to give freedom from attacks for a few days; however, the recurrence rate is high.

Surgical Treatment of Chronic Intractable Cluster Headache

The following are indications for surgery in chronic CH:

1. Total resistance to medical treatment.
2. Strictly unilateral case.
3. Stable psychologic and personality profiles, including low addiction proneness.

Over the last decades, a number of procedures have been tried for surgical treatment of CH (Table 4-4).

Radiofrequency Trigeminal Rhizotomy

Of all the procedures listed in Table 4-4, those directed toward the trigeminal nerve, particularly percutaneous radiofrequency trigeminal rhizotomy, have been the most effective. A number of related articles have appeared in the literature.[53–58] The radiofrequency trigeminal rhizotomy utilizes the thermocoagulation of the pain-carrying fibers of the trigeminal nerve. It is a stereotactic procedure.

RESULTS. Experience in many centers indicates that approximately 70% to 75% of patients obtain beneficial effects from radiofrequency trigeminal rhizotomy. In the majority, the CH attacks stop. In a smaller percentage, there is a substantial improvement, with occasional mild episodes. The results are not fully satisfactory, and failure of the procedure can occur in approximately 15% of patients.

Those who show excellent and good results continue to improve for a number of years. Long-term follow-up for more than 20 years has indicated continuing good results. Recurrence of pain is seen in approximately 20% of patients who had excellent or very good results initially. Patients who have recurrence can undergo repeat surgery, which may take place on the oppo-

Table 4-4. Surgical procedures for cluster headache

Procedures directed toward sensory trigeminal nerve

Alcohol injection into supraorbital and intraorbital nerves
Alcohol injection into Gasserian ganglion
Avulsion of infraorbital, supraorbital, and supratraochlear nerves
Retrogasserian glycerol injection
Radiofrequency trigeminal gangliorhizolysis
Gamma knife trigeminal rhizotomy
Microvascular decompression of trigeminal root (Jannetta)
Trigeminal sensory root sections

Procedures directed toward autonomic pathways

Section of greater superficial petrosal nerve
Section of nervus intermedius
Section of cocainization of sphenopalatine ganglion

site side. It is our experience that patients who have had a history of an occasional headache on the opposite side may develop recurrence on the opposite side. Therefore we recommend selecting patients with a history of strictly unilateral headache.

COMPLICATIONS. A number of relatively minor complications can occur, especially in the immediate postoperative period. These include transient diplopia, stabbing pain in the distribution of the trigeminal nerve, difficulty in chewing on the side of the lesion, and jaw deviation. These complications are usually transient, and complete recovery is the rule. A more troublesome complication is anesthesia dolorosa. The incidence of anesthesia dolorosa is very low. In our series of 98 patients on long-term follow-up, only two had moderately severe symptoms of anesthesia dolorosa. Because of corneal analgesia produced by the radiofrequency lesion, the patients must be instructed to take proper care of their eyes after surgery. Untreated corneal infections can easily result in corneal opacification because of lack of corneal sensation.

SOME OBSERVATIONS ON THE RADIOFREQUENCY PROCEDURE. In the last 17 years, some of our observations of 106 patients who have undergone radiofrequency lesions are as follows:

1. Complete analgesia is necessary for adequate beneficial effects. On the other hand, in trigeminal neuralgia, partial analgesia is all that is necessary.
2. If the pain is confined to the orbital, retroorbital, infraorbital, or supraorbital area, a lesion involving V1 and V2 divisions of the trigeminal nerve is adequate. If the pain is also in the temple and the area of the ear, a lesion of the third division is necessary because the auricular branch of the mandibular nerve supplies the temple and the ear.

Gamma knife procedure directed to the trigeminal root and ganglia is gaining acceptance in a few centers. Initial results are encouraging.[59]

REFERENCES

1. Ekbom KA. Ergotamine tartrate orally in Horten's "Histaminic Cephalalgia" (also called Harris's "Ciliary Neuralgia"). *Acta Psychiatr Scand* 1947;46:106–13.
2. Kunkle EC, Pfeiffer JB Jr, Wilhoit WM, et al. Recurrent brief headache in cluster pattern. *Transactions of the American Neurological Association* 1952;77:240–243.
3. Headache Classification Committee of the International Headache Society. Classification and diagnostic criteria for headache disorders, cranial neuralgias and facial pain. *Cephalalgia* 1988;8[Suppl 7]:1–96.
4. Manzoni GC, Prusinski A. Cluster headache: introduction. In: Olesen J, Tfelt-Hansen P, Welch KMA, eds: *The headaches*. New York: Raven Press, 1993:543–545.
5. Sanin LC, Mathew NT, Ali S. Extratrigeminal cluster headache. *Headache* 1993;33:369–371.
6. Ekbom K. Pattern of cluster headache with a note on the relation to angina pectoris and peptic ulcer. *Acta Neurol Scand* 1970; 45:225–237.
7. Kudrow L, McGinty DJ, Philips ER, et al. Sleep apnea in cluster headache. *Cephalalgia* 1984;4:33–38.

8. Mathew NT, Glaze D, Frost JR. Sleep apnea and other sleep abnormalities in primary headache disorders. In: Clifford Rose F, ed. *Migraine clinical and research advances*. London: Karger, 1985:40–49.

9. Ekbom K. Nitroglycerine as a provocative agent in cluster headache. *Arch Neurol* 1968;19:487–493.

10. Hales CA, Westphal D. Hypoxemia following the administration of sublingual nitroglycerin. *Am J Med* 1978;65:911–917.

11. Kudrow L, Kudrow DB. Association of sustained oxyhemoglobin desaturation and arrest of cluster headache attacks. *Headache* 1990;30:474–480.

12. Kudrow L, Kudrow DB. The role of chemoreceptor activity and oxyhemoglobin desaturation in cluster headache. *Headache* 1993; 33:483–484.

13. Krabbe A. The prognosis of cluster headache: a long-term observation of 226 cluster headache patients. *Cephalalgia* 1991;11 [Suppl 11]:250–251.

14. Manzoni GC, Terzano MG, Bono G, et al. Cluster headache: clinical findings in 180 patients. *Cephalalgia* 1983;3:21–30.

15. Ekbom K, Greitz T. Carotid angiography in cluster headaches. *Acta Radiol Diagn* 1970;10:177–183.

16. Waldenlind E, Ekbom K, Torhall J. MR angiography during spontaneous attacks of cluster headache: a case report. *Headache* 1993;33:291–295.

17. Drummond PD, Lance JW. Thermographic changes in cluster headache. *Neurology* 1984;34:1292–1295.

18. Goadsby PJ, Edvinsson L. Human in vivo evidence of trigeminovascular activation in cluster headache: neuropeptide changes and effects of acute attacks therapies. *Brain* 1994;117: 427–434.

19. Sicuteri F, Geppetti P, Marabini S. Pain relief by somatostatin in attacks of cluster headache. *Pain* 1984;18:359–364.

20. Moskowitz MA. Cluster headache: evidence for a pathophysiologic focus in the superior pericarotid cavernous sinus plexus. *Headache* 1988;28:584–586.

21. Hannerz J. Orbital phlebography and signs of inflammation in episodic and chronic cluster headache. *Headache* 1991;31: 540–542.

22. Hannerz J. Recurrent tolosa-hunt syndrome. *Cephalalgia* 1992; 12:45–61.

23. Leone M, Bussone G. A review of hormonal findings in cluster headache: evidence for hypothalamic involvement. *Cephalalgia* 1993;13:309–317.

24. Kudrow L. The cyclic relationship of natural illumination to cluster headache frequency. *Cephalalgia* 1987;7[Suppl 6]:76–78.

25. May A, Bahra A, Buchel C, et al. Hypothalamic activation in cluster headache attacks. *Lancet* 1998;352:275–278.

26. Watson C, Vijayan N. Evaluation of oculocephalic sympathetic function in vascular headache syndromes. Part 1: methods of evaluation. *Headache* 1982;22:192–199.

27. Mathew NT. Symptomatic cluster. *Neurology* 1993;43:1270.

28. Reik L. Cluster headache after head injury. *Headache* 1987;27: 509–511.

29. Mathew NT, Rueveni U. Cluster-like headache following head trauma. *Headache* 1988;28:297.

30. Kudrow L. Response of cluster headache attacks to oxygen inhalation. *Headache* 1981;21:1–4.
31. The Sumatriptan Cluster Headache Study Group. Treatment of acute cluster headache with sumatriptan. *N Engl J Med* 1991; 325:322–326.
32. Ekbom K, Cole JA. Subcutaneous sumatriptan in the acute treatment of cluster headache attacks. *Can J Neurol Sci* 1993;20 [Suppl 4]:F61.
33. Hardebo JE, Dahlof C. Sumatriptan nasal spray (20 mg/dose) in the acute treatment of cluster headache. *Cephalalgia* 1998;18: 487–489.
34. Goadsby PJ, Gawel M, Hardebo J, et al. Oral zolmitriptan is effective in the acute treatment of episodic cluster headache. *Neurology* 1989;52[Suppl 2]:A257.
35. Goadsby PJ, Edvinsson L. Human in vivo evidence of trigemino-vascular activation in cluster headache: neuropeptide changes and effects of acute attacks therapies. *Brain* 1994:117:427–434.
36. Ekbom K, Monstad I, Prusinski A, et al. Subcutaneous suma-triptan in the acute treatment of cluster headache: a dose com-parison study. *Acta Neurol Scand* 1993;88:63–69.
37. Ekbom K, Krabbe A, Micieli G, et al. Cluster headache attacks treated for up to three months with subcutaneous sumatriptan. *Cephalalgia* 1995;15:230–236.
38. Monstad I. Preemptive oral treatment with sumatriptan during a cluster period. *Cephalalgia* 1993;13[Suppl 13]:35.
39. Kitelle JP, Grouse DS, Seyburn ME. Cluster headache: local anesthetic abortive agents. *Arch Neurol* 1985;42:496–499.
40. Raskin NH. *Headache.* New York: Churchill Livingstone, 1988.
41. Gabal U, Spierings EL. Prophylactic treatment of cluster head-ache with verapamil. *Headache* 1989;29:167–168.
42. Muther PJ, Silberstein SD, Schulman EA, et al. The treatment of cluster headache with repetitive intravenous dihydroergota-mine. *Headache* 1991:31;25–32.
43. Mathew NT. Clinical subtypes of cluster headache and response to lithium therapy. Headache 1978;18:26–30.
44. Manzoni GC, Bono G, Lanfrenchi M, et al. Lithium carbonate in cluster headache assessment of its short term and long term therapeutic efficacy. *Cephalalgia* 1983;3:109–114.
45. Ekbom K. Lithium for cluster headache: a review of the litera-ture and preliminary results of long-term treatment. *Headache* 1981;21:132–139.
46. Hering R, Kurtz A. Sodium valproate in the treatment of cluster headache: an open trial. *Cephalalgia* 1989;9:195–198.
47. Kailasam J, Mathew NT, Meadors L, et al. Intravenous sodium valproate (Depacon) aborts migraine rapidly: a preliminary report. To be presented at AASH Annual Meeting 1999.
48. Marks DR, Rapoport A, Padia D, et al. A double-blind placebo-controlled trial of internasal capsaicin for cluster headache. *Cephalalgia* 1993;13:114–116.
49. D'Andrea G, Perini F, Granella F, et al. Efficacy of transdermal clonidine in short-term treatment of cluster headache: a pilot study. *Cephalalgia* 1995;15:430–433.
50. Leone M, Attanasio A, Grazzi L, et al. Transdermal clonidine in the prophylaxis of episodic cluster headache: an open study. *Headache* 1997;37:559–560.

51. Mathew NT. Indomethacin responsive headache syndrome. *Headache* 1980;21:147–150.
52. Anthony M. Arrest of attacks of cluster headache by local steroid injection of the occipital nerve. In: Clifford Rose F, ed. *Migraine: clinical and Research Advances.* London: Karger, 1985:169–173.
53. Maxwell RE. Surgical control of chronic migrainous neuralgia by trigeminal gangliorhizolysis. *J Neurosurg* 1982;57:459–466.
54. Onoforio BM, Campbell JK. Surgical treatment of chronic cluster headache. *Mayo Clin Proc* 1986;61:537–544.
55. Sweet WH, Wepsie JG. Controlled thermocoagulation of trigeminal ganglion and rootlets for differential destruction of pain fibers. Part 1: trigeminal neuralgia. *J Neurosurg* 1974;40:143–156.
56. Mathew NT, Hurt W. Percutaneous radiofrequency trigeminal gangliorhizolysis in intractable cluster headache. *Headache* 1988;28:328–331.
57. Taha JM, Tew JM. Long-term results of radiofrequency rhizotomy in the treatment of cluster headache. *Headache* 1995;35:193–196.
58. Waltz TA, Dalessio DJ, Ott KH, et al. Trigeminal cistern glycerol injections for facial pain. *Headache* 1985;25:354–357.
59. Ford RG, Fort DT, Swaid S, et al. Gammaknife treatment of refractory cluster headache. *Headache* 1998;38:3–9.

First or Worst Headaches

Randolph W. Evans

First or worst refers to a new type of headache that may be the first episode of a primary headache, such as migraine or cluster, or the worst headache, which could be due to a primary or secondary headache disorder. About 1% of patients presenting to the emergency department have headache of acute onset as their chief complaint. About 20% of patients presenting to the emergency department with the "worst headache of my life" have a subarachnoid hemorrhage.[1]

There are numerous possible causes of the acute severe new-onset headache (Table 5-1). The following may cause a sudden-onset headache but more often have a subacute onset: meningitis, encephalitis, sinusitis, periorbital cellulitis, cerebral vein thrombosis, optic neuritis, migraine, ischemic cerebrovascular disease, and cerebral vasculitis. An acute severe headache associated with neck rigidity raises concern about subarachnoid hemorrhage, meningitis, and systemic infections. Although many first or worst headaches are due to migraine, remember that migraine is a diagnosis of exclusion. Many secondary headaches mimic migraine. This chapter reviews headaches due to subarachnoid hemorrhage and thunderclap headache. Other types and causes of first or worst headaches are described in other chapters.

SUBARACHNOID HEMORRHAGE

Epidemiology

There are about 32,500 cases of nontraumatic subarachnoid hemorrhage (SAH) per year in the United States. About 80% are due to ruptured intracranial aneurysms (with a yearly incidence of about 10 in 100,000, resulting in 18,000 deaths) and 5% due to rupture of an intracranial arteriovenous malformation (AVM). In about 15% of cases, an arteriogram does not reveal the cause of the bleeding. In about 50% of these arteriogram-negative cases, the computed tomography (CT) scan demonstrates blood confined to the cisterns around the midbrain. Perimesencephalic hemorrhage usually indicates a ruptured prepontine or interpeduncular cistern dilated vein or venous malformation, although about 5% of the time a basilar artery aneurysm may be responsible. Other causes of SAH with a negative arteriogram include occult aneurysm, vertebral or carotid artery dissection, dural arteriovenous malformation, spinal arteriovenous malformation, mycotic aneurysm, pituitary hemorrhage, sickle cell anemia, coagulation disorders, drug abuse (methamphetamine and cocaine use), primary or metastatic intracranial or cervical tumors, infections (e.g., herpes encephalitis), and vasculitis (Table 5-2).[2]

The prevalence of intracranial saccular aneurysms is about 2%, with 93% of aneurysms ≤10 mm. Ten to 15 million people in the United States have or will have intracranial aneurysms. The mean age of rupture of aneurysms is around 50 years, with an increas-

Table 5-1. Differential diagnosis of the acute severe new-onset headache ("first or worst")

Primary headache disorders
  Migraine
  Cluster
  Benign exertional headache
  Benign orgasmic cephalgia

Posttraumatic

Associated with vascular disorders
  Acute ischemic cerebrovascular disease
  Subdural and epidural hematomas
  Parenchymal hemorrhage
  Unruptured saccular aneurysm
  Subarachnoid hemorrhage
  Systemic lupus erythematosis
  Temporal arteritis
  Internal carotid and vertebral artery dissection
  Cerebral venous thrombosis
  Acute hypertension
    Pressor response
    Pheochromocytoma
    Preeclampsia

Associated with nonvascular intracranial disorders
  Intermittent hydrocephalus
  Benign intracranial hypertension
  Post–lumbar puncture
  Related to intrathecal injections
  Intracranial neoplasm
  Pituitary apoplexy

Acute intoxications

Associated with noncephalic infection
  Acute febrile illness
  Acute pyelonephritis

Cephalic infection
  Meningoencephalitis
  Acute sinusitis

Acute mountain sickness

Disorders of eyes
  Acute optic neuritis
  Acute glaucoma

Cervicogenic
  Greater occipital neuralgia
  Cervical myositis

Trigeminal neuralgia

**Table 5-2.   Causes of nontraumatic
subarachnoid hemorrhage**

80% intracranial saccular aneurysm

5% intracranial arteriovenous malformation

15% negative arteriogram
  50% benign perimesencephalic hemorrhage
  50% other causes
    Occult aneursym
    Mycotic aneurysm
    Vertebral or carotid artery dissection
    Dural arteriovenous malformation
    Spinal arteriovenous malformation
    Sickle cell anemia
    Coagulation disorders
    Drug abuse (especially cocaine)
    Primary or metastatic intracranial tumors
    Primary or metastatic cervical tumors
    Central nervous system (CNS) infection
    CNS vasculitides

ing frequency of rupture until at least the eighth decade. Before 50
years of age, ruptured aneurysms are more common in men; after
50 years of age they are more frequent in women. In children and
young adults, aneurysmal SAH is uncommon (less than 10% in 30
years of age or younger and less than 2% of those under 18 years
of age) and SAH is more likely due to ruptured AVMs.

About 85% of aneurysms are located in the anterior circulation, most commonly at the junction of the internal carotid
artery and the posterior communicating artery, the junction of
the anterior cerebral artery and the anterior communicating
artery, or the trifurcation of the middle cerebral artery (Fig. 5-1)[3]
Posterior circulation aneurysms are most frequently located at
the bifurcation of the basilar artery or the junction of a vertebral
artery and the ipsilateral posterior inferior cerebellar artery.
About 20% to 30% of patients have multiple aneurysms (especially in mirror locations), usually two or three.

Risk factors for rupture include size and location of the
aneurysm, a history of prior SAH from a separate aneurysm (11
times higher risk), cigarette smoking (up to 11 times higher),
hypertension, a moderate to high level of alcohol consumption;
cocaine use; lean body weight; pregnancy (up to 20% of ruptures
occur during pregnancy and during the early postpartum
period), and a positive family history of aneurysms (Table 5-3).[4]

Familial disorders are associated with an increased risk of
intracranial aneurysms. Seven to 20% of those with a ruptured
aneurysm have a first- or second-degree relative with an
intracranial aneurysm. The risk of rupture of first-degree relatives (highest in siblings) of those with aneurysmal SAH is four
times greater than in the general population. Other hereditable
connective-tissue disorders associated with an increased risk of
aneurysms include polycystic kidney disease (10% have
intracranial aneurysms), Ehlers-Danlos syndrome type IV, neurofibromatosis type I, and Marfan's syndrome.

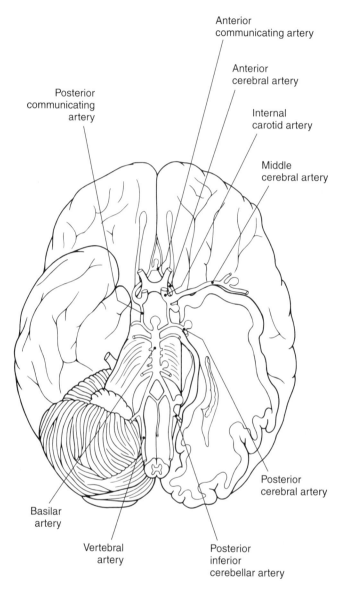

Figure 5-1.   Common sites of intracranial aneurysms on the circle of Willis at the base of the brain.

Table 5-3.   Risk factors for rupture of intracranial saccular aneurysms

Older age

Size and location of the aneurysm

History of prior subarachnoid hemorrhage from a separate aneurysm

Cigarette smoking

Hypertension

Cocaine use

Lean body mass

Moderate to high level of alcohol consumption

Pregnancy

Positive family history of intracranial aneurysms

The risk of bleeding from an unruptured aneurysm is about 1% per year. Aneurysmal rupture occurs with the following activities: one-third occur during sleep; one-third, during routine daily activities; and one-third, during strenuous activities such as bending, lifting, defecation, or sexual intercourse. Most episodes of rupture occur in the morning (9 A.M.) and evening (9 P.M.); the fewest occur during the night (3 A.M.). The rate of rupture is lowest in the summer and increases within 3 days of a substantial climatic change and within 24 hours of a large change in barometric pressure.

Headache from SAH

Headache occurs in about 90% of people with SAH.[5] The classic headache due to SAH is acute, severe, continuous, and generalized and is often associated with nausea, vomiting, meningismus, focal neurologic symptoms, and loss of consciousness. This explosive headache is typically described as the "worst headache of my life." Twelve percent report a feeling of a "burst." In a series of 42 patients with aneurysmal SAH, the onset of headache was as follows: almost instantaneous, 50%; 2 to 60 seconds, 24%; and 1 to 5 minutes, 19%.[6] The headaches, which can occur in any location, may start in one location ipsilateral to the site of the ruptured aneurysm and then generalize or persist unilaterally. The headache typically reaches maximum intensity rapidly and then decreases in intensity over hours to days. However, 8% of those with SAH describe a mild, gradually increasing headache.

Clinical Presentation of SAH

Headache and findings on examination are variable. Perhaps 50% of patients with SAHs will present with none or minimal headache and slight nuchal rigidity or moderate to severe headache with no neurologic deficit or a cranial nerve palsy. Occasionally, patients can present with a stiff neck and no headache. Meningeal irritation may also cause back pain and radicular symptoms in the extremities. A supple neck does not exclude SAH. A stiff neck is present in the following percentages at various times after aneurysm rupture: 74%, day of rupture; 85%, second day; 83%, third day; and 75%, fourth day. During the first 24 hours of aneurysmal SAH, 40% of patients are alert, 67% have normal speech, and 69% have a normal motor examination.[7] About 50% of patients have a presentation similar to meningitis with headache, stiff neck, nausea and vomiting, photophobia, and low-grade fever. Table 5-4 summarizes the presentation of SAH.

Sentinel Headache or Warning Leak

A sentinel headache (a retrospective diagnosis) or warning leak occurs in about 50% of patients before a major rupture of a saccular aneurysm. Accurate diagnosis of the headache can be lifesaving because major SAH has a morbidity and mortality of 50% to 70% and occurs in 30% to 50% of patients in the days or weeks after the sentinel headache. About 50% of the major SAHs occur within 1 week of the sentinel headache.

Sentinel headaches can be in any location and unilateral or bilateral. They typically have a sudden onset and are usually present for 1 or 2 days but can last from only several minutes to several hours or persist for 2 weeks. Associated symptoms and signs occur in about 70% of cases, including the following: nausea and vomiting in about 30% of cases; neck pain or stiffness in about 30%; visual disturbances such as blurred or double vision in about 15%; motor or sensory abnormalities in about 20%; and drowsiness, dizziness, or transient loss of consciousness, each of

Table 5-4. Presentations of subarachnoid hemorrhage

Headache present in 90%

Classic headache: sudden, severe, and continuous, often with nausea, vomiting, meningismus, focal neurologic findings, and loss of consciousness

Explosive headache: "worst headache of my life"

Feeling of a "burst" in 12%

Mild, gradually increasing headache in 8%, sudden severe in 92%

Can occur in any location, unilateral or bilateral

33% present with headache only

75% present with headache, nausea, and vomiting

66% sudden severe headache with loss of consciousness or focal deficits

50% present with none or minimal headache and slight nuchal rigidity or moderate to severe headache with no neurologic deficit or a cranial nerve palsy

Stiff neck present in 75% during first 24 hours and on fourth day after subarachnoid hemorrhage

During have first 24 hours: 40% alert, 67% have normal speech, and 69% have a normal motor examination

50% have presentation similar to meningitis: headache, stiff neck, nausea and vomiting, photophobia, and low-grade fever

Transient loss of consciousness in up to 33%

Table 5-5.   Features of sentinel headache

Any location, unilateral or bilateral

Occurs before major subarachnoid hemorrhage in 50%

Usually sudden onset

Duration usually 1 to 2 days but can last several minutes to
several hours to 2 weeks

Associated symptoms or signs in 70%
   30% nausea and vomiting
   30% neck pain or stiffness
   15% blurred or double vision
   20% motor or sensory abnormalities
   20% drowsiness
   20% dizziness
   20% transient loss of consciousness

50% of these patients see a doctor and are frequently misdiagnosed

which occurs in about 20% of cases.[8] In more than 50% of cases,
the headache may be followed by nuchal rigidity and pain and/or
nausea and vomiting, and/or transient loss of consciousness.

Perhaps 50% of those with sentinel headaches do not seek
medical attention. When these patients see doctors, they are
commonly misdiagnosed at the peril of themselves and their doctors (who are subject to malpractice suits). Common misdiag-
noses include migraine, hypertension, sinusitis, and flu. *Beware
of new-onset "migraine."* The diagnosis of sentinel headache and
SAH should be considered in every patient with sudden, severe,
and unusual headache or face pain. Features of sentinel headache are summarized in Table 5-5

CT and Magnetic Resonance Imaging Scans in SAH

A CT scan of the brain is the initial imaging study of choice to
detect SAH. During the first 24 hours, aneurysmal SAH is present
on 95% of scans but decreases to 50% by the end of the first week
(Table 5-6)[9,10] In the absence of an intracranial hematoma, the
pattern of hemorrhage helps to suggest the location of the ruptured saccular aneurysm (Table 5-7). From more than 3 to 14 days
after the hemorrhage, Magnetic resonance imaging (MRI) (using

**Table 5-6.   Approximate probability of detecting
aneurysmal hemorrhage on CT scan after the initial event**

Time	Probability (%)
First 24 hours	95
Day 3	74
1 week	50
2 weeks	30
3 weeks	Almost 0

Table 5-7. Aneurysm sites suggested by the location of subarachnoid hemorrhage

Site of aneurysm	Predominant location of SAH
Anterior communicating artery	Interhemispheric fissure and/or septum pellucidum
Middle cerebral artery	Sylvian fissure cistern
Posterior communicating artery	Suprasellar cistern
Infratentorial arteries	Posterior fossa cistern
Unknown origin	Diffuse, symmetric cisterns

the fluid-attenuated inversion recovery [FLAIR] sequence) is more sensitive than CT scan in the identification and delineation of SAH.

Lumbar Puncture and SAH

In cases of suspected SAH, a CT or MRI scan of the brain should be performed first, because lumbar puncture can result in clinical deterioration and death after SAH. *A lumbar puncture should be performed on all patients with a new-onset headache suspicious for SAH who have normal CT or MRI scans.*

Red blood cells (RBCs) are present in virtually all cases of SAH and variably clear from about 6 to 30 days. When the cerebrospinal fluid (CSF) obtained from the first lumbar puncture is bloody, the only certain way to distinguish SAH from a traumatic tap is the presence of a xanthochromia. (*Xanthochromia* literally means "yellow color" but generally refers to a colored supernatant.) Although a decrease in RBC from the first to the third test tube can be seen after a traumatic tap, a decrease may not be present or a similar decrease may be seen after a previous bleed. The presence of crenated RBC is not a reliable sign of SAH.

The breakdown of RBC in the CSF releases oxyhemoglobin from 2 to 12 hours after the SAH. Oxyhemoglobin is degraded by macrophages and other cells in the leptomeninges to bilirubin by the third to fourth day. Oxyhemoglobin and bilirubin are responsible for xanthochromia after SAH. The CSF supernatant is pink or pink-orange due to oxyhemoglobin, yellow due to bilirubin, and an intermediate color if both are present. Methemoglobin, a reduction product of hemoglobin, is found in encapsulated subdural hematomas and in old-loculated intracerebral hemorrhages. Because of the variability of the time for oxyhemoglobin release, some authorities recommend delaying the lumbar puncture for 12 hours after the ictus to avoid confusing a traumatic tap with a SAH.

Absorption spectrophotometry is more sensitive for the detection of xanthochromia than the naked eye. However, because oxyhemoglobin can form in vitro due to a traumatic tap, false-positives can occur.[11] Table 5-8 provides the probability of detecting xanthochromia by spectrophotometry at various times after SAH.[12] There are other causes of xanthochromia, including the following: CSF protein > 150 mg/dl; jaundice, usually with a total

Table 5-8.   The probability of detecting xanthochromia with spectrophotometry in the cerebrospinal fluid at various times after a subarachnoid hemorrhage

12 hours	100%
1 week	100%
2 weeks	100%
3 weeks	over 70%
4 weeks	over 40%

plasma bilirubin of 10 to 15 mg/dl; dietary hypercarotenemia; oral intake of rifampin; malignant melanomatosis; and an earlier traumatic lumbar puncture (Table 5-9).

Cerebral Arteriography, Magnetic Resonance Angiography, and Spiral CT Angiography[13]

If the CT or MRI scan and/or lumbar puncture demonstrate a SAH, a four-vessel cerebral arteriogram should be performed to try to identify the source of the bleed and to exclude multiple aneurysms that can occur in 20% to 30% of cases.

In up to 16% of cases, the initial arteriogram may fail to identify the aneurysm, especially of the anterior communicating artery. Potential reasons for the false-negative study include vasospasm, thrombosis of the aneurysm, observer error, and technical factors such as inadequate oblique views. Indications for a repeat arteriogram after about 2 weeks include the following: findings of vasospasm; an aneurysmal pattern of blood on the initial CT scan; and thin or thick subarachnoid blood, particularly with a great deal of blood in the basal frontal interhemispheric fissure, when a CT scan performed within 4 days after the SAH.

Magnetic resonance (MR) angiography can detect up to 90% of saccular aneurysms with a size of ≥5 mm. False-positive studies can occur, and confirmation with cerebral arteriography is necessary. MR angiography is very useful as a screening procedure. The treatment of incidental aneurysms, particularly those less than

Table 5-9.   Causes of cerebrospinal fluid xanthochromia

Subarachnoid hemorrhage
   Breakdown of red blood cells produces xanthochromia
   Oxyhemoglobin is released after 2–12 hours: pink or pink-orange color
   Bilirubin is produced by the third or fourth day: yellow color
CSF protein > 150 mg/dl
Total plasma bilirubin of 10–15 mg/dl
Dietary hypercarotenemia
Malignant melanomatosis
Oral intake of rifamin
Earlier traumatic lumbar puncture

Table 5-10. Causes of thunderclap headache

Primary causes
  Migraine
  Benign thunderclap headache
  Benign orgasmic headache
Secondary causes
  Unruptured intracranial saccular aneurysm
  Cerebral vasospasm
  Cerebral venous thrombosis
  Carotid artery or vertebral artery dissection
  Pituitary apoplexy
  Occipital neuralgia
  Erve virus

10 cm in diameter with no prior history of aneurysmal rupture, is controversial.[14] Spiral (helical) CT angiography can detect about 85% of intracranial saccular aneurysms. Spiral CT can be very useful instead of or as an alternative to MR angiography for patients with contraindications to MRI such as pacemakers, intracranial ferromagnetic clips, and severe claustrophobia. However, in addition to contrast allergy, there is additional risk of intravenous contrast in patients with renal insufficiency, dehydration, and diabetes.

THUNDERCLAP HEADACHES

A sudden severe headache with maximal onset within 1 minute without evidence of SAH is termed a *thunderclap headache*. A small percentage of these patients will have unruptured aneurysms, cerebral vasospasm, cerebral venous thrombosis, carotid artery or vertebral artery dissections, pituitary apoplexy, occipital neuralgia, and possibly Erve virus (Table 5-10). Most cases are due to primary disorders: benign thunderclap headache, migraine, and benign orgasmic headache.

Further investigations should be considered when the initial scan and CSF examinations are normal. A normal CT scan does not mean the absence of pathology because the various secondary causes of thunderclap headache can be easily missed. An MRI scan including MR angiography can detect unruptured aneurysms, cerebral venous sinus thrombosis (a MR venogram may also be indicated), carotid or vertebral artery dissections, and pituitary hemorrhage. A spiral CT angiogram is another noninvasive alternative for detection of aneurysms. However, as noted, aneurysms can be missed on MR and CT angiograms. Aneurysmal mechanisms of thunderclap headache include aneurysmal expansion, thrombosis, and intramural hemorrhage.

REFERENCES

1. Morgenstern LB, Luna-Gonzales H, Huber JC, et al. Worst headache and subarachnoid hemorrhage: prospective, modern computed tomography and spinal fluid analysis. *Ann Emerg Med* 1998;32:297–304.
2. Khajavi K, Chyatte D. Subarachnoid hemorrhage. In: Gilman S, Goldstein GW, Waxman SG, ed. *Neurobase*. San Diego: Arbor, 2000.

3. Schievink WI. Intracranial aneurysms. *N Engl J Med* 1997;336: 28–40.
4. Becker K. Epidemiology and clinical presentation of aneurysmal subarachnoid hemorrhage. *Neurosurg Clin N Am* 1998;9:435–444.
5. Weir B. Headaches from aneurysms. *Cephalalgia* 1994;14:79–87.
6. Linn FHH, Rinkel GJE, Algra A, et al. Headache characteristics in subarachnoid haemorrhage and benign thunderclap headache. *J Neurol Neurosurg Psychiatry* 1998;65:791–793.
7. Kassell NF, Torner JC, Haley EC, et al. The international cooperative study on the timing of aneurysm surgery. Part 1: overall management results. *J Neurosurg* 1990;73:18–36.
8. Hauerberg J, Anderssen BB, Eskesen V, et al. Importance of the recognition of a warning leak as a sign of a ruptured intracranial aneurysm. *Acta Neurol Scand* 1991; 83:61–64.
9. Adams HP, Kassell NF, Torner JC, et al. CT and clinical correlations in recent aneurysmal subarachnoid hemorrhage: a preliminary report of the cooperative aneurysm study. *Neurology* 1983;33:981–988.
10. Van Gijn J, Van Dongen KG. The time course of aneurysmal hemorrhage on computed tomograms. *Neuroradiology* 1982;23: 153–156.
11. Beetham R, Fahie-Wilson MN, Park D. What is the role of CSF spectrophotometry in the diagnosis of subarachnoid haemorrhage? *Ann Clin Biochem* 1998;35:1–4.
12. Vermeulen M, Hasan D, Blijenberg BG, et al. Xanthochromia after subarachnoid haemorrhage needs no revisitation. *J Neurol Neurosurg Psychiatry* 1989;52:826–828.
13. Baxter AB, Cohen WA, Maravilla KR. Imaging of intracranial aneurysms and subarachnoid hemorrhage. *Neurosurg Clin N Am* 1998;9:445–462.
14. Caplan LR. Should intracranial aneurysms be treated before they rupture? *N Engl J Med* 1998;339:1774–1775.

Posttraumatic Headaches

Randolph W. Evans

Headaches commonly occur following head and neck injuries. This chapter will review mild head injury and the postconcussion syndrome and whiplash injuries that are two of the most controversial topics in medicine. The types of headaches due to other neck injuries are similar to those following whiplash injuries.

MILD HEAD INJURY AND THE POSTCONCUSSION SYNDROME

Epidemiology

Mild head injury accounts for 75% or more of all brain injuries. Mild closed head injury is typically defined by the following criteria: a duration of loss of consciousness of 30 minutes or less or being dazed without loss of consciousness; an initial Glasgow Coma Scale score of 13 to 15 without subsequent deterioration; and absence of focal neurologic deficits without evidence of depressed skull fractures, intracranial hematomas, or other neurosurgical pathology. The annual incidence of mild head injury in the United States is about 140 in 100,000. The causes of head injuries are as follows: motor vehicle accidents, 45%; falls, 30%; occupational accidents, 10%; recreational accidents, 10%; and assaults, 5% (Table 6-1). Motor vehicle accidents are more common in the young, and falls are more common in the elderly. Men are more frequently injured than women by a factor of 2 to 1. About one-half of all patients with mild head injury are between the ages of 15 and 34. Perhaps 50% of patients with mild head injury will develop the postconcussion syndrome. About 20% to 40% of people with mild head injuries in the United States do not seek treatment.

Clinical Manifestations

The postconcussion syndrome follows usually mild head injury and comprises one or more of a large constellation of symptoms and signs, including the following categories: headaches, cranial nerve symptoms and signs, psychologic and somatic complaints, cognitive impairment, and rare sequelae (Table 6-2).[1] The most

Table 6-1. Causes of head trauma in the United States (estimated)

Motor vehicle accidents	45%
Falls	30%
Occupational injuries	10%
Recreational accidents	10%
Assaults	5%

Table 6-2.   Sequelae of mild head injury

Headache types and causes
   Tension type
      Cranial myofascial injury
   Secondary to neck injury (cervicogenic)
      Myofascial injury
      Intervertebral discs
      Cervical spondylosis
      C2–3 facet joint (third occipital headache)
   Greater and lesser occipital neuralgia
   Secondary to temporomandibular joint injury
   Migraine
      Without and with aura
      Footballer's migraine
   Mixed
   Cluster
   Supraorbital and infraorbital neuralgia
   Due to scalp lacerations or local trauma
   Low-CSF-pressure headache
   Dysautonomic cephalgia
   Orgasmic cephalgia
   Carotid or vertebral artery dissection
   Subdural or epidural hematomas
   Hemorrhagic cortical contusions
   Hemicrania continua
Cranial nerve symptoms and signs
   Dizziness
   Vertigo
   Tinnitus
   Hearing loss
   Blurred vision
   Diplopia
   Convergence insufficiency
   Light and noise sensitivity
   Diminished taste and smell
Psychologic and somatic complaints
   Irritability
   Anxiety
   Depression
   Personality change
   Fatigue
   Sleep disturbance
   Decreased libido
   Decreased appetite
   Posttraumatic stress disorder
Cognitive impairment
   Memory dysfunction
   Impaired concentration and attention
   Slowing of reaction time
   Slowing of information-processing speed

Table 6-2. *Continued.*

Uncommon and rare sequelae
  Subdural and epidural hematomas
  Cerebral venous thrombosis
  Second impact syndrome
  Seizures
  Nonepileptic seizures (pseudoseizures)
  Transient global amnesia
  Tremor
  Dystonia

common complaints are headaches, dizziness, fatigue, irritability, anxiety, insomnia, loss of concentration and memory, and noise sensitivity. Loss of consciousness does not have to occur for the postconcussion syndrome to develop.

Headache Types

Headaches are variably estimated as occurring in 30% to 90% of those who are symptomatic following mild head injury. Paradoxically, headache prevalence and lifetime duration are greater in those with mild head injury than in those with more severe trauma. Posttraumatic headaches are more common in people with a history of headache. According to the International Headache Society criteria, the onset of the headache should be less than 14 days after the injury, although some experts suggest within 3 months.[2] Many patients have more than one type of headache or have headaches with tension and migraine features. Neck injuries commonly accompany head trauma and can produce headaches. Headaches from neck trauma are discussed in the next section on whiplash injuries.

Tension Type

Eighty-five percent of posttraumatic headaches are of the tension type. The headaches can occur in a variety of distributions, including generalized, nuchal-occipital, bifrontal, bitemporal, caplike, or headband. The headache, which may be constant or intermittent with variable duration, is usually described as a feeling of pressure, tightness, or dull aching. The headache may be present on a daily basis. Temporomandibular joint injury can be caused either by direct trauma or jarring associated with the head injury. Patients may complain of jaw pain and hemicranial or ipsilateral frontotemporal aching or pressure headaches.

Occipital Neuralgia

The term *occipital neuralgia* is in some ways a misnomer because the pain is not necessarily from the occipital nerve and does not usually have a neuralgic quality. Greater occipital neuralgia is a common type of posttraumatic headache but frequently is seen without injury as well. The aching, pressure, stabbing, or throbbing pain may be in a nuchal-occipital and/or parietal, temporal, frontal, or periorbital or retroorbital distribution. Occasionally, a true neuralgia may be present with paroxysmal, shooting pain. The headache may last for minutes to hours to days and can be unilateral or bilateral. Lesser occipital neuralgia can similarly occur, with pain generally referred more laterally over the head.

The headache may be due to an entrapment of the greater occipital nerve in the aponeurosis of the superior trapezius or semispinalis capitis muscle, or it can be referred without nerve compression from trigger points in these or other suboccipital muscles. Digital pressure over the greater occipital nerve at the mid-superior nuchal line (halfway between the posterior mastoid and the occipital protuberance) reproduces the headache (Fig. 6-1). However, pain referred from the C2–3 facet joint or other upper cervical spine pathology and posterior fossa pathology may produce a similar headache.

Migraine

Recurring attacks of migraine[3] with and without aura can result from mild head injury. Impact can also cause acute migraine episodes often in adolescents with a family history of migraine. This was originally termed *footballer's migraine* to describe young men playing soccer who had multiple migraine with aura attacks triggered only by impact.[4] Similar attacks can be triggered by mild head injury in any sport. The most famous example involved the running back of the Denver Broncos and was witnessed by hundreds of millions of people around the world during the 1998 Super Bowl. Terrell Davis, who had preexisting migraine, developed a migraine with aura after a ding on the head at the end of the first quarter. After successfully using dihydroergotamine (DHE) nasal spray, he was able to return for the third quarter, scored the winning touchdown, set a Super Bowl rushing record, and was voted most valuable player.

Following minor head trauma, children, adolescents, and young adults can develop a variety of transient neurologic sequelae that are not always associated with headache and may be due to vasospasm. Four clinical types can cause hemiparesis; somnolence, irritability, and vomiting; transient blindness, often precipitated by occipital impacts; and brain stem signs.[5]

Cluster Headaches

Rarely, cluster headaches can be due to mild head injuries.

Supraorbital and Infraorbital Neuralgia

Injury of the supraorbital branch of the first trigeminal division as it passes through the supraorbital foramen just inferior to the medial eyebrow can cause supraorbital neuralgia. Similarly, infraorbital neuralgia can result from trauma to the inferior orbit. Shooting, tingling, aching, or burning pain along with decreased or altered sensation and sometimes decreased sweating in the appropriate nerve distribution may be present. The pain can be paroxysmal or fairly constant. A dull aching or throbbing pain may also occur around the area of injury.

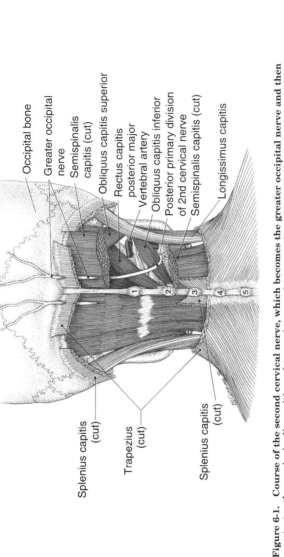

Occipital bone

Greater occipital nerve

Semispinalis capitis (cut)

Obliquus capitis superior

Rectus capitis posterior major

Vertebral artery

Obliquus capitis inferior

Posterior primary division of 2nd cervical nerve

Semispinalis capitis (cut)

Longissimus capitis

Splenius capitis (cut)

Trapezius (cut)

Splenius capitis (cut)

Figure 6-1. Course of the second cervical nerve, which becomes the greater occipital nerve and then penetrates the semispinalis capitis and trapezius muscles to continue beneath the scalp. Entrapment can occur where the nerve passes through the semispinalis muscle. Note the vertebral artery in the suboccipital triangle, which is bounded by the rectus capitis posterior major and the obliqui capitis superior and inferior muscles. (From Travell JG, Simons DG. *Myofascial pain and dysfunction: the trigger point manual.* Baltimore: Williams & Wilkins, 1983:313, with permission.)

Scalp Lacerations and Local Trauma

Dysesthesias over scalp lacerations occur frequently. In the presence or absence of a laceration, an aching, soreness, tingling, or shooting pain over the site of the original trauma can develop. The symptoms may persist for weeks or months but rarely for more than 1 year.

Subdural Hematomas

Tearing of the parasagittal bridging veins (which drain blood from the surface of the hemisphere into the dural venous sinuses) leads to hematoma formation within the subdural space. Even minor injuries without loss of consciousness such as bumps on the head or riding a roller coaster can result in this tearing. Falls and assaults are more likely to cause subdurals than motor vehicle accidents.

Subdural hematomas are usually located over the hemispheres, although other locations such as between the occipital lobe and tentorium cerebelli or between the temporal lobe and base of the skull can occur. A subdural hematoma becomes subacute between 2 and 14 days after the injury, when there is a mixture of clotted and fluid blood, and becomes chronic when the hematoma is filled with fluid more than 14 days after the injury. Rebleeding can occur in the chronic phase. Most patients with chronic subdural hematomas are in late middle age or are elderly. Subdural hematomas can be present with a normal neurologic examination.

The headaches associated with subdurals are nonspecific and range from mild to severe and paroxysmal to constant. Unilateral headaches are usually due to ipsilateral subdural hematomas. Headaches associated with chronic subdural hematomas have at least one of the following features present in 75% of cases: sudden onset; severe pain; exacerbation with coughing, straining, or exercise; and vomiting and/or nausea.

Epidural Hematomas

Bleeding into the epidural space from a direct blow to the head produces an epidural hematoma. The source of the bleeding is variable and can be arterial, venous, or both. In the supratentorial compartment, bleeding can result from the following origins: middle meningeal artery (50%), middle meningeal veins (33%), dural venous sinus (10%), and other sources, including hemorrhage from a fracture line (7%). Most epidural hematomas in the posterior fossa are due to dural venous sinus bleeding. The locations of epidurals are as follows: temporal region—usually under a fractured squamous temporal bone (70%), frontal convexity (15%), parietooccipital (10%), parasagittal or posterior fossa (5%). Ninety-five percent of epidurals are unilateral.

Epidural hematomas usually occur between the ages of 10 and 40 and much less frequently in those under 2 or over 60. Motor vehicle accidents or falls are the most common causes. Trivial trauma without loss of consciousness can be a cause.

Forty percent of patients with an epidural hematoma present with a Glasgow Coma Score of 14 or 15. Less than one-third of patients have the classic "lucid interval" (initially unconscious, then recovery, and then unconscious again).

Up to 30% of epidural hematomas are of the chronic type. The patient is often a child or young adult who sustains what appears to be a trivial injury often without loss of consciousness. A persistent headache then develops, often associated with nausea, vomiting, and memory impairment, which might seem consistent with a postconcussion syndrome. After the passage of days to weeks, focal findings develop. The headaches of acute and chronic epidural may be unilateral or bilateral and can be nonspecific.

Low-Cerebrospinal-Fluid-Pressure Headache

Trauma can cause a cerebrospinal fluid (CSF) leak through a dural root sleeve tear or a cribiform plat fracture and result in a low-CSF-pressure headache with the same features as a post–lumbar puncture headache.

Dysautonomic Cephalalgia

This is a rare headache due to injury of the anterior triangle of the neck or carotid sheath. Acute local pain and tenderness in anterior triangle can be followed weeks or months later by severe unilateral frontotemporal headache, ipsilateral increased sweating of the face, dilation of the ipsilateral pupil, blurred vision, ipsilateal photophobia, and nausea. The headache can occur a few times per month and last hours to days.

Other Types

New-onset orgasmic cephalalgia can follow mild head trauma within 3 to 4 weeks. The headaches associated with carotid and vertebral artery dissections are discussed in Chapter 11. Hemorrhagic cortical contusions can cause a headache due to subarachnoid hemorrhage. Rarely, hemicrania continua can result from mild head injury.[5a]

Cranial Nerve Symptoms and Signs

Various cranial nerve symptoms and signs can occur following mild head injury. Within 1 week of injury, about 50% of patients report dizziness. Central and peripheral pathologies include labyrinthine concussion, perilymph fistula, and benign positional vertigo. Fourteen percent of patients report blurred vision, usually due to convergence insufficiency. Optic nerve contusions can result in decreased visual acuity and hue discrimination. Diplopia due to cranial nerve III, IV, and VI palsies can result. Light and noise sensitivity are reported by about 10% of patients.

Psychologic and Somatic Complaints

Within 3 months of injury, up to 84% of patients have posttraumatic psychologic symptoms. The prevalence of depression is at least 34%. Posttraumatic stress disorder may be present in about 25% of patients 6 months after the injury. Fatigue is a common complaint, reported by 29% of patients at 4 weeks and by 23% of patients 6 months after the trauma. Sleep disturbance is also frequent.

Cognitive Impairment

Four weeks following mild head injury, about 20% of patients complain of loss of memory and about 20% complain of difficulty with concentration. Neuropsychologic testing can document deficits in information-processing speed, attention, reaction time, and memory for new information.

Rare Sequelae

A variety of other problems can occur uncommonly or rarely. Subdural and epidural hematomas each occur following up to 1% of mild head injuries. Subdural and epidural hematomas can occur after an initially normal computed tomography (CT) scan, but this is rare. Cerebral venous thrombosis is rarely caused by mild head injury.

Diffuse cerebral swelling is a rare complication of mild head injury; it usually occurs in children and adolescents and results in death or a persistent vegetative state. When diffuse cerebral swelling occurs after a second concussion when an athlete is still symptomatic from an earlier concussion, the term *second-impact syndrome* is used. Although the second-impact syndrome is a rare complication and somewhat controversial, guidelines have been suggested for return to play after concussion.[6]

Occasionally, mild head injuries result in a posttraumatic seizure disorder. Nonepileptic seizures or pseudoseizures usually follow mild rather than more severe degrees of head injury and typically present during the first year after the injury.

Rarely, mild head injury triggers transient global amnesia, which in children may actually be due to confusional migraine. An essential-type tremor can also result from mild head injury. Finally, multiple episodes of mild head injury can result in Parkinson's syndrome (e.g., Muhammad Ali).

Biologic Basis[7]

Mild head injury may result in cortical contusions due to coup and contrecoup injuries and diffuse axonal injury resulting from sheer and tensile strain damage. Subdural and epidural hematomas occasionally result. Release of excitatory neurotransmitters—including acetylcholine, glutamate, and aspartate—may be a neurochemical substrate for mild head injury. Neuroimaging studies—including magnetic resonance imaging (MRI), single photon emission computerized tomography (SPECT), and positron emission tomography (PET)—can show structural and functional deficits. Neuropsychologic testing can reveal cognitive deficits.

There can be a different basis for each complaint. The cause of posttraumatic migraine is unknown but could be due to neurochemical abnormalities. Local extracerebral injury can lead to other symptoms such as benign positional nystagmus (caused by the shifting of position of free debris within the semicircular canals that is traumatically dislodged from the otolith organs) and occipital neuralgia.

The basis for persistent postconcussion syndrome is controversial. Most physicians believe that there is a neuropathologic substrate. However, others differ and suggest nonorganic causes, especially in cases involving litigation dealing with such matters as secondary pain, malingering, and conversion disorder. Psychologic factors and such common symptoms as headaches, dizziness, and memory complaints that would have been present anyway are misattributed to the mild head injury. Each patient needs to be individually evaluated to try and determine the best explanation for persistent problems.

Diagnostic Evaluation

The judicious use of testing needs to be individualized for each patient. CT and MRI scans may be appropriate to evaluate many cases of mild head injury, particularly to exclude subdural and epidural hematomas. MRI is more sensitive than CT scanning for the detection of brain contusions and diffuse axonal injury. Occasionally, MRI detects isodense subdural and vertex epidural hematomas that may not be evident on CT scan.

Neuropsychologic testing may be appropriate for patients with prominent cognitive and psychologic complaints. However, there are numerous problems with test sensitivity, specificity, reliability, and confounding subject characteristics.[8] The physician should be wary: Patients are often misdiagnosed as brain injured. The psychologist also needs to be familiar with findings in malingering and exaggerated memory deficits.

Evaluation by an ear, nose, and throat physician, including an audiogram and electronystagmogram, may be warranted for those with persisting vertigo or complaints of hearing loss. Patients with visual complaints may benefit from ophthalmologic examination. Electroencephalographic studies are generally not indicated unless there is a suspicion of a seizure disorder.

Management

Treatment should be individualized after the patient's particular problems are diagnosed. Tension and migraine headaches can be treated with the usual symptomatic and preventive medications. The physician should be concerned about the potential for medication rebound headaches with the frequent use of over-the-counter medications such as acetaminophen, aspirin, and combination products containing caffeine and prescription drugs that also contain narcotics, butalbital, and benzodiazepines. Habituation is also a concern with narcotics, butalbital, and benzodiazepines. Posttraumatic chronic daily headache may respond to an intravenous DHE regimen.

Occipital neuralgia may improve with local anesthetic nerve blocks, which can be effective alone or combined with an injectable corticosteroid (e.g., 3 ml of 1% xylocaine or 2.5 ml of 1% xylocaine and 3 mg of betamethasone). Before injection, the physician should aspirate to avoid inadvertent injection into the occipital or vertebral artery. Nonsteroidal antiinflammatory drugs and muscle relaxants may also be of benefit. If there is a true occipital neuralgia with paroxysmal lancinating pain, baclofen, carbamazepine, and gabapentin may help. Physical therapy and transcutaneous electrical nerve stimulation (TENS) may help some headaches.

For patients with cognitive dysfunction, the efficacy of cognitive retraining has not yet been established by prospective studies. Those with prominent psychologic symptoms may benefit from supportive psychotherapy and the use of antidepressant and antianxiety medications. Tricyclic antidepressants such as amitriptyline and nortriptyline may be particularly useful in patients with posttraumatic headaches, depression, and sleep disturbance.

One of the most important roles for the physician is education of the patient and family members, other physicians, and, when appropriate, employers, attorneys, and representatives of insurance companies. There is widespread ignorance about the potential effects of mild head injury due to what Evans has termed the "Hollywood head injury myth."[9] Most people's knowledge of the sequelae of mild head injuries is largely the result of movie magic. Some of the funniest scenes in slapstick comedies and cartoons depict the character sustaining single or multiple head injuries, looking dazed, and then recovering immediately. In cowboy, action and detective, and boxing and martial arts films, seemingly serious head trauma is often inflicted by blows from guns and heavy objects, motor vehicle accidents, falls, fists, and kicks, all without lasting consequences. Our experience is minimal compared with the thousands of simulated head injuries seen in the movies and on television.

The physician can provide education by summarizing the literature and can use vivid examples from sports. The public is very familiar with dementia pugilistica, or punch-drunk syndrome of cumulative head injury in boxers. The examples of Joe Louis and Muhammad Ali are well known. Many have witnessed powerful punches resulting in dazed, disoriented boxers, or knockouts. In other sports, there is also growing awareness of the effects of cumulative concussions in professional football (e.g., quarterbacks Steve Young, Troy Aikman, and Stan Humphries) and hockey (e.g., Pat Lafontaine).

Prognosis

Risk Factors

The persistence and severity of symptoms and neuropsychologic deficits are not predicted by a loss of consciousness of less than 1 hour as compared with a patient being just dazed. Lesions present on MRI scanning, usually in the frontal and temporal lobes, have prognostic value for deficits of frontal lobe functioning and memory. Significant predictors for return to work by 3 months after mild head injury include older age; higher level of education, employment, and socioeconomic status; and greater income. High-IQ patients recover faster than low-IQ patients. Age over 40 years is a risk factor for increased duration and number of postconcussion symptoms. Persistent symptoms occur more often in women. Prior head injury is a risk factor for persistence and number of postconcussion symptoms, consistent with the neuropathologic concept of cumulative diffuse axonal injuries and contusions. A history of alcohol abuse may increase amount of symptomatology. Multiple trauma can cause additional functional impairment, depression, anxiety, and stress.

Symptoms

Most patients will recover within a few months. However, a significant minority have persistent problems. Outcome studies have found persistence of symptoms in various percentages of patients (Table 6-3).

Table 6-3. Range of percentages of patients in different studies with persistence of symptoms at various times following mild head injury

Symptom	1 week	1 month	6 weeks	2 months	3 months	6 months	1 year	2 years	3 years	4 years
Headache	36–71	31–90	25	32	47–78	22–27	8–35	22–24	20	24
Dizziness	19–53	12–35	15	23	22	13–22	5–26	18	16	18
Memory problems		19	8		59	15–20	4			19
Irritability		25	9			20	5			

Effect of Litigation

Patients with litigation are quite similar to those without in the following aspects: symptoms that improve with time, types of headaches, cognitive test results, and response to migraine medications. Symptoms usually do not resolve with the settlement of litigation. In one study of 50 patients with posttraumatic headaches an average of 23 months after settlement, all 50 patients continued to report persistent headaches with an improvement in the headaches in only four patients.[10] Pending litigation may increase the level of stress for some claimants and may result in an increased frequency of symptoms after settlement. Skepticism of physicians may also accentuate the level of stress and compel some patients to exaggerate so that doctors will take them seriously.

However, there certainly are some patients with persistent complaints due to secondary gain, malingering, and psychologic disorders. Potential indicators of malingering following mild head injury include the following: premorbid factors (antisocial and borderline personality traits, poor work record, and prior claims for injury); behavioral characteristics (uncooperative, evasive, or suspicious); neuropsychologic test performance (missing random items, giving up easily, inconsistent test profile, or frequently stating, "I don't know"); postmorbid complaints (describing events surrounding the accident in great detail or reporting an unusually large number of symptoms); and miscellaneous items (engaging in general activities inconsistent with reported deficits, having significant financial stressors, resistance, and exhibiting a lack of reasonable follow-through on treatments).[11]

WHIPLASH INJURIES

Whiplash in an acceleration/deceleration mechanism of energy transfer to the neck that may result from rear-end or side-impact motor vehicle collisions.

An injury may or may not result. Whiplash is best used only as a description of the mechanism of trauma and not as a description of the sequelae. The term *whiplash* was first used in 1928.

Epidemiology

In 1997 the National Safety Council estimated that there were 13.8 million motor vehicle accidents, including 3.9 million rear-end collisions in the United States. As many as 1 million people in the United States may have whiplash injuries yearly. Rear-end collisions are responsible for about 85% of all whiplash injuries.

Whiplash injuries occur more often in females, especially in the 20- to 40-year age group, with an overall male-to-female ratio of about 3:7. The greater susceptibility of females might be due to a narrower neck with less muscle mass supporting a head of roughly the same volume or a narrower spinal canal compared with men.

Clinical Manifestations

Table 6-4 lists the sequelae of whiplash injuries, which include neck and back injuries, headaches, dizziness, paresthesias,

Table 6-4.   Sequelae of whiplash injuries

Neck and back injuries
  Myofascial
  Fractures and dislocations
  Disc herniation
  Spinal cord compression
  Spondylosis
  Radiculopathy
  Facet joint syndrome
  Increased development of spondylosis
Headaches
  Tension type
  Greater occipital neuralgia
  Temporomandibular joint disorder
  Migraine
  Third occipital headache
Dizziness
  Vestibular dysfunction
  Brain stem dysfunction
  Cervical origin
  Barré syndrome
  Hyperventilation syndrome
Paresthesias
  Trigger points
  Thoracic outlet syndrome
  Brachial plexus injury
  Cervical radiculopathy
  Facet joint syndrome
  Carpal tunnel syndrome
  Ulnar neuropathy at the elbow
Weakness
  Radiculopathy
  Brachial plexopathy
  Entrapment neuropathy
  Reflex inhibition of muscle contraction by painful cutaneous
    stimulation
Cognitive, somatic, and psychologic sequelae
  Memory, attention, and concentration impairment
  Nervousness and irritability
  Sleep disturbance
  Fatiguability
  Depression
  Personality change
  Compensation neurosis
Visual symptoms
  Convergence insufficiency
  Oculomotor palsies
  Abnormalities of smooth pursuit and saccades
  Horner's syndrome
  Vitreous detachment

continued

Table 6-4. *Continued*

Rare sequelae
  Torticollis
  Tremor
  Transient global amnesia
  Esophageal perforation and descending mediastinitis
  Hypoglossal nerve palsy
  Superior laryngeal nerve paralysis
  Cervical epidural hematoma
  Internal carotid and vertebral artery dissection

weakness, cognitive, somatic and psychologic problems visual symptoms, and rare sequelae.[12,13]

Neck Pain

About 60% of patients presenting to the emergency room after a whiplash injury complain of neck pain. The onset of neck pain is within 6 hours in 65%, within 24 hours in an additional 28%, and within 72 hours in the remaining 7%. Neck pain is usually due to myofascial or facet (zygapophyseal) joint injury. Cervical disc herniations, cervical spine fractures, and dislocations are uncommon.

Facet joint injury at different levels can produce characteristic patterns of referred pain over various parts of the occipital, posterior cervical, shoulder girdle, and scapular regions (Fig. 6-2).

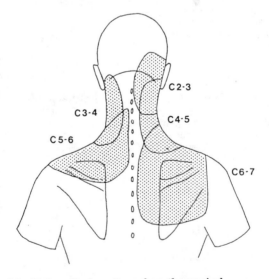

Figure 6-2.   Referred pain patterns from the cervical zygapophyseal joints. (From Dwyer A. April C. Bogduk N. Cervical zygapophyseal joint pain patterns: a study in normal volunteers. *Spine* 1990;15:453–457, with permission.)

Neck pain may arise from at least one facet joint in 54% of patients with chronic pain from whiplash injuries.

Headaches

Up to 80% of patients complain of headaches following a whiplash injury with the following locations and frequency: occipital, 46%; generalized, 34%; other, 20%. The headaches are usually of the tension type and are often associated with greater occipital neuralgia. Trigger points in muscles such as those in the suboccipital area (semispinalis capitis, obliquus capitis superior, splenius capitis, rectus capitis), splenius cervicis, upper trapezius, sternocleidomastoid, masseter, temporalis, and occipitofrontalis can also produce referred pain in the head (Figs. 6-3 and 6-4).[14] Jaw pain associated with headache can be due to temporomandibular joint injury. Occasionally, whiplash injuries precipitate recurring migraine with and without aura and basilar migraines de novo.

Headache may be referred from injury of the C2–3 facet joint that is innervation by the third occipital nerve, "third occipital headache."[15] C2–3 facet joint injury can result in pain complaints in the upper cervical region and extending at least onto the occiput and at times toward the ear, vertex, forehead, or eye. Fifty percent of those with persistent headaches after whiplash injury have this type of headache.[16]

Dizziness

Half of patients with persistent neck pain and headaches for 4 months or longer after the injury complain of vertigo. Table 6-4 lists the various causes of the dizziness. Hyperventilation syndrome can also occur in patients who are in pain and anxious, producing dizziness and paresthesias periorally and/or of the extremities either bilaterally or unilaterally.[17]

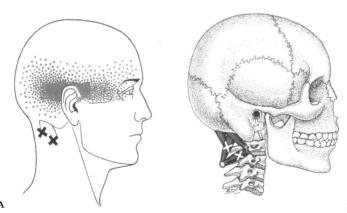

A   B

Figure 6-3.   Referred pain pattern (A) of trigger points (Xs) in the right suboccipital muscles (B). (From Travell JG, Simons DG. *Myofascial pain and dysfunction: the trigger point manual.* Baltimore: Williams & Wilkins, 1983:322, with permission.)

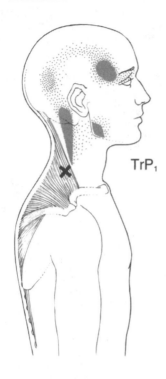

TrP₁

Figure 6-4. Referred pain pattern and location (Xs) of trigger point 1 in the upper trapezius muscle. Solid shading shows the essential referred pain zone; stippling map shows the spillover zone. (From Travell JG, Simons DG. *Myofascial pain and dysfunction: the trigger point manual.* Baltimore: Williams & Wilkins, 1983:184, with permission.)

Paresthesias

About one-third of patients report upper-extremity paresthesias that can be referred from trigger points, brachial plexopathy, facet joint syndrome, entrapment neuropathies, cervical radiculopathy, and spinal cord compression. Carpal tunnel syndrome can be caused by acute hyperextension of the wrist on the steering wheel.

Thoracic outlet syndrome is a common cause of aching, numbness, tingling, and burning pain usually going down the ulnar aspect of the arm and forearm into the fourth and fifth fingers. The ratio of women to men is 4:1. Following whiplash injuries, 85% of cases of thoracic outlet syndrome are of the nonspecific neurogenic type with no objective evidence of neural compression. The neurogenic type demonstrates dysfunction due to compression of the lower trunk of the brachial plexus. The nonspecific type may actually be a myofascial pain syndrome with referred pain from the scalene muscles in the anterior neck or from the pectoralis minor in the shoulder area.

The nonspecific type of thoracic outlet syndrome is a diagnosis of exclusion. Findings on physical exam that are consistent with this diagnosis include reproduction of the symptoms with the following: digital pressure on the scalene muscles; the 90-degree abduction external rotation test (the arm is abducted to a right angle and externally rotated with the forearm flexed at 90 degrees while the head is turned to the opposite side); the exaggerated military maneuver (the patient is asked to brace the shoulders downward and backward forcefully, with the chest thrust forward and the chin slightly elevated); and the hyperabduction test (the arms are brought together above the head). A positive Adson's test is often not helpful because more than 50% of normal, asymptomatic people will have a positive test.

Weakness

Complaints of upper-extremity weakness, heaviness, or fatigue are common even when there is no evidence of cervical radiculopathy, myelopathy, brachial plexopathy, or entrapment neuropathy. The nonspecific type of thoracic outlet syndrome can produce these complaints. Patients can also report a sensation of heaviness or weakness because of reflex inhibition of muscle due to pain that can be overcome by more central effort.

Psychologic and Cognitive Symptoms

Patients often report nervousness and irritability, cognitive problems, sleep disturbances, fatiguability, and depression after whiplash injuries. These symptoms are nonspecific and are common in patients with postconcussion syndrome, chronic pain disorders, depression, and anxiety.

It is controversial whether persistent neuropsychologic deficits following whiplash injury are evidence for mild traumatic brain injury. Subjective cognitive complaints may be due to chronic pain, depression, stressful life events, and malingering.

Other Symptoms

A variety of other problems may follow whiplash injuries. About one-third of patients complain of interscapular and low-back pain. Patients often report visual symptoms, especially blurred vision, which can be due to convergence insufficiency, although oculomotor palsies occasionally occur. Rare sequelae are listed in Table 6-4.

Biologic Mechanisms

Animal and human studies have demonstrated structural damage from whiplash-type injuries, including muscle damage, rupture of the anterior longitudinal and other ligaments, avulsion of disc from the vertebral body, retropharyngeal hematoma, intralaryngeal and esophageal hemorrhage, cervical sympathetic nerve damage, and even various brain injuries, such as hemorrhages and contusions of brain and brain stem. Autopsy series have demonstrated clefts in the cartilage plates of the intervertebral discs, posterior disc herniations through a damaged annulus fibrosis, and hemarthrosis in facet joints.

The acute whiplash syndrome with complaints of neck stiffness, aching, and headaches is well accepted by physicians and the public. However, as the symptoms persist for months or years, some physicians argue that sprain should heal within a few months and there must be another reason that patients continue to complain. Nonorganic explanations offered for persistent complaints include emotional or psychologic problems; exposure to social or medical fashions that perpetuate pain; a culturally conditioned and legally sanctioned illness, a man-made disease; a result of social and peer copying; secondary gain and malingering; and insistence on an explanation outside the realm of organic psychiatry and neurology. In addition, persistent complaints of those involved in low-speed rear-end collisions are not seen in volunteer subjects exposed to speed changes from 4 to 14 km/hour.

Diagnostic Evaluation

Cervical spine series are often obtained to exclude the occasional fracture or subluxation. In patients with abnormal neurologic examinations or persistent complaints suggesting the possibility of radiculopathy or myelopathy, a cervical spine MRI study may be indicated. A cervical myelogram followed by CT scan may be useful if the MRI study demonstrates equivocal findings or if the MRI cannot be done. CT scan/myelography may be more sensitive than MRI in some cases for nerve root compression. Electromyogram and nerve conduction velocity studies can provide evidence of radiculopathy, brachial plexopathy, carpal tunnel syndrome, or ulnar neuropathy at the elbow.

Because asymptomatic radiographic findings are common, it is often difficult to determine which findings are new and which are preexisting. Cervical spondylosis and degenerative disc disease occur with increasing frequency with older age and are often asymptomatic. Cervical disc protrusions are also common in the general population. Asymptomatic disc protrusions occur in 20% of those 45 to 54 years of age and 57% of those older than 64 years.

Management

Neck pain is often treated initially with ice; then it is treated with heat, nonsteroidal antiinflammatory drugs, muscle relaxants, and pain medications. Soft cervical collars can be used during the first 2 to 3 weeks and then avoided. Range-of-motion exercises, physical therapy, trigger point injections, and TENS units may be helpful for patients with persistent complaints.

In many cases, pain from trigger points may be reduced or even eliminated by trigger point injections. The injections can be performed using a local anesthetic (e.g., 3 ml of 1% lidocaine), dry needling without any injection, sterile water, or sterile saline. An injectable corticosteroid produces no more improvement than a local anesthetic alone. Headaches due to greater occipital neuralgia may respond to local anesthetic blocks with or without an injectable corticosteroid.

Persistent headaches and neck pain may benefit from tricyclic antidepressants such as amitriptyline and nortriptyline. The chronic, frequent use of narcotics, benzodiazepines, butalbital, and carisprosodol should be recommended sparingly because of the potential for habituation and medication rebound headaches.

Increasingly, treatment of chronic pain arising from facet joints is being studied. The symptomatic facet joint is first identified by anesthetic blocks. Percutaneous radiofrequency neurotomy with multiple lesions of target nerves can provide at least 50% relief for a median duration of 263 days, compared with similar relief for 8 days in the control group.[18]

Alternative Medicine Therapies

Patients with chronic complaints seek out a multitude of treatments such as chiropractic adjustments, acupuncture, prolotherapy, and pain clinics where the evidence for efficacy is suboptimal. The litigation process can also generate unnecessary consultations, testing, and treatment. In the United States, 34% of the adult population uses unconventional therapy yearly. Many of these people seek treatment for posttraumatic and other headaches. In some cases, patients will not reveal their use of alternative treatments to physicians because they anticipate being lectured or chastised. Alternative medicine users find these approaches to be more congruent with their own values, beliefs, and philosophic orientations toward health and life.[19] Physicians who wish to learn more about specific alternative treatments and evidence for efficacy can refer to Cassileth's book.[20] (For example, craniosacral therapy consists of gentle massage over the bones of the head, spine, and pelvis to increase the flow of CSF. The practitioner may also claim to emit no-touch healing energy to the client.) Informed physicians can do their patients a service by providing unbiased information. Many alternative medicine treatments may have merit. Rather than getting hung up with the terms *alternative* or *conventional,* we need to understand that some medical approaches work and others do not. As Angell and Kassirer write, "Alternative treatments should be subjected to scientific testing no less rigorous than that required for conventional treatments."[21]

A compassionate, sympathetic approach by the physician may result in greater patient satisfaction and reduce unnecessary expenditures from patients' therapeutic quests. Nothing stimulates further therapeutic quests more than being told by a physician that there are no objective findings and there is no reason to complain of pain. If this argument is extended to nontraumatic headaches such as migraine and tension type, then no one should have headaches at all. Even if you believe that there is no scientific basis for chronic pain complaints following whiplash trauma, can you read a person's mind and determine that he or she does not really have any pain? This type of physician response is the ultimate arrogance.

Prognosis[22]

Risk Factors

There are a variety of risk factors for persistent symptoms (Table 6-5). Prospective studies have demonstrated that psychosocial factors, negative affectivity, and personality traits are not predictive of persistent symptoms.

Symptoms

Numerous studies have shown persistence of symptoms in a minority of patients. Table 6-6 summarizes the results of a well-designed 2-year prospective study.[23,24] Five percent of patients were disabled 1 year after the accident. Other studies have shown even higher percentages of patients with persistent symptoms. Neck pain present 2 years following the injury is still present after 10 years.

Table 6-5. Risk factors for persistent symptoms after whiplash injuries

Accident mechanisms
   Inclined or rotated head position
   Unpreparedness for impact
   Car stationary when hit

Occupant's characteristics
   Older age
   Female gender
   Stressful life events unrelated to the accident

Symptoms
   Intensity of initial neck pain or headache
   Occipital headache
   Interscapular or upper back pain
   Multiple symptoms or paresthesias at presentation

Signs
   Reduced range of movement of the cervical spine
   Objective neurologic deficit

Radiographic findings
   Preexisting degenerative osteoarthritic changes
   Abnormal cervical spine curves
   Narrow diameter of the cervical spinal canal

Table 6-6. Percentages of patients with persistence of neck pain and headaches following a whiplash injury

Symptom	1 week	3 months	6 months	1 year	2 years
Neck pain	92	38	25	19	16
Headache	57	35	26	21	15

Effect of Litigation

Most patients who are symptomatic when litigation is settled continue to be symptomatic; they are not cured by a verdict. Litigants and nonlitigants have similar recovery rates and similar response rates to treatment for facet joint pain. However, just as with postconcussion syndrome, there are patients with pain complaints due to secondary gain, exaggeration, malingering, and psychosocial factors. The clinician should evaluate the merits of each case individually. The literature does not support bias against patients just because they have pending litigation.

REFERENCES

1. Evans RW. The postconcussion syndrome and the sequelae of mild head injury. In: Evans RW, ed. *Neurology and trauma.* Philadelphia: WB Saunders, 1996:91–116.

2. Haas DC. Chronic post-traumatic headaches classified and compared with natural headaches. *Cephalalgia* 1996;16:486–493.
3. Solomon S. Posttraumatic migraine. *Headache* 1998;38:772–778.
4. Matthews WB. Footballer's migraine. *BMJ* 1972;2:326–327.
5. Weinstock A, Rothner AD. Trauma-triggered migraine: a cause of transient neurologic deficit following minor head injury in children. *Neurology* 1995;45[Suppl 4]:A347–A348.
5a. Lay CL, Newman LC. Posttraumatic hemicrania coninua. *Headache* 1999;39:275–279.
6. Practice parameter: the management of concussion in sports (summary statement). Report of the Quality Standards Subcommittee. *Neurology* 1997;48:581–585.
7. Graham DI, McIntosh TK. Neuropathology of brain injury. In: Evans RW, ed. *Neurology and trauma.* Philadelphia: WB Saunders, 1996:53–90.
8. Report of the Therapeutics and Technology Assessment Subcommittee of the American Academy of Neurology. Assessment: neuropsychological testing of adults. Considerations for neurologists. *Neurology* 1996;47:592–599.
9. Evans RW. The post-concussion syndrome. In: Evans RW, Baskin DS, Yatsu FM, eds. *Prognosis of neurological disorders,* 2nd ed. New York: Oxford University Press, 2000.
10. Packard RC. Posttraumatic headache: permanence and relationship to legal settlement. *Headache* 1992;32:496–500.
11. Ruff RM, Wylie T, Tennant W. Malingering and malingering-like aspects of mild closed head injury. *J Head Trauma Rehabil* 1993; 8:60–73.
12. Evans RW. Whiplash injuries. In: Evans RW, ed. *Neurology and trauma.* Philadelphia: WB Saunders, 1996:439–547.
13. Evans RW. Whiplash injuries. In: Gilman S, Goldstein GW, Waxman SG, eds. *Neurobase,* 2nd ed. San Diego: Arbor, 2000.
14. Travell JG, Simons DG. Myofascial pain and dysfunction: the trigger point manual. Baltimore: Williams & Wilkins, 1983.
15. Bogduk N, Marsland A. On the concept of third occipital headache. *J Neurol Neurosurg Psychiatry* 1986;49:775–780.
16. Lord SM, Barnsley L, Wallis BJ, Bogduk N. Chronic cervical zygapophysial joint pain after whiplash: a placebo-controlled prevalence study. *Spine* 1996;21:1737–1745.
17. Evans RW. Neurological manifestations of hyperventilation syndrome. *Semin Neurol* 1995;15:115–125.
18. Lord SM, Barnsley L, Wallis BJ, et al. Percutaneous radio-frequency neurotomy for chronic cervical zygapophyseal-joint pain. *N Engl J Med* 1996;335:1721–1726.
19. Astin J. Why patients use alternative medicine: results of a national study. *JAMA* 1998;279:1548–1553.
20. Cassileth BR. *The alternative medicine handbook: the complete reference guide to alternative and complementary therapies.* New York: Norton, 1998.
21. Angell M, Kassirer JP. Alternative medicine-the risks of untested and unregulated remedies. *N Engl J Med* 1998;339: 839–841.
22. Evans RW. Whiplash injuries. In: Evans RW, Baskin DS, Yatsu FM, eds. *Prognosis of neurological disorders,* 2nd ed. New York: Oxford University Press, 2000.

23. Radanov BP, Sturzenegger M, Di Stefano G, et al. Relationship between early somatic, radiological, cognitive and psychosocial findings and outcome during a one-year follow-up in 117 patients suffering from common whiplash. *Br J Rheumatol* 1994; 33:442–448.
24. Radanov BP, Sturzenegger M, Di Stefano G. Long-term outcome after whiplash injury: a 2-year follow-up considering features of injury mechanism and somatic, radiologic, and psychosocial findings. *Medicine* 1995;74:281–297.

Headaches During Childhood and Adolescence

Randolph W. Evans

Headaches are common in children and teenagers. By 7 years of age, 40% of children have had headaches, with 2.5% having frequent nonmigraine types and 1.4% having migraine.[1] By 15 years of age, 75% have had headaches: 15.7% with frequent tension type, 5.3% with migraines, and 54% with infrequent nonmigraine headaches.

The evaluation of the child with headaches is similar to the basic approach in adults, which is described in Chapter 1. A complete history is essential. Information from parents and other family members or caregivers, especially for younger children, is vital. In some adolescents, it is helpful to obtain the history from the child without family members present and then from family members. A psychosocial history is also important. For recurring or chronic headaches, what is the impact of the headaches on the child's life? Has school been missed, has homework gone undone, or have other activities been curtailed? Because of the frequent familial nature of migraine, family history is also important. When you ask the parents about their own headaches, often you will diagnose their migraines for the first time. A general physical and neurologic examination is also necessary. General indications for diagnostic testing are discussed in Chapter 1, with Table 1-8 giving general indications for neuroimaging and Table 1-9 focusing on indications in children.

This chapter covers the following topics: migraine, episodic tension-type headaches, chronic nonprogressive headaches, acute headaches, and chronic progressive headaches. Cluster headaches, the subject of Chapter 4, are not separately discussed because the onset usually occurs after 20 years of age and these headaches are rare in children. Some other causes of secondary headaches in children and adolescents, such as posttraumatic, ophthalmologic causes, and pseudotumor cerebri, are also reviewed in other chapters.

MIGRAINE

Introduction

A variety of migraine types can occur in children and teenagers.[2] Individuals may have just one type or they may have different types. In addition to obtaining the usual history, ask about possible triggers; it is also helpful to ask about a history of motion sickness or somnambulism (sleepwalking), both of which occur much more often in migraineurs. Motion sickness is reported by 45% of children with migraine and 5% of controls.[3] Sleepwalking occurs in 28% of children with migraine and 5% of controls.[4]

Epidemiology

The onset of migraine frequently occurs during childhood: 20% before 10 years of age and 45% before 20 years of age. Until puberty, the prevalence of migraine is the same in boys and girls. After puberty, the ratio of females to males is 3:1. The peak of new cases of migraine, the incidence, occurs during childhood (Table 7-1).[5] The onset of migraine with aura is earlier than that of migraine without aura. Migraine also begins earlier in males than in females. By 15 years of age, 5% of children have had migraines. Of these, about 1.5% have migraine with aura. The risk of a child developing migraine is 70% when both parents have migraine and 45% when one parent is affected.

Clinical Manifestations

Migraine Without Aura

As in adults, migraine without aura is the most common type. However, childhood migraine can be somewhat different. The duration of headache is often much less and can last as little as 1 hour. Pediatric migraine is more often bilateral, frontal and temporal, than unilateral (35% versus 60% in adults). Finally, there is a higher incidence of light or noise sensitivity alone than is found in adults. To reflect these differences, there is a proposed revision of the IHS classification (Table 7-2).[6]

Migraine with Aura

About 20% of children will report the gradual onset of a visual aura before or during the onset of the headache. Descriptions include spots, colors, dots, or lights which are usually found in both eyes but about 7% of the time occur only in one eye. The aura usually lasts less than 30 minutes. There can even be distortion of vision in which objects may appear larger and smaller ("Alice in Wonderland" syndrome). Table 7-2 provides criteria for diagnosis.

Rarely, benign occipital epilepsy can mimic migraine with aura in children and adolescents. Visual symptoms, such as amaurosis, phosphenes (flashes of light), illusions, and visual hallucinations, may be followed by usually hemiclonic movements. Other types of seizure activity can occur, such as simple partial, complex partial,

Table 7-1.   The peak incidence of migraine with and without aura in males and females

Gender	Incidence (per 1000 person-years)	Peak age (years)
Male		
With aura	6.6	5
Without aura	10	10–11
Females		
With aura	14.1	12–13
Without aura	18.9	14–17

Table 7-2. Proposed diagnostic criteria (revised IHS classification) for pediatric migraine

Migraine without aura

A. At least five attacks fulfilling B–D

B. Headache attack lasting 1 to 48 hours

C. Headache has at least two of the following:
    1. Bilateral (frontal/temporal) or unilateral location
    2. Pulsating quality
    3. Moderate to severe intensity
    4. Aggravation by routine physical activity

D. During headache, at least one of the following:
    1. Nausea and/or vomiting
    2. Photophobia and/or phonophobia

Migraine with aura

A. At least two attacks fulfilling B

B. At least three of the following:
    1. One or more fully reversible aura symptoms indicating focal cortical and/or brain stem dysfunction
    2. At least one aura developing gradually over more than four minutes, of two or more symptoms occurring in succession
    3. No auras lasting more than 60 minutes
    4. Headache following within less than 60 minutes (Headache usually lasts 1 hour to 48 hours)

and partial with secondary generalization. Headache, nausea, vomiting, and vertigo can be pre- and postictal symptoms. The EEG usually shows occipital discharges.

Familial Hemiplegic Migraine

Familial hemiplegic migraine,[7] a rare variant, is migraine with aura that includes hemiplegia or hemiparesis. At least one first-degree relative has migraine with at least one hemiparetic attack. The inheritance is autosomal dominant on chromosome 19. The gene defect is a mutation in a brain-specific P/Q calcium channel subunit.

Attacks may occur on the same or different side from prior episodes. The face, arm, and leg typically become paretic with a slow, spreading progression. There may be an associated alteration in consciousness that ranges from confusion to coma. When the dominant hemisphere is involved, aphasia may also be present. Episodes may be triggered by minor head trauma and can occur without associated headache. The headache can be ipsilateral to the paresis in one-third of cases. The hemiparesis may last from less than 1 hour to days or weeks. Complete recovery usually occurs. Triptans and dihydroergotamine (DHE) should not be used during the neurologic deficit because of the potential for vasoconstriction and stroke. Beta-blocker medications might be avoided because of anecdotal reports of migraine-induced stroke. Verapamil and valproic acid can be used as preventive agents.

Depending on the availability of a family history, the evaluation is similar to that of stroke in the young and may include magnetic resonance imaging (MRI) with magnetic resonance angiography (MRA) and sometimes magnetic resonance venography, blood studies (complete blood count, with platelets, anticardiolipin antibodies, lupus anticoagulant, antithrombin III, protein S and C, factor V mutation, and others, depending on the clinical context), and cardiac evaluation, such as two-dimensional echocardiography. There are numerous causes of hemiparesis and headache, including partial seizures, congenital heart disease, acquired heart disease, infectious/inflammatory disease (e.g., HIV and varicella encephalitis), systemic vascular dysfunction (e.g., venous sinus thrombosis and hypertension), vascular disorders (e.g., carotid artery dissection; homocystinuria; mitochondrial encephalomyopathy, lactic acidosis, and strokelike episodes [MELAS] syndrome; and connective-tissue disorders), hematologic disorders (e.g., hemoglobinopathies, disseminated intravascular coagulation, and antiphospholipid antibody syndrome), cerebrovascular malformations (arteriovenous malformations, aneurysms, and Sturge-Weber syndrome), and head trauma.

Basilar Migraine[8]

Migraine with aura symptoms originating from the brain stem or from both occipital lobes is known as basilar migraine (Table 7-3). The aura of basilar migraine usually lasts from 5 to 60 minutes but can last up to 3 days. Visual symptoms—including blurred vision, teichopsia (shimmering colored lights accompanied by blank spots in the visual field), scintillating scotoma, graying of vision, or total loss of vision—may start in one visual field and spread to become bilateral. Diplopia may be present in up to 16% of cases. Vertigo (which can be present with tinnitus),

Table 7-3. IHS diagnostic criteria for basilar migraine (migraine with aura symptoms clearly originating from the brain stem or from both occipital lobes)

A. Fulfills criteria for migraine with aura

B. Two or more aura symptoms of the following types:

Visual symptoms in both the temporal and nasal fields of both eyes
Dysarthria
Vertigo
Tinnitus
Decreased hearing
Double vision
Ataxia
Bilateral paresthesias
Bilateral paresis
Decreased level of consciousness

dysarthria, gait ataxia, and paresthesias (usually bilateral but may alternate sides with a hemidistribution) may be present alone or in various combinations. In 50% of cases, bilateral motor weakness occurs. Impairment of consciousness often occurs, including obtundation, amnesia, syncope, and rarely, prolonged coma.

A severe throbbing headache is present in 96% of cases, usually with a bilateral occipital location. Nausea and vomiting typically occur, with light and noise sensitivity occurring in up to 50%.

The differential diagnosis and diagnostic evaluation are similar to those in hemiplegic migraine. Partial seizures, especially of occipital and temporal lobe origin, can have features similar to basilar migraine. An electroencephalogram (EEG) study may be considered as part of the evaluation. EEG abnormalities are found in less than 20% of cases. Children and adolescents may have interictal occipital spike-slow-wave or spike-wave activity.

Basilar migraine is an uncommon disorder. The onset is typically before 30 years of age (although the first attack occasionally occurs in those over 50 years of age) with a female preponderance following puberty of 3:1, as in other forms of migraine. The age of onset peaks during adolescence. Children may also have this migraine type. Those with basilar migraine may also have other types of migraine, although the basilar type is the predominant one in 75% of cases.

The frequency of basilar migraine decreases as patients enter their 20s and 30s. Stroke is a rare complication. As with other forms of migraine, triggers should be avoided if possible. Although analgesics or nonsteroidal antiinflammatory drugs can be used for the pain, triptans, ergotamine, and DHE should not be used at all because of the potential for vasoconstriction and stroke. Beta-blockers should be avoided because of the potential for stroke, but verapamil and valproic acid can be tried as preventive agents.

Ophthalmoplegic Migraine

Patients with ophthalmoplegic migraine present complaining of migraine headache and diplopia. This is a rare condition. Onset is often during adolescence, although it may occur during infancy.

As the intensity of an ipsilateral severe headache subsides after a day or more, paresis of one or more of cranial nerves III, IV, and VI occurs. The third cranial nerve is involved in about 80% of cases, initially with ptosis and then with oculomotor paresis that is usually complete but may be partial. Dilation of the pupil, mydriasis, is present in more than 50% of cases. Recovery of nerve function may occur in a week to 4 to 6 weeks. Recovery may be incomplete after multiple attacks.

The diagnosis is made by excluding, as appropriate, such conditions as Tolosa-Hunt syndrome (granulomatous inflammation in the cavernous sinus), parasellar lesions, diabetic cranial neuropathy, collagen vascular disease, and orbital pseudotumor (an idiopathic infiltration of orbital structures with chronic inflammatory cells). MRI with MRA is usually adequate, although a cerebral arteriogram may be necessary in some cases.

Benign Paroxysmal Vertigo of Childhood

The onset of benign paroxysmal vertigo of childhood[9] usually occurs between 2 and 5 years of age but can be before 1 year of age or as late as 12 years of age. Unprovoked stereotypical episodes of true vertigo (with a sensation of movement as described by verbal children) usually last for seconds or minutes but may last for hours. The child becomes pale, cannot maintain an upright posture, and wishes to remain absolutely still. There is no complaint of headache or alteration of consciousness, although nausea or other abdominal discomfort may follow the vertigo. Because the episodes are so brief, treatment is not usually needed.

As the child becomes older, the episodes of vertigo may be associated with migraine headache or may become less severe and disappear. Other types of migraine may then occur in 21% of these patients.[10]

Other causes of vertigo in children should be considered. A single prolonged episode could be due to infection of the labyrinth or vestibular nerve. Partial seizures can also produce true vertigo.

Abdominal Migraine

Criteria suggested for abdominal migraine (cyclical vomiting) include a family history of migraine; a history of migraine with or without aura; recurrent identical attacks of abdominal pain; no abdominal symptoms between attacks; onset of attacks of abdominal pain in early childhood or early adult life (before 40 years of age), mainly in females; episodes lasting from 1 to several hours; and pain usually located in the upper abdomen.[11] The episodes may be associated with nausea and vomiting and pallor or flushing. The prevalence peaks at ages 5 to 9 years. As with all migraine types, this is a diagnosis of exclusion. If there is alteration of consciousness, a seizure disorder should be considered. Other disorders in the differential diagnosis include urogenital disorders, ornithine transcarbamylase deficiency, peptic ulcer disease, cholecystitis, Meckel's diverticulum, partial duodenal obstruction, gastroesophageal reflux, Crohn's disease, and irritable bowel syndrome. Drugs used for migraine prevention and symptomatic treatment may be helpful.

Confusional Migraine

Confusional migraine is migraine with a headache, which can be minimal, associated with a confusional state that can last from 10 minutes to 2 days. The patient may be agitated and have impaired memory. There may be inattention, distractibility, and difficulty maintaining coherent speech or action. The diagnosis is made by excluding, as appropriate, the numerous causes of an acute encephalopathy, including partial complex seizures, metabolic disorders, infection, and subarachnoid hemorrhage (SAH).

"Footballer's" Migraine

As discussed in Chapter 6, acute minor head trauma can trigger migraine in children and adolescents. In a study of children with a mean age of 7.4 years who had mild head injuries, a history of motion sickness, migraines, and migraine in other family members is highly predictive of vomiting after a mild head injury.[12]

MELAS Syndrome

Mitochondrial encephalomyopathy, lactic acidosis, and stroke-like episodes, a rare disorder, can present as episodic migraine early in the course of the disease. The following features must be present: strokelike episodes before 40 years of age; encephalopathy with seizures, dementia, or both; and evidence of a mitochondrial myopathy with lactic acidosis, ragged-red fibers, or both. At least two of the following should be present: normal early development, recurrent headache, and recurrent vomiting. Most patients have exercise intolerance, limb weakness, short stature, hearing loss, and elevated cerebrospinal fluid (CSF) protein.

The cause of 90% of cases is an A-to-G point mutation in the mitochondrial gene encoding for $tRNA^{[Leu(UUR)]}$ at nucleotide position 223243. The other 10% are due to seven other mitochondrial DNA point mutations. All children of mothers with MELAS are affected because of maternal transmission of mitochondrial DNA.

Management

Nonmedication Approaches

Identification and avoidance of migraine triggers are important. Missing meals, stress, and sleep deprivation can be particularly important triggers. Elimination of caffeinated beverages can be helpful in some cases. Biofeedback, stress management, and progressive relaxation training may be beneficial.[13] Education about migraine for the patient and parents or caretakers is well worthwhile.

Pharmacologic Treatments

Acute or symptomatic and preventive medications are available. Many of the recommendations in this section are anecdotal because of the lack of well-designed studies of treatment of childhood and adolescent migraine.

ACUTE HEADACHES. Aspirin should be avoided before 15 years of age because of the potential for Reye's syndrome. Headaches in children 6 years of age and younger are typically brief and resolve with acetaminophen and/or sleep. For children over 6 years of age, acetaminophen alone (10 to 15 mg/kg) or with the addition of pseudoephedrine (30 mg tablet) may be effective (Table 7-4).[14]

Other options include nonsteroidal antiinflammatory drugs such as ibuprofen (10 mg/kg),[15] naproxen sodium (10 mg/kg); isometheptene mucate (65 mg), dichloralphenazone (100 mg), and acetaminophen (325 mg) (Midrin, one capsule); butalbital (50 mg), acetaminophen (325 mg), and caffeine (40 mg) (Fioricet, 6 to 9 years, one-half tablet; 9 to 12 years, three-fourths tablet; and more than 12 years, one tablet).

Children with significant nausea and/or vomiting may benefit from the use of metoclopramide 0.2 mg/kg orally or promethazine 0.5 mg/kg orally or in suppository form. Some children and adolescents also benefit from a combination of codeine and acetaminophen or acetaminophen, butalbital, and caffeine.

Table 7-4. Symptomatic treatment for migraine in children and adolescents

Medication	Dosage
Acetaminophen	10–15 mg/kg po
Pseudoephedrine HCL	30 mg po
Ibuprofen	10 mg/kg po
Naproxen sodium	10 mg/kg po
Butalbital 50 mg, acetaminophen 325 mg, caffeine 40 mg	6–9 yr, ½ tablet
	9–12 yr, ¾ tablet
	>12 yr, 1 tablet
Isometheptene mucate, dichloralphenazone 100 mg, and acetaminophen 325 mg	6–12 yr, 1 capsule
	>12 yr, 1–2 capsules
Sumatriptan	0.06 mg/kg SC
	25–50 mg po
	5 or 20 mg NS
DHE	IV (see Table 7-6)

Total weekly doses of symptomatic medications and caffeine should be carefully monitored because of the potential for causing rebound headaches. There are restrictions on the use of certain acute and preventive medications in hemiplegic and basilar migraine as detailed earlier.

Additional treatments are available for severe migraines in children and adolescents ages 6 and over who do not respond to these medications. In a study of 50 children between the ages 6 and 18, Linder administered sumatriptan (Imitrex) subcutaneously (dose of 0.06 mg/kg) and reported efficacy in 78%.[16] In responders, the migraine recurrence rate was 6%. Adverse events, usually transient and mild, occur in 80%.

Oral triptans, such as sumatriptan (Imitrex, 25 to 50 g),[7] are often effective in adolescents of 12 years of age and over. Sumatriptan nasal spray (5 mg or 20 mg, depending on size of the patient, efficacy, and adverse events) can also be effective. Anecdotally, triptans may be effective in children over 6 years of age. Side effects of triptans are discussed in Chapter 2. Triptans are not approved by the Food and Drug Administration (FDA) for those under 18 years of age.

Alternatively, as in adults, children and adolescents with prolonged migraine often respond to an inpatient protocol of an antiemetic, metoclopramide, and DHE (Table 7-5), as reported by Linder.[18] The oral metoclopramide and IV DHE can be given every 6 hours for a maximum of eight doses. When the headache ceases, one additional dose can be given. The dose of DHE may be increased by 0.05 mg/dose up to the point at which the patient has mild abdominal discomfort. The protocol should be continued at the dose prior to the onset of the abdominal discomfort.

Table 7-5. Dosing of metoclopramide and DHE for severe intractable migraine

Age in years	Metoclopramide*	DHE
6–9	0.2 mg/kg	0.1 mg/dose
9–12	0.2 mg/kg	0.15 mg/dose
12–16	0.2 mg/kg	0.2 mg/dose

*Administered orally 30 minutes prior to administration of IV DHE. Maximum dose of 20 mg.

Triptans and DHE should not be given within less than 24 hours of each other.

These medications can have significant side effects. If metoclopramide causes an extrapyramidal syndrome, diphenhydramine can be given (1 mg/kg, maximum dose of 50 mg) orally, intramuscularly, or intravenously (IV). Metoclopramide can also cause nausea and vomiting. For subsequent DHE doses, ondansetron 0.15 mg/kg IV 30 minutes prior to the DHE dose can be given as an alternative, if necessary, to prevent nausea and vomiting, which can be a side effect of DHE or part of the migraine. Side effects of DHE include a flushed feeling, tingling in the extremities, leg cramping, and a transient increase in headache. DHE is not FDA approved for use in those under 18 years of age.

PREVENTIVE MEDICATIONS. Preventive medications[19] should be considered for children and adolescents with frequent migraines that are not responsive to symptomatic medications or that significantly interfere with school or home activities (Table 7-6).

Table 7-6. Preventive medications for migraine in children and adolescents

Medication	Dosage
Propanolol	<14 yr, initial dose 10 mg po bid. May increase by 10 mg/day/each week to 20 mg TID maximum >14 yr, initial dose 20 mg po BID. May increase by 20 mg/day each week up to 240 mg/day. Equivalent long-acting doses may be used.
Cyproheptadine HCl	≥6 yr, 4 mg po hs. May be slowly increased to 12 mg po hs or 8 mg po hs and 4 mg po q a.m.
Amitriptyline or nortriptyline	10 mg po hs. May be increased every 2 weeks to 50 mg po hs <12 yr and 100 mg po hs >12 yr
Divalproex sodium	>10 yr, 125–250 mg po hs, slowly increase to 500–1,000 mg in two divided doses

In general, preventive medications are started at low doses and are increased slowly.

Beta-blockers such as propranol may be effective. The initial dose for children 8 years of age or older is 10 mg two times a day, which can be increased, depending on response, by 10 mg per week or slower to a maximum of 20 mg three times a day for children under 14 years of age. Adult doses (Table 7-6) can be given to those 14 years of age and older. Those on higher doses of propranolol can be switched to or started on the long-acting preparation. Among the numerous possible side effects, beta-blockers can occasionally exacerbate asthma, cause hypotension, and cause depression. Propranolol given to diabetic children on insulin can mask symptoms of hypoglycemia. Congestive heart failure, atrioventricular conduction defects, and renal insufficiency are also contraindications to use. In some patients, nadolol or atenolol may be better tolerated, with fewer side effects, such as depression or asthenia, than propranolol.

Cyproheptadine (Periactin), an antihistamine, can also be an effective preventive medication in single doses of from 4 to 12 mg at bedtime or in divided doses, such as morning and evening for children 6 years and older (e.g., starting at 4 mg at bedtime [hs] and, depending on effect, slowly increasing after several weeks to 8 mg hs, and later, if necessary, to 12 mg hs or 8 mg hs and 4 mg in the morning). The dose for children under 6 years of age is 1 mg hs, slowly increasing to 2 mg hs and 2 mg in the morning. Common side effects include weight gain and drowsiness. Cyproheptadine may be the preventive of first choice for those with frequent migraines and atopic allergies or sinus disease.

Tricyclic antidepressants, such as amitriptyline (Elavil) and nortriptyline (Pamelor), can also be used. For children over 8 years of age, the starting dose of either is 10 mg/day at bedtime. Depending on the response and side effects, the total daily dose can be increased by 10 mg every 1 to 2 weeks or slower. Effective daily dosage is typically 50 mg or less in younger children and 100 mg or less in adolescents. Common side effects include sedation, weight gain, and dry mouth. Nortriptyline is less sedating than amitriptyline. The tricylics are often the preventive of choice for those with frequent migraine and tension-type headaches, chronic daily headaches, or associated depression or sleep disturbance. If a tricyclic is ineffective, a trial of trazodone (1 mg/kg a day divided into three doses) might be considered.[20]

Valproic acid may also be effective for migraine prevention in children and adolescents. Divalproex sodium (Depakote), the enteric coated form, is commonly used to minimize gastrointestinal side effects. According to data from adult studies, there may be efficacy for migraine prevention at doses lower than those used for epilepsy. A starting dose of about 125 to 250 mg given at bedtime may be used and then slowly increased at 2-week intervals or slower. The total daily effective dose, given at bedtime and in the morning, is often 500 mg/day or less in younger children and 500 to 1,000 mg/day in adolescents. This total daily dose may be less than that used for the treatment of epilepsy. There are numerous side effects, as described in Chapter 2, most commonly weight gain, tremor, hair loss, and nausea. Tremor and hair loss are fully reversible after discontinuing the medication. If nausea is persistent, the sprinkle formulation may be better tolerated. This drug can be the one of choice for those with epilepsy and migraines.

The rare complication of fatal hepatotoxicity almost always occurs in children under 10 years of age. (This complication has been reported for children taking the medication for epilepsy. The risk for those on polytherapy is 1:8,307 and on monotherapy, 1:16,317.) Therefore divalproex sodium should be avoided in children under 10 years of age unless routine medications have failed, in which case it should be used as monotherapy.[21]

Prognosis

Migraine with onset before 7 years of age more commonly remits in boys than in girls. By 22 years of age, 50% of men and 60% of women still have migraine. In those with severe migraine beginning between the ages of 7 and 15, 20% are migraine-free by 25 years of age and 50% continue to have it into their 50s and 60s.[22]

EPISODIC TENSION-TYPE HEADACHES

The most common recurrent headache in children and adolescents is episodic tension type. Tension-type headaches typically have the following characteristics: duration of 30 minutes to many days; bilateral with a pressing or tightening quality; mild to moderate intensity; and not worsened by routine physical activity. Although nausea is absent, light or noise sensitivity may be present.

When symptomatic medication is necessary, acetaminophen, ibuprofen, or naproxen sodium may be effective. Frequent use of these or other symptomatic drugs or caffeine can lead to medication rebound headaches.

If the headaches are frequent, adequate sleep, regular exercise, and avoidance of caffeine may be beneficial. Biofeedback, stress management, and progressive relaxation training may also be helpful. Psychologic or psychiatric evaluation may be worthwhile in some cases where school or family problems, stress, depression, or anxiety is prominent. If there is a significant muscle contraction contribution, treatments such as a short-term course of muscle relaxants, nonsteroidal antiinflammatory drugs, physical therapy, and a trial of a transcutaneous nerve stimulator unit may be warranted. Preventive medications such as amitriptyline, nortriptyline, and paroxetine (Paxil 10 to 20 mg daily) can be effective.

CHRONIC NONPROGRESSIVE HEADACHES[23]

Frequent nonmigrainous headaches occur in 2.5% of children by 7 years of age and in 15.7% by 15 years of age. The headache may be present on awakening and last all day. The history, examination, and neuroimaging, as indicated, exclude secondary headaches. Chronic pansinusitis should be considered as the cause of chronic headaches even when sinus symptoms are not present.

Depending on the specifics, the headache may be classified as chronic tension type, mixed (both distinct migraine and tension headaches or headaches with features of both), transformed migraine (a history of episodic migraine transforming into daily or near daily headaches), or caused by medication rebound.[24]

Medication rebound headache is important to identify because discontinuing the analgesics alone can produce great improvement.[25] These patients typically have a history of migraine and/or tension-type headache. Without a definite precipitating event or following an injury or illness, the headaches may increase in frequency; then a pattern develops of daily or almost daily analgesic use. The daily analgesic use, in susceptible individuals, can cause daily bilateral or unilateral headaches with tension and migraine features. Frequent use of caffeine may also cause or contribute to daily headaches. Episodic migraine headaches may also occur. The headaches may persist for months or years. Preventive medications may be less effective in this setting.

Medications that can cause rebound headaches include the following: acetaminophen; ibuprofen and other nonsteroidal antiinflammatory drugs; combination drugs with such agents as butalbital, acetaminophen, caffeine, aspirin, and codeine; propoxyphene; and ergotamine. In some cases, frequent triptan use can also cause rebound headaches. The number of doses of analgesics taken per week, in the largest study with patients from ages 5 to 17 years, ranged from 8 to 84.[26] Acetaminophen and ibuprofen were the most commonly overused medications. Discontinuing daily analgesics and taking amitriptyline 10 mg orally daily reduced the frequency of headaches by 80%.

If headaches persist despite medication withdrawal or if chronic tension-type or mixed headaches are present, a psychologic or psychiatric evaluation should be considered to evaluate the presence of home and school problems, other stressors, or depression, which may contribute to headaches. Biofeedback, stress management training, relaxation training, and behavioral contingency management may be helpful in reducing the headaches. The preceding section on tension-type headaches describes preventive medications that may be effective. Divalproex sodium can also be helpful in some cases. A 3-day intravenous DHE protocol administered every 8 days can be indicated for some refractory cases (Table 7-5).

New daily, persistent headaches can also occur without a history of increasingly frequent tension- and/or migraine-type headaches. The headache develops over less than 3 days. In many cases, the etiology is unknown. Other cases may reflect a postviral syndrome.

Acute infectious mononucleosis should be considered, especially when there are accompanying complaints of sore throat and findings of cervical adenopathy. (The term *infectious mononucleosis* was first used in 1920 to describe medical students at Johns Hopkins with the condition who were found to have atypical mononuclear cells.) The typical picture is a 7-day prodromal illness followed by a 4-day to 3-week acute illness with fever, headache, malaise, pharyngitis, cervical lymphadenopathy, and mononuclear leukocytosis with atypical lymphocytes.[27] Transient hepatic dysfunction and splenic and hepatomegaly may be present. The monospot or heterophile antibody test is positive. Longer-duration chronic headaches can be present with persistent Epstein-Barr infection.[28]

ACUTE HEADACHES

Epidemiology

Chapter 5 reviews first or worst headaches in adults. In children and adolescents, the epidemiology is different. In a study of 150 consecutive children presenting to the emergency department with a chief complaint of acute headache, the diagnoses were as follows: viral upper respiratory infection, 39%; migraine, 18%; sinusitis, 9%; streptococcal pharyngitis, viral meningitis, and undetermined cause, each 7%; posterior fossa tumor, 2.5%; ventriculoperitoneal shunt malfunction, 2%; intracranial hemorrhage and seizure, each 1.5%; post–lumbar puncture and post-concussion, each 1%.[29] Upper-respiratory infections with fever accounted for 54% of the cases. Viral meningitis can present without fever and with a supple neck and normal neurologic examination.

In children and adolescents, aneurysmal SAH is uncommon: fewer than 2% of cases occur in those under 18 years of age. SAH is more likely due to ruptured arteriovenous malformations, which outnumber aneurysms by nearly 10 to 1 in childhood.

Brain Abscess

Brain abscess in children has a peak incidence of 4 to 7 years. Twenty-five percent of these children have cyanotic congenital heart disease with a right-to-left shunt resulting in hematogenous spread of infection. Otogenic abscesses also occur in children. Brain abscesses due to frontal or sphenoid sinusitis occur in children ages 10 and older because of the late development of these sinuses.[30] Emissary veins spread infection into the brain from the paranasal sinuses, mastoids, and middle ear.

About 75% of patients with brain abscess present with symptoms of less than 2 weeks' duration. The classic clinical triad of headache, fever, and focal neurologic signs occurs in only a minority of patients. Headache is present in about 75% of patients, and nausea and vomiting are found in about 50%. Signs are present as follows: fever, less than 50%; seizures, 33%; nuchal rigidity, 25%; and papilledema, 25%.[31]

CHRONIC PROGRESSIVE HEADACHES

The epidemiology of chronic progressive headaches is also different in children and adolescents from that in adults (Table 7-7).[32] Causes include brain tumors, hydrocephalus, brain abscess, hematomas, pseudotumor cerebri, malformation, hypertension, and medication rebound. Pseudotumor cerebri (Chapter 12) may be present without papilledema. The diagnosis can only be made with lumbar puncture and measurement of the opening pressure. This section will review brain tumors and hydrocephalus. The remaining causes are discussed elsewhere in this book.

Brain Tumors

Although parents and children often fear that their headache is due to a brain tumor, brain tumors uncommonly occur. The clinical presentation depends on the type and location of tumor. Posterior fossa tumors that result in hydrocephalus can produce the classic brain tumor headaches with nausea, early-morning

Table 7-7. Causes of chronic progressive headaches in children and adolescents

Neoplasms
  Medulloblastoma
  Cerebellar astrocytoma
  Brain stem glioma
  Ependymoma
  Pineal region tumors
  Craniopharyngioma
  Supratentorial astrocytoma
Hydrocephalus
  Obstructive
  Communicating
Brain abscess
Chronic subdural and epidural hematomas
Pseudotumor cerebri
Malformations
  Chiari malformation
  Dandy Walker cyst
Hypertension
Medication rebound

vomiting, and headaches. Headaches from supratentorial tumors are less specific.

In a study of 74 children with primary brain tumors from England, headache was present in 64%, vomiting in 65%, and changes in personality in 47%.[33] Only 34% of headaches were always associated with vomiting, and only 28% occurred in the early morning. Misdiagnosis was common: migraine was diagnosed in 24% and a psychologic etiology was found in 15%. Additional features of headaches due to brain tumors are discussed in Chapter 12.

Brain metastases in children and adolescents most often arise from sarcomas and germ cell tumors. A variety of primary brain tumors can occur. About 60% of primary brain tumors are infratentorial (posterior fossa) and 40% supratentorial. The annual incidence of pediatric primary brain tumors is about two or three out of 100,000.

Medulloblastoma

Medulloblastomas (primitive neuroectodermal tumors), the most common, account for 20% of childhood brain tumors and 30% to 40% of posterior fossa childhood tumors. The tumor may occur at any time of life, including adulthood, but is most common in the first decade, with peaks at 3 to 4 years of age and 8 to 10 years. Medulloblastomas usually arise from the cerebellar vermis. Symptoms and signs are due to obstruction of the fourth ventricle and hydrocephalus, infiltration of cerebellar tissue, and leptomeningeal spread. By the time of diagnosis, 90% of patients have papilledema, headaches, vomiting (especially morning vomiting), and lethargy. Ataxia is often present early in the course of the disease.

Cerebellar Astrocytoma

The classic, or juvenile, pilocytic cerebellar astrocytoma is a slow-growing lesion arising from the lateral cerebellar hemispheres. This astrocytoma is the second most common tumor of the posterior fossa, accounting for 30% to 40% of cases and comprises 10% to 20% of all childhood brain tumors. The peak ages of incidence are the latter half of the first decade and the first half of the second decade of life. Initially, appendicular cerebellar symptoms may be present for weeks to months. As the tumor extends to the midline and obstructs the fourth ventricle resulting in hydrocephalus, the classic brain tumor symptoms of early-morning vomiting and headaches may be present.

Brain Stem Glioma

Brain stem gliomas constitute 10% to 20% of all childhood brain tumors and are the third most common posterior fossa tumor. The median age of occurrence is between 5 and 9 years. The neurologic presentation depends on the location of the tumor. The classic present is a triad of cranial neuropathies, ataxia, and long tract signs. About one-third of patients have headache, nausea, and vomiting.

Ependymoma

Ependymomas comprise 5% to 10% of childhood primary brain tumors. Two-thirds arise in the posterior fossa and are usually benign, whereas one-third arise supratentorially and are usually malignant. Infratentorial ependymomas arise from the floor, roof, or lateral recesses of the fourth ventricle. By the time of diagnosis, most of the infratentorial tumors have blocked the third or fourth ventricle, producing hydrocephalus. Headaches, nausea, and vomiting will then occur. Depending on location of the tumor, supratentorial ependymomas can produce focal neurologic findings and seizures. By the time of diagnosis, most patients have headaches and other signs and symptoms of increased intracranial pressure.

Pineal Region Lesions

Pineal region lesions include germinomas (1% of childhood primaries), pineoblastomas, glial neoplasms, meningiomas, lymphomas, and pineal cysts. Growth of the tumor causes compression of the aqueduct of Sylvius and hydrocephalus. The typical picture of hydrocephalus can occur with headaches, nausea, and vomiting. Involvement of the superior colliculus can lead to Parinaud's syndrome with paralysis of upgaze, near-light dissociation, and convergence-retraction nystagmus.

CRANIOPHARYNGIOMA. Craniopharyngiomas are benign tumors located in the parasellar region. Although they can occur at any age, the onset is before 15 years of age in 50% of cases. These are the third most common primary in children after medulloblastomas and gliomas. Growth failure is the most common sign at presentation. Visual dysfunction is present in up to 70% of patients at the time of presentation because of the prechiasmal location. Fifty percent of patients complain of severe headaches.

ASTROCYTOMA. Supratentorial astrocytomas can produce focal neurologic findings and seizures (in about 25% of cases). Low-grade gliomas can produce a very gradual onset of symptoms, including headache and/or subtle neurobehavioral changes. Increased difficulty with school work can be blamed on social or psychologic factors. Malignant astrocytomas are more commonly seen in adults.

Hydrocephalus[34]

There are two categories of hydrocephalus, which is a heterogenous disorder. *Obstructive,* or noncommunicating, *hydrocephalus* is due to a blockage of CSF pathways at or proximal to the outlet foramina of the fourth ventricle, the foraminas of Luschka and Magendie. *Communicating hydrocephalus* is due to a blockage of CSF in the basal subarachnoid cisterns, in the subarachnoid spaces over the brain surface, or within the arachnoid granulations.

Table 7-8 lists the various causes of hydrocephalus in children and adults. Diagnostic testing helps to define the features of hydrocephalus, including the site of blockage of CSF, the etiology, and whether the condition is arrested or progressive.

Clinical Manifestations

Small children may present with symptoms and signs of raised intracranial pressure, including headaches, vomiting, irritability, lethargy, and poor feeding. Acute hydrocephalus in older children can result in headaches, often worse in the morning; vomiting; cranial nerve VI palsies; papilledema; and altered levels of consciousness. Headaches due to hydrocephalus are often bilateral and are made worse by coughing, sneezing, straining, or head movement.

Table 7-8. Causes of hydrocephalus

Noncommunicating	Communicating
Aqueductal stenosis	Chiari malformation
Chiari malformation	Dandy-Walker malformation
Dandy-Walker malformation	Encephalocele
Atresia of the foramen of Monroe	Benign cysts
Skull bases anomalies	Incompetent arachnoid villi
Neoplasms	Leptomeningeal inflammation
Benign intracranial cysts	Viral infection
Inflammatory ventriculitis	Bacterial infection
Hemorrhage	Subarachnoid hemorrhage
Infection	Chemical arachnoiditis
Chemical meningitis	Carcinomatous meningitis
Ruptured arachnoid cyst	

From Kinsman SL. Hydrocephalus. In: Gilman S, Goldstein GW, Waxman SG, eds. *Neurobase.* San Diego: Arbor, Publishing, 2000. Modified, with permission.

Ventriculoperitoneal shunts are appropriate treatment for many cases of hydrocephalus. Acute hydrocephalus due to shunt failure can result in headaches, vomiting, altered consciousness, and seizures. Physicians who care for children with shunts should be aware of the rare complication of slit ventricle syndrome.

Symptoms and signs of intermittent intracranial hypertension develop in a patient who has been stable for months to years with a shunt. A scan of the brain shows a smaller than normal ventricular system that could be due to acquired rigidity of the ventricular system. There are numerous other complications of shunts, including infections, subdural hematomas, and seizures.

Colloid Cysts of the Third Ventricle

Colloid cysts of the third ventricle are benign cysts that can move in and out of the foramen of Monro on its pedicle, producing intermittent obstruction of CSF. Colloid cysts are rarely diagnosed during childhood. The cysts can produce severe paroxysmal headaches that can be mistaken for migraine and can lead to sudden death in about 5% of cases.[35]

Dandy-Walker Malformation

Dandy-Walker malformation is a developmental disorder characterized by partial or complete absence of the cerebellar vermis and cystlike dilatation of the fourth ventricle. Other features often present include hydrocephalus; enlargement of the posterior fossa; elevation of the tentorium, transverse sinus, or both; and lack of patency of the foramina of Luschka, Magendie, or both. The incidence is about one in 30,000 live births. There are a variety of clinical presentations, including mental retardation in about 50%, ataxia, brain stem dysfunction, and symptoms and signs due to hydrocephalus, which is present in about 80% of cases by 1 year of age. The initial presentation can occur as late as adulthood, with such complaints as headache, cerebellar ataxia, and progressive spastic weakness of all four extremities.

Acknowledgements. The assistance of Drs. Steven Linder, Paul Winner, and Robert Zeller in discussing their approaches to migraine management, and Drs. Ian Butler and Raymond Kahn in reviewing this chapter is appreciated.

REFERENCES

1. Bille B. Migraine in school children. *Acta Pediatr Scand* 1962;51 [Suppl 136]:1–151.
2. Kandt RS. Childhood migraine. In: Gilman S, Goldstein GW, Waxman SG, eds. *Neurobase.* San Diego: Arbor, 2000.
3. Jan MMS. History of motion sickness is predictive of childhood migraine. *J Paediatr Child Health* 1998;34:483–484.
4. Giroud M, Nivelon JL, Dumas R. [Somnambulism and migraine in children: a non-fortuitous association]. *Arch Fr Pediatr* 1987; 44:263–265.
5. Stewart WF, Linet MS, Celentano DD, et al. Age and sex-specific incidence rates of migraine with and without visual aura. *Am J Epidemiol* 1993:34:1111–1120.

6. Winner P, Wasiewski W, Gladstein J, et al. Multicenter prospective evaluation of proposed pediatric migraine revisions to the IHS criteria. *Headache* 1997;37:545–548.

7. Welch KMA. Hemiplegic migraine. In: Gilman S, Goldstein GW, Waxman SG, eds. *Neurobase.* San Diego: Arbor, 2000.

8. Welch KMA. Basilar migraine. In: Gilman S, Goldstein GW, Waxman SG, eds. *Neurobase.* San Diego: Arbor, 2000.

9. Davidoff RA. Benign paroxysmal vertigo of childhood. In: Gilman S, Goldstein GW, Waxman SG, eds. *Neurobase.* San Diego: Arbor, 2000.

10. Lindskog U, Ödkvist L, Noaksson L, et al. Benign paroxysmal vertigo in childhood: a long-term follow-up. *Headache* 1999;39: 33–37.

11. Lundberg PO. Abdominal migraine. *Triangle* 1978;17:81–84.

12. Jan MM, Camfield PR, Gordon K, et al. Vomiting after mild head injury is related to migraine. *J Pediatr* 1997;130:134–137.

13. Sartory G, Muller B, Metsch J, et al. A comparison of psychological and pharmacological treatment of pediatric migraine. *Behav Res Ther* 1998;36:1155–1170.

14. Linder S. Acute management of migraine in children and adolescents. American Academy of Neurology Annual Courses, Minneapolis, 1998.

15. Hamalainen ML, Hoppo K, Valkeila E, et al. Ibuprofen or acetaminophen for the acute treatment of migraine in children: a double-blind, randomized, placebo-controlled crossover study. *Neurology* 1997;48:103–107.

16. Linder S. Subcutaneous sumatriptan in the clinical setting: the first fifty consecutive patients with acute migraine in a pediatric neurology office practice. *Headache* 1996;36:419–422.

17. Winner P, Prensky A, Linder S, et al. Efficacy and safety of oral sumatriptan in adolescent migraines. Presentation. *Headache* 1996;36.

18. Linder S. Treatment of childhood headache with dihydroergotamine mesylate. *Headache* 1994;34:578–580.

19. Winner P. Pharmacologic management of childhood migraine. Part B: Analgesics, anti-emetics, and prophylactic agents. American Academy of Neurology Annual Courses, Minneapolis, 1998.

20. Battistella PA, Ruffilli R, Cernetti R, et al. A placebo-controlled crossover trial using trazadone in pediatric migraine. *Headache* 1993;33:36–39.

21. Silberstein SD. Divalproex sodium in headache: literature review and clinical guidelines. *Headache* 1996;36:547–555.

22. Bille B. A 40-year follow-up of school children with migraine. *Cephalalgia* 1997;17:488–491.

23. Jensen VK, Rothner AD. Chronic non-progressive headaches in children and adolescents. American Academy of Neurology Annual Courses, Minneapolis, 1998.

24. Gladstein J, Holden EW. Chronic daily headache in children and adolescents: a 2-year prospective study. *Headache* 1996;36: 349–351.

25. Symon DN. Twelve cases of analgesic headache. *Arch Dis Child* 1998;73:555–556.

26. Vasconcellos E, Piña-Garza JE, Millan EJ, et al. Analgesic rebound headache in children and adolescents. *J Child Neurol* 1998;13:443–447.

27. Roos KL. Chapter 41. Viral infections. In: Goetz CG, Pappert EJ, eds. *Textbook of clinical neurology*. Philadelphia: WB Saunders, 1998:819–841.
28. Vanast WJ. New daily persistent headaches: definition of a benign syndrome. *Headache* 1987;26:318.
29. Lewis DW. Acute "organic" headache in childhood and adolescence. American Academy of Neurology Annual Courses Syllabus, Minneapolis, 1998.
30. Giannoni C, Sulek M, Friedman EM. Intracranial complications of sinusitis: a pediatric series. *Am J Rhinol* 1998;12:173–178.
31. Greenlee JE. Brain abscess. In: Gilman S, Goldstein GW, Waxman SG, eds. *Neurobase*. San Diego: Arbor, 2000.
32. Lewis DW. Chronic progressive headache in childhood and adolescence. American Academy of Neurology Annual Course Syllabi, Minneapolis, 1998.
33. Edgeworth J, Bullock P, Bailey A, et al. Why are brain tumours still being missed? *Arch Dis Child* 1996;74:148–151.
34. Kinsman SL. Hydrocephalus. In: Gilman S, Goldstein GW, Waxman SG, eds. *Neurobase*. San Diego: Arbor, 2000.
35. Aronica PA, Ahdab-Barmada M, Rozin L, et al. Sudden death in an adolescent boy due to a colloid cyst of the third ventricle. *Am J Forensic Med Pathol* 1998;19:119–122.

Headaches in Women

Randolph W. Evans

Women have headaches more commonly than men. The prevalence of migraine is 18% of women and 6% of men. This gender ratio increases from menarche, peaks at 42 years of age, and then declines. For females the incidence of migraine with aura peaks between the ages of 12 and 13 (14.1/1,000 person-years), and migraine without aura peaks between the ages of 14 and 17 (18.9/1,000 person-years).[1] Table 8-1 provides the lifetime prevalence of various headaches in women and men.

Estrogen levels are a key factor in the increased prevalence of migraine in women. Evidence includes the following: migraine prevalence increases at menarche; estrogen withdrawal during menstruation is a common migraine trigger; estrogen administration in oral contraceptives and hormone replacement therapy can trigger migraines; migraines typically decrease during the second and third trimesters of pregnancy, when estrogen levels are high; migraines are common immediately post partum, with the precipitous drop in estrogen levels; and migraines generally improve with physiologic menopause. Exactly how changes in estrogen levels influences migraine is not understood. Among numerous effects, fluctuations in estrogen levels can result in changes in prostaglandins and the uterus, prolactin release, opioid regulation, and melatonin secretion. These fluctuations can also cause changes in neurotransmitters, including the catecholamines, noradrenaline, serotonin, dopamine, and endorphins.[2]

This chapter reviews some important headache issues for women, including menstrual migraine, menopause and migraine, oral contraceptive use in migraineurs, and headaches during pregnancy and the post partum.

MENSTRUAL MIGRAINE

The reported prevalence of menstrual migraine varies from 4% to 73%, depending on the criteria used for the timing of the

Table 8-1. Lifetime prevalence of headaches in women and men

Type	Women	Men
Any headache	99%	93%
Migraine	25%	8%
Tension	88%	69%

Data from Rasmussen BK, Jensen R, Schroll M, et al. Epidemiology of headache in a general population—a prevalence study. *J Clin Epidemiol* 1991;44: 1147–1157.

attack. MacGregor proposes the following definition: attacks of migraine without aura that occur regularly on day 1 of menstruation ± 2 days and at no other time.[3] Using this definition, 7% of female migraineurs have only menstrual migraine. Menstruation is a trigger for about 60% of migraineurs. Symptoms of the premenstrual syndrome, which occurs during the luteal phase, include depression, anxiety, crying spells, difficulty thinking, lethargy, backache, breast tenderness, swelling, and nausea. Both migraine and tension-type headaches can be associated.

Management

The symptomatic treatment is the same as for other migraines and includes nonsteroidal antiinflammatory drugs, ergotamine, dihydroergotamine, and triptans (Chapter 2).[3a] Triptans are just as effective for menstrual migraine. Women with frequent migraines, including menstrual migraine, may benefit from preventive treatment (Chapter 2). Increasing the dose perimenstrually can be helpful in some cases.

When menstrual migraine is the only migraine or the most severe and prolonged, a variety of short-term preventive treatments may be effective starting 3 days premenstrually and continuing during the menses for women with regular cycles (Table 8-2).[4,5] Nonsteroidal antiinflammatory drugs (NSAID) can be especially helpful when migraine occurs with dysmenorrhea or menorrhagia.[6] Some patients may respond to one class of NSAID and not another.

Hormonal treatments that may be effective include transdermal estradiol (Table 8-2), bromocriptine 2.5 mg three times a day (continuous treatment more effective than interval),[7] danazol

Table 8-2.   Options for interval preventative treatment of menstrual migraine starting 2–3 days before and continuing during the menses

Medication	Dose
Amitriptyline or nortriptyline	25 mg hs
Propanolol long-acting	60–80 mg qd
Nadolol	40 mg qd
NSAIDs	
Naproxen sodium	550 mg bid
Naproxen	500 mg bid
Ibuprofen	400 mg tid
Mefenamic acid	500 mg bid
Ketoprofen	75 mg tid
Ergotamine	1 mg bid
DHE	1 mg SC or IM bid
Sumatriptan	50 mg qd
Transdermal estradiol	100 µg on day −3 replaced on days −1 and +2

Table 8-3.   Treatment of estrogen replacement headache

Reduce estrogen dose

Change estrogen type from conjugated estrogen (Premarin) to pure
    estradiol (Estrace) to synthetic estrogen (Estinyl) to pure estrone
    (Ogen)

Convert from interrupted to continuous dosing

Convert from oral to parenteral dosing (Alora, Climara, Estraderm,
    or Vivelle-Dot)

Add androgens

From Silberstein SD, Merriam G. Sex hormones and headache. *J Pain Symptom Manage* 1993;8:98–114, modified with permission.

200 mg two or three time a day, and tamoxifen 5 to 15 mg daily
for days 7 to 14 of the luteal cycle. (There are concerns about use
because of an increased risk of uterine cancer.[8]) Some women
may respond to a short, tapering dose of corticosteroids or chlorpromazine 10 to 50 mg twice a day for 4 to 7 days. Oral magnesium (360 mg of magnesium pyrrolidone carboxylic acid) may
also be effective.[9] Hysterectomy is not recommended for the
management of menstrual migraine.

MENOPAUSE AND MIGRAINES

Two-thirds of women with prior migraine improve with physiologic menopause. By contrast, surgical menopause results in
worsening of migraine in two-thirds of cases.

Estrogen Replacement Therapy

Hormone replacement therapy has a variable effect on
migraine frequency: 45% improve, 46% worsen, and 9% are
unchanged.[10] Table 8-3 provides changes in hormone replacement therapy that may be helpful when migraines increase.[10a]
The usual abortive and prophylactic migraine medications can
also be used (Chapter 2).

ORAL CONTRACEPTIVE USE AND MIGRAINE

Influence on Onset and Frequency

Migraines may occur for the first time following oral contraceptive (OC) use. The effect of OC use is quite variable: migraines
may increase, decrease, or stay the same. Much of the data on this
topic is from older studies of the use of high-dose estrogen contraception, which often increased migraine frequency. Low-estrogen-
dose OCs usually have no effect or may improve migraine. When
new-onset migraine occurs or migraine frequency increases, 30%
to 40% of this group may improve when OCs are discontinued.
However, improvement may not occur for up to 1 year.

Risk of Stroke[11]

Since the 1970s, there has been concern that OCs in
migraineurs may increase the risk of stroke. Review of the risk
of stroke in young women, in female migraineurs, and in those
using OCs helps to clarify this issue.

Table 8-4. Approximate incidence of ischemic stroke (strokes per 100,000 women per year) in women with and without migraine who do not use oral contraceptives

		Migraine	
Age	Without migraine	Without aura	With aura
25–34	1.3	4	8
35–44	3.6	11	22

Data from Becker WJ. Migraine and oral contraceptives. *Can J Neurol Sci* 1997;24:16–21.

Stroke in Young Women

The annual incidence of cerebral infarction in young women is low: about four in 100,000 for women aged 25 to 34 and 11 in 100,000 in women aged 35 to 44. For women who do not have migraine and do not take OCs, the annual incidence is perhaps 1.3 in 100,000 for women aged 25 to 34 and 3.6 in 100,000 for women aged 35 to 44.

Hypertension, diabetes, cigarette smoking, and cocaine use are significant risk factors.

Stroke and Migraine

There is an increased risk of stroke in women with migraine.[12,13] Using a variety of assumptions, Becker has calculated the approximate risk of stroke in young women not on OC with and without migraine (Table 8-4).[11]

Stroke and Use of OCs

Stroke and the use of OCs is a controversial topic because studies of low-dose estrogens have yielded conflicting results.[13a] The risk of stroke associated with OCs may vary with the estrogen dose. Based on numerous studies, OCs with different estrogen doses have an increased risk of thromboembolic stroke (odds ratio) as follows: more than 50 mg, 8 to 10; 50 mg, 2 to 4; and 30 to 40 mg, 1.5 to 2.5.[2] However, recent studies have not shown an increased risk of stroke in women who use low-estrogen-dose OCs.[14–16] OCs containing only progesterone do not increase the risk of stroke.[17]

Use of OCs in Migraineurs

There is some evidence to suggest that OC use in migraineurs increases the risk of stroke. Tzourio et al. reported the odds ratio (increase of relative risk) of ischemic stroke in young women using low-estrogen-dose OCs as follows: without migraine, 3.5, and with migraine, 13.9.[12] The significance of this finding is uncertain in view of the more recent OC use and stroke studies showing no increased risk.

Most women with migraine without aura can safely take low-dose-estrogen OCs when there are no other contraindications to OC use. Similarly, those with migraine with auras such as visual symptoms lasting less than 1 hour can use OCs. Women with aura symptoms such as hemiparesis or dysphasia or prolonged focal neurologic symptoms and signs lasting more than 1 hour might best avoid starting low-dose-estrogen OCs and stop the medication if they are already taking it. In addition, the physician should consider other factors in prescribing OCs, such as older age, cigarette smoking, and comorbidity such as diabetes, uncontrolled hypertension, and coronary artery disease. Progesterone-only OCs and the many other contraceptive options can be considered.

HEADACHES DURING PREGNANCY AND POST PARTUM

About 90% of headaches occurring during pregnancy and the postpartum period are benign. The frequency of tension-type headaches generally does not change. Migraine headaches usually occur less often. Management of frequent benign headaches can be challenging because of restrictions on medication use. Life-threatening causes of headache that can occur during this time include preeclampsia and eclampsia, subarachnoid hemorrhage, intracerebral hemorrhage, and cerebral venous thrombosis. There are numerous other secondary causes, including pseudotumor cerebri, brain tumors (including choriocarcinoma), and infections such as those arising from *Listeria*.

Neuroimaging[18]

When there are appropriate indications (Chapter 1), neuroimaging should be performed during pregnancy. With the use of lead shielding, a standard computed tomography (CT) scan of the head exposes the uterus to less than 1 mrad. A radiation dose of ≥15 rad is necessary to result in deformities that might justify termination of the pregnancy. CT scan is the study of choice for the evaluation of head trauma or acute subarachnoid hemorrhage. Magnetic resonance imaging (MRI) is more sensitive for disorders that may occur during pregnancy, such as pituitary apoplexy, cerebral venous sinus thrombosis (with the addition of magnetic resonance venography), and metastatic choriocarcinoma. There is no known risk of MRI during pregnancy, but there is some controversy because the magnets induce an electric field and raise the core temperature slightly (less than 1 degree centigrade). Although there is no known risk of intravenous contrast for CT scan or gadolinium for MRI, contrast should be avoided if possible. The radiation dose to the uterus for a typical cervical or intracranial arteriogram is less than 1 mrad.

Migraine

Epidemiology

The new onset of migraine has been variably reported as occurring in 1% and 10% of migraineurs during pregnancy, usually during the first trimester. During pregnancy, preexisting migraine improves or disappears in about 60%, is unchanged in 20%, and grows more frequent in 20%. Improvement often occurs during the second or third trimester. In one study, menstrual migraine disappeared or improved in 85% and worsened in 7%, in contrast to nonmenstrual migraine, which disappeared or improved in 60% and worsened in 15%.[19] When improvement occurs with the first pregnancy, improvement also occurs during subsequent pregnancies in about 50%, whereas an increased frequency occurs in the other 50%.[20] Migraineurs do not have an increased risk of miscarriages, toxemia, congenital anomalies, or stillbirth.

One study reported that 38% of women had headaches during the first postpartum week, especially between days 3 and 6.[21] These headaches occurred more often in women with either a personal or family history of migraine. Many of the women described a mild to moderately severe bifrontal pain associated with photophobia and nausea. These headaches may be triggered by rapidly falling estrogen levels. In another study, 4.5% of women had the new onset of migraine during the postpartum period.[22]

Management[23–26a]

Fortunately, migraines usually improve or disappear during pregnancy. Nonmedication approaches include avoidance of triggers, ice, sleep, and biofeedback.

Before prescribing medication, the patient should be advised of the potential risk during pregnancy. For many drugs there is insufficient knowledge about the risks of birth defects despite the fact that 67% of women take medications during pregnancy and 50% take them during the first trimester.[27] The Food and Drug Administration (FDA) drug risk ratings provide some guidance for medication during pregnancy. If nonobstetricians (such as neurologists or internists) are managing the migraines, they should confer with the obstetrician about medication use.

SYMPTOMATIC MEDICATIONS. Many migraineurs want to take medication during pregnancy, especially for moderate to severe migraines. Concerns include not only the potential of risk for the fetus, but also medication rebound headaches from overuse as well as habituation with the overuse of butalbital and narcotics.

Acetaminophen, which is an FDA Class B drug (no evidence of risk in humans, but there are no controlled human studies), is the medication of choice because there is no evidence of any teratogenic effect. Aspirin is rated Class C (risk to humans has not been ruled out) during the first and second trimesters and Class D (positive evidence of risk to humans from human or animal studies) during the third trimester. Although there is no definite evidence of teratogenicity, there are multiple possible adverse effects, including the following: inhibition of uterine contraction, longer gestation and labor, increased maternal and newborn bleeding, narrowing of the ductus arteriosus, and hyperbilirubinemia. Low-dose daily aspirin is generally safe when used to prevent preeclampsia or for the treatment of antiphospholipid antibody syndrome, although there may be an increased risk of abruptio placentae.

Caffeine in small doses of less than 300 mg a day is Class B and probably safe. Although butalbital is Class C, there has been no evidence of an association with malformations. However, prolonged overuse can result in fetal dependence and severe neonatal withdrawal. If acetaminophen alone is ineffective, some patients will benefit from the addition of butalbital (Phrenillin) or butalbital and caffeine (Fioricet), which can also be combined with codeine.

Codeine in reasonable amounts is probably safe. However, indiscriminate use of codeine (Class C) during the first and second trimesters has a potential for risk because defects such as cleft lip or palate and hip dislocation have been reported. Meperidine, methadone, and butorphanol (all Class C) are probably not teratogenic.

Nonsteroidal antiinflammatory drugs such as ibuprofen and naproxen are Class B during the first two trimesters but should be avoided during the third trimester because of the potential of inhibiting labor, prolonging the length of the pregnancy, and decreasing amniotic fluid volume. There is also concern about the possibility of causing pulmonary hypertension or premature closure of the ductus arteriosus.

Ergotamine and dihydroergotamine (both Class X, contraindicated in pregnancy) should not be used during pregnancy although the actual risk is not clear. Triptans such as sumatriptan (Imitrex) are Class C. Although there is no evidence of teratogenicity at this time, the use of triptans during pregnancy should be avoided.

Antiemetics may be necessary if the headache is associated with prominent nausea or vomiting and their use may prevent dehydration that can pose a risk to both the mother and fetus. Prochlorperazine, promethazine, and chlorpromazine (available orally, parenterally, and by suppository) are all Class C. Metoclopramide is Class B. These drugs are generally considered reasonably safe during pregnancy, especially with occasional use. No congenital malformations have been reported with the use of metoclopramide.

Prolonged migraine may be treated with 10 mg of prochlorperazine intravenously and intravenous (IV) fluids. The addition of parenteral narcotics may help some patients. Migraine status may respond to the administration of intravenous corticosteroids such as dexamethasone 4 mg IV.

PREVENTIVE MEDICATIONS. Frequent severe migraines associated with nausea and vomiting may justify the use of preventive medications.

Valproic acid, which is Class D (positive evidence of risk to humans from human or animal studies), should be avoided because of the 1% to 2% risk of neural tube defects when taken between day 17 and day 30 after fertilization.

Beta-blockers, routinely used during pregnancy for the treatment of hypertension, are the preventive of choice if medical contraindications are not present. Atenolol, nadolol, propranolol, metoprolol, and timolol are all Class C. Although there is no evidence of teratogenicity, there may be an increased incidence of small-for-gestational-age infants. Propranolol may cause fetal and neonatal toxicity.

Antidepressants might be considered in some cases. The class rating of some tricyclic antidepressants are as follows: amitriptyline, Class B; nortriptyline, Class D; and doxepin and protriptyline, Class C. These drugs are associated with a low risk of harm to the fetus, if any. Tricyclics should be stopped at least 2 weeks before the due date. There are reports of infants with respiratory distress and feeding difficulties born to women who took tricyclics through delivery. Fluoxetine (Class C), a selective

**Table 8-5. Drug therapy in lactating
women: questions and options**

1. Is the drug therapy really necessary? Consultation between the
   pediatrician and the mother's physician can be most useful.
2. Use the safest drug—for example, acetaminophen rather than
   aspirin for analgesia.
3. If there is a possibility that a drug may prevent a risk to the
   infant, consideration should be given to measurement of blood
   concentrations in the nursing infant.
4. Drug exposure to the nursing infant may be minimized by
   having the mother take the medication just after she has
   breastfed the infant and/or just before the infant is due to have
   a lengthy sleep period.

From The American Academy of Pediatrics Committee on Drugs. The transfer
of drugs and other chemicals into human milk. *Pediatrics* 1994;93:137–150.

serotonin reuptake inhibitor (SSRI), is questionably effective for
migraine prevention, but there is evidence of efficacy for chronic
daily headache. Fluoxetine might be considered in a patient with
frequent headaches and depression.

Another option is the calcium channel blocker verapamil
(Class C), which is probably safe during pregnancy. This drug is
preferable to beta-blockers for prevention of migraine with prolonged aura. In addition, verapamil can also be considered in
women with hypertension and frequent migraines who cannot
take beta-blockers.

BREASTFEEDING AND MIGRAINE MANAGEMENT. The American
Academy of Pediatrics Committee on Drugs has made recommendations based on their review of drug use during lactation
(Table 8-5).[28] Ergotamine is contraindicated during breastfeeding. Drugs whose effect on nursing infants is unknown but may
be of concern include such antidepressants as amitriptyline and
fluoxetine. Their use is probably safe because there are no
reported adverse effects.

Maternal medications usually compatible with breastfeeding
include the following: acetaminophen; barbiturates (which may
cause infant sedation); caffeine (which may cause irritability or
poor sleeping pattern if the mother uses a lot of it); nonsteroidal
antiinflammatory drugs, such as ibuprofen and naproxen; beta-
blockers, such as propranolol and nadolol; narcotics, including
codeine, morphine, and butorphanol; valproic acid; and verapamil. Triptans (which are not listed in the report) should be
used with caution.

Preeclampsia and Eclampsia[29]

Epidemiology

Preeclampsia occurs in up to 7% of pregnancies, and eclampsia is found in up to 0.3%. The criteria for preeclampsia include
the following: proteinuria of more than 300 mg/day or two spot
urines with more than 1 g protein/liter collected more than 6

hours apart; edema; hypertension persistently greater than 140/90 or relative hypertension with a rise over a first-trimester baseline blood pressure of at least 30 mm Hg systolic or 15 mm Hg diastolic; and onset after the twentieth week of gestation up until 48 hours post partum. Eclampsia occurs with the additional complications of seizures or coma. As many as 45% of cases of eclampsia have an onset post partum, with a mean of 6 days and up to 4 weeks.

Risk factors for preeclampsia in primigravida are prepregnancy hypertension, obesity, multiple abortions or miscarriages, and cigarette smoking. The incidence of pregnancy-induced hypertension is greater in first or multiple pregnancies and in younger and older women. Black women have twice the incidence of whites.

Clinical Manifestations

Nonneurologic complications include the following: renal dysfunction with oliguria, casts, and elevated serum uric acid, urea, and creatinine; pulmonary edema; vomiting and epigastric pain; subcapsular hepatic hemorrhage; and hemolysis, elevated liver enzymes, and low platelets (HELLP syndrome), which can be further complicated by disseminated intravascular coagulation (DIC) in up to 40% of patients.

Neurologic complications consist of the following: headaches that are typically bilateral; dizziness; tinnitus; altered consciousness or coma; seizures; and visual disturbances, including diplopia, scotomas, blurring, and blindness. Blindness, which can occur in up to 15% of eclamptics, may be due to retinal hemorrhages, edema, or detachment or occipital ischemia.

Subarachnoid Hemorrhage

Nontraumatic subarachnoid hemorrhage (SAH) during pregnancy has an incidence of about 20 per 100,000 deliveries. This is the third most common cause of nonobstetric mortality, accounting for 5% to 10% of all maternal deaths. This risk is five times higher than that outside pregnancy. SAH is due to ruptured saccular aneurysms and arteriovenous malformations with equal frequency. Up to 20% of aneurysmal ruptures occur during pregnancy or in the early postpartum period. The risk of aneurysmal SAH is highest during the late third trimester, during delivery, and in the puerperium.[30] The most common time for hemorrhage from an arteriovenous malformation (AVM) is between 16 and 20 weeks' gestation or during parturition. About 25% of pregnant women who have already bled from an AVM will rebleed during the same pregnancy. Chapter 5 reviews the clinical manifestations of SAH.

Other causes of intracranial hemorrhage during pregnancy and the puerperium include eclampsia, cerebral venous thrombosis, choriocarcinoma, bacterial endocarditis, drug abuse, DIC, moyamoya disease, hematologic disorders, tumor, ruptured spinal cord vascular malformations, and arterial hypertension.

Stroke and Cerebral Venous Thrombosis[31]

The risk of ischemic stroke is 13 times higher during pregnancy and the puerperium than expected outside of pregnancy.

Either ischemic or hemorrhagic stroke occurs in up to 19 in 100,000 deliveries. Arterial occlusions account for 60% to 80% of these strokes. The headaches that can be associated with stroke are described in Chapter 11.

There are numerous causes of arterial ischemic strokes, including cardioembolic disorders (rheumatic heart disease, prosthetic heart valves, atrial fibrillation, bacterial and nonbacterial endocarditis, peripartum cardiomyopathy, mitral valve prolapse, and paradoxical embolus), cerebral angiopathies (atherosclerosis; arterial dissection; fibromuscular dysplasia; cerebral vasculitis, such as systemic lupus erythematosus, Takayasu's disease, periarteritis nodosa, and isolated angiitis of the brain; and postpartum cerebral angiopathy), hematologic disorders (sickle cell anemia; Sneddon's syndrome; antiphospholipid antibodies; thrombotic thrombocytopenic purpura; homocystinuria; deficiency of antithrombin II, protein C, and protein S; and DIC), and other causes (eclampsia, choriocarcinoma, amniotic fluid embolism, air embolism, fat embolism, drug abuse, and Sheehan's syndrome).

The only three pregnancy specific disorders are eclampsia, choriocarcinoma, and amniotic fluid embolism. Postpartum cerebral angiopathy and peripartum cardiomyopathy have also been reported apart from pregnancy.

Pregnancy and the puerperium are associated with an increased risk of cerebral venous thrombosis (Chapter 11). Ninety percent of cases occur during the puerperium, most commonly in the second or third weeks post partum.

Sheehan's syndrome is the spontaneous ischemic necrosis of the pituitary gland in the postpartum period, resulting in hypopituitarism. Most cases are due to hypotension and shock from acute blood loss, resulting in ischemia of a hypertrophied pituitary gland of pregnancy. About 1% to 2% of women who have a significant postpartum hemorrhage will have this syndrome. In contrast to pituitary apoplexy (Chapter 12), headaches and cranial nerve abnormalities are not usually associated.

Pseudotumor Cerebri

Although pregnancy is not a risk factor, pseudotumor cerebri can develop or worsen during pregnancy. Visual outcome is the same for pregnant and nonpregnant patients. Subsequent pregnancy does not increase the risk of recurrent pseudotumor cerebri. This disorder is further discussed in Chapter 12.

Brain Tumors

Pregnancy does not increase the risk of developing a primary brain tumor. Meningiomas may increase in size during pregnancy and then regress post partum. Twenty-five percent of macroprolactinomas will expand enough to cause problems during pregnancy.

Choriocarcinoma is due to malignant transformation of the trophoblast. Although choriocarcinomas usually follow a molar pregnancy, they can also follow term delivery, abortion, and ectopic pregnancy. Brain metastases occur in 20% of cases.

Trophoblasts can invade blood vessels and result in thrombosis and cerebral infarctions. Neoplastic aneurysms and cerebral hemorrhage can also occur.

Infections

Pregnancy is a state of relative immunosuppression. Coccid-
iomycosis, tuberculosis, listeriosis, and malaria have an
increased risk of spread to the central nervous system when
acquired during pregnancy. Headache can certainly be a presenting or prominent symptom.

ACKNOWLEDGMENT

The assistance of Dr. Brian Kirshon in reviewing this chapter
is appreciated.

REFERENCES

1. Lipton RB, Stewart SW. Epidemiology and comorbidity of
   migraine. In: Goadsby PJ, Silberstein SD. *Headache.* Boston:
   Butterworth-Heinemann, 1997:75–96.
2. Silberstein SD, Merriam GR. Sex hormones and headache. In:
   Goadsby PJ, Silberstein SD, eds. *Headache.* Boston: Butterworth-Heinemann, 1997:143–176.
3. MacGregor EA. Menstruation, sex hormones, and migraine.
   Neurol Clin 1997;15:125–141.
3a. Boyle CA. Management of menstrual migraine. *Neurology* 1999;
   53(4 Suppl I):S14–18.
4. Newman LC, Lipton RB, Lay CL, et al. A pilot study of oral
   sumatriptan as intermittent prophylaxis of menstruation-
   related migraine. *Neurology* 1998;51:307–309.
5. Moore KL. Headache associated with hormonal fluctuations.
   In: Gilman S, Goldstein GW, Waxman SG, eds. *Neurobase.* San
   Diego: Arbor, 2000.
6. Nattero G, Allais G, De Lorenzo C, et al. Biological and clinical
   effects of naproxen sodium in patients with menstrual
   migraine. *Cephalalgia* 1991; 11[Suppl 11]:201–202.
7. Herzog AG. Continuous bromocriptine therapy in menstrual
   migraine. *Neurology* 1997;48:101–102.
8. O'Dea JP, Davis EH. Tamoxifen in the treatment of menstrual
   migraine. *Neurology* 1990;40:1470–1471.
9. Facchinetti F, Sances G, Borella P, et al. Magnesium prophylaxis of menstrual migraine: effects on intracellular magnesium. *Headache* 1991;31:298–301.
10. MacGregor EA. Is HRT giving you a headache? *Br Migraine
   Assoc Newsletter* 1993:19–24.
10a. Fettes I. Migraine in the menopause. *Neurology* 1999;53 (4
   Suppl I):S29–33.
11. Becker WJ. Migraine and oral contraceptives. *Can J Neurol Sci*
   1997;24:16–21.
12. Tzourio C, Tehindrazanarivelo A, Iglesias S, et al. Case-control
   study of migraine and risk of ischaemic stroke in young women.
   BMJ 1995;310:830–833.
13. Welch KMA, Tatemichi TK, Mohr JP. Migraine and stroke. In:
   Barnett JHM, Mohr JP, Stein BM, Yatsu FM, eds. *Stroke: pathophysiology, diagnosis, and management.* New York: Churchill
   Livingstone, 1998:845–868.
13a. Zeitouh K, Carr PR. Is there an increased risk of stroke associated with oral contraceptives? *Drug SAF* 1999;20:467–473.
14. Petitti DB, Sidney S, Berstein A, et al. Stroke in users of low-
   dose oral contraceptives. *N Engl J Med* 1996;335:8–15.

15. Schwartz SM, Siscovick DS, Longstreth WT, et al. Use of low-dose oral contraceptives and stroke in young women. *Ann Intern Med* 1997;127(8,Pt 1):596–603.
16. Hannaford PC, Kay CR. The risk of serious illness among oral contraceptive users: evidence from the RCGP's oral contraceptive study. *Br J Gen Pract* 1998;48:1657–1662.
17. Lidegaard O. Oral contraception and risk of a cerebral thromboembolic attack: results of a case-control study. *BMJ* 1993;306:956–963.
18. Silberstein SD, Lipton RB, Goadsby PJ. Pregnancy, breast feeding and headache. In: *Headache in clinical practice.* Oxford: Isis, 1998.
19. Bousser MG, Ratinahirana H, Darbois X. Migraine and pregnancy: a prospective study in 703 women after delivery. *Neurology* 1990;40:437.
20. Maggioni F, Alessi C, Maggino T, et al. Headache during pregnancy. *Cephalalgia* 1997;17:765–769.
21. Stein GS. Headache in the first postpartum week and their relationship to migraine. *Headache* 1981;21:201–205.
22. Granella F, Sances G, Zanferrari C, et al. Migraine without aura and reproductive life events: a clinical epidemiological study in 1300 women. *Headache* 1993:33:385.
23. Hainline B. Headache in Neurologic complications of pregnancy. *Neurol Clin* 1994;12:443–459.
24. Silberstein SD. Migraine and pregnancy. *Neurol Clin* 1997;15: 209–231.
25. Pfaffenrath V, Rehm M. Migraine in pregnancy: what are the safest treatment options? *Drug Saf* 1998;19:383–388.
26. Gilmore J, Pennell PB, Stern BJ. Medication use during pregnancy for neurologic conditions. *Neurol Clin* 1998;16:189–206.
26a. Aube M. Migraine in pregnancy. *Neurology* 1999;53(4 Suppl I):S26–28.
27. Moore KL. Headache associated with hormonal fluctuation. In: Gilman S, Goldstein GW, Waxman SG, eds. *Neurobase.* San Diego: Arbor, 2000.
28. Committee on Drugs. The transfer of drugs and other chemicals into human milk. *Pediatrics* 1994;93:137–150.
29. Pleasure JR. Neurologic problems in pregnancy. In: Rosenberg RN, Pleasure DE, eds. *Comprehensive neurology,* 2nd ed. New York: John Wiley, 1998:825–847.
30. Stoodley MA, Macdonald L, Weir BKA. Pregnancy and intracranial aneurysm. *Neurosurg Clin N Am* 1998;9:549–556.
31. Mas J-L, Lamy C. Stroke in pregnancy and the puerperium. *J Neurol* 1998;245:305–313.

Headaches Over the Age of 50

Randolph W. Evans

The prevalence of headache decreases with older age (Table 9-1).[1] Although 90% of headaches in younger patients are of the primary type, only 66% of those in the elderly are primary.[2]

There are numerous causes of new-onset headaches in those over 50 years of age (Table 9-2).[3] Although new-onset tension-type headaches are fairly common, migraine and cluster-type headaches uncommonly begin after 50 years of age. Temporal arteritis, hypnic headache, and headache of Parkinson's disease are secondary headaches occurring with much greater frequency in this population.

Causes of secondary headache disorders beginning in later life include the following: neoplasms; subdural and epidural hematomas; head trauma; cerebrovascular disease; temporal arteritis; trigeminal neuralgia; postherpetic neuralgia; medication-related headache, including those caused by specific medications and medication rebound; systemic disease, such as infections, acute hypertension, hypoxia, or hypercarbia; and other metabolic disorders, such as hypercalcemia, severe anemia, hyponatremia, and chronic renal failure; diseases of the cranium, neck, eyes, ears, and nose, including cervicogenic headache, glaucoma, otitis, sinusitis, and dental infections; Parkinson's disease; and angina, which may rarely present with exertional headache without chest pain.

In a study of 193 patients 65 years of age and over seen by a neurology service with new-onset headaches, the most frequent diagnoses were tension type (43%) and trigeminal neuralgia (19%).[4] Only one patient met migraine criteria. Fifteen percent had secondary headaches due to conditions such as stroke, temporal arteritis, or intracranial neoplasm. The risk of serious disorders causing headache increased 10 times after age 65, compared with younger patients.

This chapter reviews the primary headaches and some of the secondary headaches, including temporal arteritis, postherpetic neuralgia, and Parkinson's disease. The other secondary head-

Table 9-1. Prevalence of headaches at various ages

Age	Women	Men
21–34	92%	74%
55–74	66%	53%
75+	55%	22%

**Table 9-2.   New-onset headaches
occurring over 50 years of age**

Primary headaches
  Migraine
  Tension
  Cluster
  Hypnic
Secondary headaches
  Neoplasms
  Subdural and epidural hematomas
  Head trauma
  Cerebrovascular disease
  Temporal arteritis
  Trigeminal neuralgia
  Postherpetic neuralgia
  Mediation related
  Systemic disease
  Diseases of the cranium, neck, eyes, ears, and nose
  Parkinson's disease
  Exertional headache due to angina

aches are covered in Chapters 3 (medication related), 6 (subdural
and epidural hematomas), 10 (trigeminal neuralgia), and 12.

PRIMARY HEADACHES

Migraine

Only 2% of migraineurs have the new onset after 50 years of
age. Migraine prevalence decreases with older age. The prevalence is 5% in women and 2% in men past 70 years of age. When
migraine criteria are met, computed tomography (CT) or magnetic resonance imaging (MRI) scans have a very low yield in
this population.[5]

Medication use presents a variety of problems in older
patients. Ergotamine, dihydroergotamine (DHE), and triptans
should not be used in patients with coronary artery disease,
cerebrovascular disease, or peripheral vascular disease. Some
patients without such a history may require screening, especially if they have risk factors such as diabetes, a positive family history, smoking, or hyperlipidemia. Older patients may be
more sensitive to anticholinergic, hypotensive, sedative, cognitive, and cardiac side effects of preventive medications. For
example, patients with prostatism, glaucoma, or cardiac
arrhythmias may need to avoid tricyclic antidepressants,
whereas those with congestive heart failure, diabetes, or
bronchial asthma may need to avoid beta-blockers. Drugs used
for other indications, such as estrogen replacement therapy or
nitrates, may trigger migraines. A variety of other medications
can cause headaches, including nifedipine and nonsteroidal
antiinflammatory drugs (also see Chapter 3).

Late-Life Migraine Accompaniments

Fisher described late-life migrainous accompaniments,[6,7] which are transient visual, sensory, motor, or behavioral neurologic manifestations that are similar or identical to the auras of migraine with aura.[8] Headache is associated with only 50% of cases and may be mild. These accompaniments occur more often in men than in women.

Table 9-3 provides the features of this disorder. The complaints occur as follows, from most to least common: visual symptoms (transient blindness, homonymous hemianopsia, and blurring of vision); paresthesias (numbness, tingling, pins-and-needles sensation, or a heavy feeling of an extremity); brain stem and cerebellar dysfunction (ataxia, clumsiness, hearing loss, tinnitus, vertigo, and syncope); and disturbances of speech (dysarthria or dysphasia).

Other causes of transient cerebral ischemia should be considered, especially when the patient is seen after the first episode or if there are unusual aspects. The usual diagnostic evaluation for transient ischemic attacks (TIAs) or seizures (such as CT scan, MRI and magnetic resonance angiography of the brain, carotid ultrasound, electroencephalography, cardiac evaluation, and blood studies) is performed.

The following features help to distinguish migraine from TIAs: a gradual buildup of sensory symptoms, a march of sensory paresthesias, serial progression from one accompaniment to another, longer duration (90% of TIAs last for less than 15 minutes), and multiple stereotypical episodes.

If the episodes are frequent, preventive treatment can be considered with medications such as verapamil, aspirin, ticlopidine, or clopidigrel. Beta-blockers should be avoided because of the potential for worsening vasospasm. For acute treatment, ergotamine, DHE, and triptans should be avoided because of the risk of increasing cerebral vasospasm.

Table 9-3.   Late-life migraine accompaniments

1. Gradual appearance of focal neurologic symptoms with spread or worsening over a period of minutes.

2. Headache is only present in 50% of cases and may be mild

3. Positive visual symptoms such as scintillating scotoma, flashing or bright lights

4. A history of similar episodes associated with a more severe headache

5. Serial progression from one accompaniment to another (e.g., from flashing lights to paresthesias, paresis, or dysphasia)

6. Diagnosis facilitated with the occurrence of two or more identical episodes

7. A duration of 15 to 25 minutes

8. A characteristic "flurry" of accompaniments

9. A usually benign natural history, without permanent sequelae

10. Another cause not shown by diagnostic testing that is performed when indicated

Tension-Type Headaches

About 10% of those with tension-type headaches have an onset after 50 years of age. When new-onset tension-type headaches occur, the diagnosis is one of exclusion. Over the age of 65 years, the prevalence of tension-type headaches is 27%. The patient and physician should be aware of the potential for medication-overuse headaches.

Medications for tension-type headaches are the same as those for younger people. It is often prudent to start with lower doses and to be cautious about an increased susceptibility to side effects in the elderly. Physical therapy can be helpful for cervicogenic headache.

Cluster Headaches

Cluster headaches are a rare disorder with a 5:1 male-to-female preponderance. Although the age of onset is typically between the ages of 20 and 50 years, onset can occur in the 70s.

Hypnic Headache

Hypnic headache is a rare disorder originally described by Raskin in 1988,[9] which has since been reported in men and women from the ages of 40 to 79 years. The headache only occurs during sleep when the sufferer is awakened at a consistent time. Nausea is infrequent and autonomic symptoms are rarely associated. The headache can be unilateral or bilateral, throbbing or nonthrobbing, and mild to severe in intensity. The headache can last 15 minutes to 6 hours and can occur frequently, as often as nightly, for many years. Medications that may be effective include caffeine (1 or 2 cups of caffeinated coffee or a 40- to 60-mg caffeine tablet before bedtime), lithium carbonate (300 mg at bedtime), indomethacin, atenolol, cyclobenzaprine, and flunarizine (not available in the United States).[10,11]

The diagnosis is one of exclusion because secondary causes of nocturnal headaches include drug withdrawal, temporal arteritis, sleep apnea, oxygen desaturation, pheochromocytomas, primary and secondary neoplasms, communicating hydrocephalus, subdural hematomas, and vascular lesions.[12]

Migraine, cluster, and chronic paroxysmal hemicrania are other primary headaches that can cause awakening from sleep. Migraine typically has associated symptoms and occurs very uncommonly only during sleep. Cluster headaches have autonomic symptoms and may occur during the day as well as during sleep. Chronic paroxysmal hemicrania occurs both during the day and at night, lasts for less than 30 minutes, and occurs 10 to 30 times a day.

SECONDARY HEADACHES

Temporal Arteritis

Epidemiology

Temporal (giant cell) arteritis (TA) is a systemic panarteritis that selectively involves arterial walls with significant amounts of elastin. Approximately 50% of patients with TA have polymyalgia rheumatica, and about 15% of patients with polymyalgia rheumatica have TA. Both conditions occur almost exclusively in patients over the age of 50, with a mean age of onset of about 70. The ratio of women to men is 3:1. The disorder is more common in Scandinavia and the northern United States, and is more common in whites than in other ethnic groups. The annual incidence is about 18 in 100,000 over 50 years of age.

Clinical Manifestations[13]

Headaches are the most common symptom reported by 60% to 90% of patients. The pain is most often throbbing, although many patients describe a sharp, dull, burning, or lancinating type of pain. The pain may be intermittent or continuous and is more often severe than moderate or slight. For some patients, the pain may be worse at night when lying on a pillow, while combing the hair, or when washing the face. Tenderness or decreased pulsation of the superficial temporal arteries is present on physical examination in about half of the patients with TA.

The location of the headache is variable. In one series, 65% of patients presented with temporofrontal headache.[14] In another series, the following percentages of patients reported the distribution of pain in these categories: 25%, only the temple; 54%, the temple, either exclusively or inclusively; 29%, not involving the temple at all; and 8%, generalized.[15] When headaches were limited to or included the temple, the headaches were bilateral in 50% of the patients. Intermittent jaw claudication was reported by 38%. Other studies have reported one-sided pain in 2%; 8% reported pain affecting the face or neck.

Temporal arteritis can present as occipital neuralgia. In a study of 46 patients with biopsy-proven TA, 17% of the patients had an initial presentation with occipital pain, which was unilateral in 38%.[16] Two of the patients with unilateral pain exactly similar to greater occipital neuralgia had normal sedimentation rates but abnormal superficial temporal artery biopsies. Tenderness over the greater occipital nerve can be explained by inflammation of the occipital artery, which is adjacent to the greater occipital nerve in the suboccipital region. TA should be considered in patients over 50 years of age who present with new-onset "occipital neuralgia," even with normal sedimentation rates, especially when they do not respond to the usual treatments.

Neurologic manifestations of TA are common. One series found evidence of neurologic disease in 31% of the patients, including ophthalmologic findings, 20%; mononeuropathies and peripheral neuropathies, 14%; carotid distribution transient ischemic events or stroke, 7%; vertebrobasilar distribution transient ischemic events or stroke, 2%; otologic findings, 7%; tremor, 4%; psychiatric findings, 3%; tongue numbness, 2%; and transverse myelopathy, <1%.[17] Depression and confusion can be associated with temporal arteritis.

There is a broad spectrum of neuroophthalmologic manifestations of TA.[18] Visual loss may occur because of anterior and posterior ischemic optic neuropathy; central and branch retinal artery occlusion; anterior segment ischemia; and prechiasmal, perichiasmal, and postchiasmal field defects. Ophthalmoparesis can be due to the following: oculomotor, abducens, and trochlear nerve palsies; orbital constriction resulting from orbital cellulitis and cavernous sinus thrombosis; and oculomotor synkinesis. Autonomic dysfunction may be caused by Horner's syndrome and parasympathetic pupillary light dysfunction/near-dissociation. Rarely, complex visual hallucinations occur after infarction of the tertiary visual association cortex.

Diagnostic Evaluation

According to the American College of Rheumatology 1990 criteria, the diagnosis of TA can be established by fulfilling three out of five criteria (Table 9-4).[19] The presence of three or more of the five criteria is associated with a sensitivity of 93.5% and a specificity of 91.2%.

The diagnosis is based on clinical suspicion that is usually but not always confirmed by laboratory testing.[19a] The three best tests are the Westergren erythrocyte sedimentation rate (ESR), the C-reactive protein (CRP), and temporal artery biopsy. Elevation of plasma viscosity has a sensitivity and specificity similar to that of the ESR. Mild normochromic normocytic anemia, elevation of liver enzymes (especially alkaline phosphatase), and decreased alpha$_2$-globulin levels are fairly common.

Color duplex ultrasonography of the superficial temporal arteries is a promising new approach to diagnosis based on several studies, including a prospective one of 30 patients.[20] In 73% of patients, ultrasonography showed a dark halo around the lumen of the superficial temporal arteries that may be due to edema of the artery wall. The dark halo disappeared after a mean of 16 days of treatment with corticosteroids. Eighty percent of the patients had stenoses or occlusions of temporal artery segments, and 93% had stenoses, occlusions, or a halo.

For elderly patients, the ESR range of normal may vary from <20 mm/h to 40 mm/h. A formula for the upper limits of normal for the ESR that includes 98% of healthy people is as follows: age in years divided by 2 for men and age in years plus 10 divided by 2 for women.[21] Elevation of the ESR is not specific for TA. Elevation can be seen in any infectious, inflammatory, or rheumatic disease. The level can even be affected by the length of time between the venipuncture and the laboratory testing.[22] TA with a normal ESR has been reported in 10% to 36% of patients. Repeating the ESR may be helpful in some cases where the ESR is initially normal and then rises. When abnormal, the ESR averages 70 to 80 and may reach 120 or even 130 mm/h. When the

Table 9-4. Criteria for the diagnosis of TA of the American College of Rheumatology

Three out of the following five criteria should be satisfied:
1. Age at least 50 years
2. New onset of localized headache
3. Temporal artery tenderness or decreased pulse
4. Erythrocyte sedimentation rate of at least 50 mm/h
5. Positive histology

ESR is elevated at the time of diagnosis, it can be followed to help guide the dosage of corticosteroid medication.

CRP is an acute-phase plasma protein from the liver. As with the ESR, elevation is nonspecific and can be seen with numerous disorders. The CRP is not influenced by various hematologic factors or age and is more sensitive than the ESR for the detection of TA. The ESR and CRP combined give the best specificity, 97%.

The diagnosis is made with certainty when the superficial temporal artery biopsy demonstrates necrotizing arteritis characterized by a predominance of mononuclear cell infiltrates or a granulomatous process with multinucleated giant cells. The false-negative rate of temporal artery biopsies in various series ranges from 5% to 44%. Biopsy negative cases may have a more benign course than biopsy positive cases.[22a]

Possible reasons for negative temporal artery biopsies include noncontinuous pathologic findings or skip lesions, choice of site and length of the biopsy, examination of an incomplete number of sections, involvement of other vascular territories, and initiation of corticosteroid therapy prior to the biopsy. When the biopsy is negative, a biopsy of the contralateral superficial temporal artery increases the positive yield by 5% to 15%. Pathologic evidence of TA persists for at least 4 to 5 days after the start of corticosteroid treatment.

Since temporal artery biopsy is a simple, low-risk procedure, a case can be made for obtaining a biopsy in every suspected patient. However, when three or four of the American College of Rheumatology criteria are met (Table 9-4), a strong argument can be made for treatment without biopsy. The result of the CRP and/or color duplex ultrasonography may also influence the decision.

In patients in which the clinical presentation is somewhat suspicious or when there is a very high probability of corticosteroid side effects (e.g., a type I diabetic), a biopsy should be obtained. In the occasional patient with a normal or only slightly elevated ESR and a negative biopsy, the same consideration may apply in a decision to biopsy the contralateral artery.

Management

When contraindications are not present, treatment is typically started with prednisone at a dosage of 40 to 80 mg/day.[23] The headache will often improve within 24 hours. The initial dose is maintained for about 4 weeks and then slowly reduced over many months, depending on the clinical effect, the ESR, and occurrence of side effects. Since TA is active for at least 1 year and an average of 3 to 4 years in some series, long-term treatment is usually required. There are numerous complications of long-term steroid treatment.[24] Some physicians give calcium and vitamin D supplementation or etidronate to help prevent osteoporosis due to long-term corticosteroid use, especially in women.

Postherpetic Neuralgia[25,26]

Epidemiology

Acute herpes zoster occurs when the dormant varicella zoster virus (from a previous chickenpox infection) is reactivated in the trigeminal, geniculate, or dorsal root ganglion. The annual incidence of acute herpes zoster is approximately 400 in 100,000. The incidence dramatically increases with older age. According to various studies, the incidence ranges from 40 to 160 in 100,000 for those under 20 years of age to 450 to 1,100 in 100,000 for those 80 years of age or older. There are more than a million cases per year in the United States, most in the elderly. The lifetime risk of developing acute herpes zoster for those who live into their 70s and 80s is as high as 40%. The lifetime risk of a second or third attack in healthy people is about 5%.

Postherpetic neuralgia (PHN) is the most common neurologic complication of varicella zoster infection and occurs in about 10% to 15% of those with acute zoster. PHN develops in some 50% of those older than 50 years of age and in 80% of those older than 80. Up to 200,000 people in the United States have PHN, which can persist for years. Zoster involving the face nearly doubles the risk of developing PHN, which lasts longer than PHN in other locations.

Clinical Manifestations

Radicular pain is the most common complication of zoster and may precede the eruption of grouped vesicles (shingles) by days to weeks. Zoster occurs in a trigeminal distribution, usually in the ophthalmic division, in 23% of cases. Uncommonly, an extraocular muscle paresis may be associated as a result of involvement of the third, fourth, or sixth cranial nerves. Reactivation of virus in the geniculate ganglion can result in vesicles in the external auditory canal and a facial palsy known by the eponym of Ramsay-Hunt syndrome. Occasionally, pain occurs without a rash (zoster sine herpete). The pain is usually sharp or stabbing. Typically, the vesicles crust, the skin heals, and the pain resolves within 3 to 4 weeks of the onset of the rash. However, in many people the pain can persist.

Postherpetic neuralgia is the persistence of pain after the initial rash for more than 1 to 6 months. (There are different opinions about the definition in the literature.) The involvement of the head is typically unilateral in the distribution of the ophthalmic or maxillary divisions of the trigeminal nerve or at the occipitocervical junction. Three types of pain may be present: a constant burning or deep aching; an intermittent spontaneous pain with a jabbing or lancinating quality; and a superficial, sharp, or radiating pain or itching provoked by light touch (allodynia). The types of pains vary from person to person. Allodynia is present in 90% of individuals with PHN. The pain often interferes with sleep.

Management

For the treatment of acute zoster, oral corticosteroids (prednisone starting at 60 mg/day and tapering off over 2 weeks) may reduce acute pain but may not reduce the risk of PHN. Use of oral acyclovir may decrease the acute pain but only modestly decreases the risk of PHN. Famciclovir[27] (500 mg every 8 hours for 1 week) and valacyclovir (1 g every 12 hours for 1 week) are more effective in reducing the incidence and duration of PHN. (The doses of both drugs are reduced in renal insufficiency.) Although nerve blocks are a highly effective treatment for acute pain, it is uncertain if this approach will reduce the risk of PHN.

A variety of treatments are available for PHN with varying efficacies. Tricyclic antidepressants, including amitriptyline, nortriptyline, and desipramine, are effective treatments. Start with a low dose and then slowly increase to an optimal dose with the most pain relief and tolerable side effects. Up to 61% of patients may have pain relief with tolerable side effects. Some patients may benefit from the addition of a phenothiazine medication such as fluphenazine. Gabapentin is also effective in the treatment of pain and sleep interference associated with PHN.[28] Anecdotally, other antidepressants such as fluoxetine may also be effective.

Topical agents, including capsaicin, lidocaine, aspirin, and nonsteroidal antiinflammatory drugs, may be useful. The 0.075% capsaicin cream may be more effective than lower concentrations. Some patients may have burning pain on application of the cream, which limits use.

Opioids such as sustained-release oxycodone (10 mg every 12 hours, slowly increasing as necessary to 30 mg every 12 hours)[29] and oral levorphanol may be effective when other drugs fail or cannot be tolerated. Transcutaneous electrical nerve stimulation (TENS), with the electrodes placed above and below the involved area, may help about one third of patients. Because efficacy has not been demonstrated in properly designed studies, neural destructive treatments such as neurolytic nerve blocks, nerve sectioning, and dorsal root entry zone lesions are not recommended.

Cervicogenic Headache

Cervical spondylosis and muscle spasm may cause headache in older patients. The headache may be unilateral or bilateral. Digital pressure in the suboccipital area may reproduce the headache. The headache may be due to occipital neuralgia, myofascial pain with trigger points, or referred from neck structures such as the upper cervical facets (Chapter 6). Beneficial treatments include nonsteroidal antiinflammatory drugs, muscle relaxants, tricyclic antidepressants, and physical therapy. Occipital nerve blocks and trigger point injections may be helpful in appropriate cases.

Parkinson's Disease

Headache associated with muscle rigidity may occur more often in Parkinson's disease. Tricyclic medications such as amitriptyline or nortriptyline may be effective. Amantidine and L-Dopa, drugs for the treatment of Parkinson's, can cause headaches in some people.

REFERENCES

1. Waters WE. The Pontypridd headache survey. *Headache* 1974; 14:81–90.
2. Solomon GD, Kunkel RS, Frame J. Demographics of headache in elderly patients. *Headache* 1990;30:273–276.

3. Geriatric headache. In: Silberstein SD, Lipton RB, Goadsby PJ. *Headache in clinical practice.* Oxford: Isis, 1998:201–212.
4. Pascual J, Berciano J. Experience in the diagnosis of headaches that start in elderly people. *J Neurol Neurosurg Psychiatry* 1994;57:1255–1257.
5. Cull RE. Investigation of late-onset migraine. *Scott Med J* 1995;40:50–52.
6. Fisher CM. Late-life migraine accompaniments as a cause of unexplained transient ischemic attacks. *Can J Neurol Sci* 1980; 7:9–17.
7. Fisher CM. Late-life migraine accompaniments: further experience. *Stroke* 1986;17:1033–1042.
8. Meyer JS, Terayama Y, Konno S, et al. Late-life migrainous accompaniments. In: Gilman S, Goldstein GW, Waxman SG, eds. *Neurobase.* San Diego: Arbor, 2000.
9. Raskin NH. The hypnic headache syndrome. *Headache* 1988; 28:534–536.
10. Dodick DW, Mosek A, Campbell JK. The hypnic ("alarm clock") headache syndrome. *Cephalalgia* 1998;18:152–156.
11. Ivanez V, Soler R, Barreiro P. Hypnic headache syndrome: a case with good response to indomethacin. *Cephalalgia* 1998;18: 225–226.
12. Gould JD, Silberstein SD. Unilateral hypnic headache: a case study. *Neurology* 1997;49:1749–1750.
13. Myklebust G, Gran JT. A prospective study of 287 patients with polymyalgia rheumatica and temporal arteritis: clinical and laboratory manifestations at onset of disease and at the time of diagnosis. *Br J Rheumatol* 1996;35:1161–1168.
14. Jonasson F, Cullen JF, Elton RA. Temporal arteritis: a 14-year epidemiological, clinical and prognostic study. *Scot Med J* 1979; 24:111–117.
15. Solomon S, Cappa KG. The headache of temporal arteritis. *J Am Geriatr Soc* 1987;35:163–165.
16. Jundt JW, Mock D. Temporal arteritis with normal erythrocyte sedimentation rates presenting as occipital neuralgia. *Arthritis Rheum* 1991;34:217–219.
17. Caselli RJ, Hunder GG, Whisnant JP. Neurologic disease in biopsy-proven giant cell (temporal) arteritis. *Neurology* 1988; 38:352–358.
18. Mehler MR, Rabinowich L. The clinical neuro-ophthalmologic spectrum of temporal arteritis. *Am J Med* 1988;85:839–844.
19. Hunder GG, Bloch DA, Beat AM, et al. The American College of Rheumatology 1990 criteria for the classification of giant cell arteritis. *Arthritis Rheum* 1990;33:1122–1128.
19a. Lee AG, Brazis PW. Temporal arteritis: a clinical approach. *J Am Geriatr Soc* 1999;47:1364–1370.
20. Schmidt WA, Kraft HE, Voker L, et al. Color duplex ultrasonography in the diagnosis of temporal arteritis. *N Engl J Med* 1997;337:1336–1342.
21. Miller A, Green M, Robinson D. Simple rule for calculating normal erythrocyte sedimentation rate. *BMJ* 1983;286:266.
22. Hayreh SS, Podhajsky PA, Raman R, et al. Giant cell arteritis: validity and reliability of various diagnostic criteria. *Am J Ophthalmol* 1997;123:285–296.

22a. Duhant P, Pinede I, Bornet H, at al. Biopsy proven and biopsy negative temporal arteritis: differences in clinical spectrum at the onset of the disease. *Ann Rheum Dis* 1999;58:335–341.

23. Nesher G, Rubinow A, Sonnenblick M. Efficacy and adverse effects of different corticosteroid dose regimens in temporal arteritis: a retrospective study. *Clin Exp Rheumatol* 1997;15: 303–306.

24. Machkhas H, Harati Y. Side effects of immunosuppressant therapies used in neurology. *Neurol Clin* 1998;16:171–188.

25. Kost RG, Straus SE. Postherpetic neuralgia-pathogenesis, treatment, and prevention. *N Engl J Med* 1996;335:32–42.

26. Cluff RS, Rowbotham MC. Pain caused by herpes zoster infection. *Neurol Clin* 1998;16:813–832.

27. Dworkin RH, Boon RJ, Griffin DR, et al. Postherpetic neuralgia: impact of famciclovir, age, rash severity, and acute pain in herpes zoster patients. *J Infect Dis* 1998;178[Suppl 1]:S76–S80.

28. Rowbotham M, Harden N, Stacey B, et al. Gabapentin for the treatment of postherpetic neuralgia: a randomized controlled trial. *JAMA* 1998;280:1837–1842.

29. Watson CP, Babul N. Efficacy of oxycodone in neuropathic pain: a randomized trial in postherpetic neuralgia. *Neurology* 1998; 50:1837–1841.

Short-Lasting Head Pains

Ninan T. Mathew

A number of headache conditions are fairly rapid in their onset but short-lived. A great majority of them are variants of cluster headache and cranial neuralgias. Others include cough headache, headache related to sexual activity, and thunderclap headache, related to warning leaks of intracranial aneurysms, which are dealt with in Chapters 5 and 13. Variants of cluster headache are listed in Table 10-1. Features of short-lasting headache are described in Table 10-2.

PAROXYSMAL HEMICRANIAS

The paroxysmal hemicranias (PH) are a group of rare, benign headache disorders that clinically resemble cluster headache but fail to remit with standard anticluster therapy. Chronic paroxysmal hemicranias (CPH),[1,2] with an unremitting course, was the first entity described in this group; later, an episodic variety (with remissions) was reported, and the term *episodic paroxysmal hemicrania* (EPH) was given.[3] CPH can evolve from EPH.

Unlike cluster headache (CH), CPH demonstrates a female preponderance. To date, 68 women and 32 men with the disorder have been reported—a female-to-male ratio of about 2:1. The paroxysmal hemicranias typically begin during adulthood, with a mean age of onset of approximately 33 years (range, 6 to 81 years).

Table 10-1. Cluster headache variants

A. Those that differ in frequency, duration, location, or treatment response
   Paroxysmal hemicranias
      Episodic (EPH)
      Chronic (CPH)
   Hemicrania continua
   Short-lasting unilateral, neuralgiform headache with conjunctival injection and tearing (SUNCT)
   Hypnic headache
   Extratrigeminal cluster headache*
B. Those with mixed features of cluster headache and another primary headache disorder
   Cluster-migraine syndrome
   Cluster-tic syndrome
   Icepick headache (idiopathic stabbing headache)
C. Those with an underlying organic pathologic process
   Symptomatic cluster headache

*See Sanin LC, Mathew NT. Extratrigeminal cluster headache. *Headache* 1993;33:369–371

Table 10-2. Differential diagnosis of short-lasting headache

Feature	Cluster headache	Chronic paroxysmal hemicrania	Episodic paroxysmal hemicrania	SUNCT	Idiopathic stabbing headache	Trigeminal neuralgia
Gender (M:F)	9:1	1:3	1:1	8:1	F>M	F>M
Pain Type	Boring	Throbbing/boring	Throbbing	Stabbing	Stabbing	Stabbing
Severity	Very severe	Very severe	Very severe	More severe	Severe	Very severe
Location	Orbital Temporal	Orbital Temporal	Orbital Temporal	Orbital Temporal	Any part	V2/V3
Attack duration	15–180 min	2–45 min	1–30 min	5–250 s	<1 s	<1 s
Attack frequency	1–8/day	1–40/day	3–30/day	1/day to 30h	Few to many/day	Few to many/day
Autonomic features	+	+	+	+	–	–
Alcohol PPT	+	+	+	+	–	–
Indomethacin	±	+	+	–	+	–

From Silberstein SD, Lipton RB, Goadsby PJ. *Headache in clinical practice.* Oxford: Isis, Medical Media, 1998:132, with permission.

Abbreviations: F = female; M = male; V1 = ophthalmic; V2 = maxiliary; V3 = mandibular divisions of the trigeminal innervation; + = precipitates headaches; ± = effect not consistent; – = no effect on headache.

A family history of CPH or EPH was not at all common. In 21% of reported cases, there was a documented family history of migraine. Only one patient reported a positive family history for CH.[4]

The pain is strictly unilateral and without side-shift in the vast majority of patients. The maximum pain is experienced in the ocular, temporal, maxillary, and frontal regions: nuchal, occipital, and retroorbital pain has less often been described. The pain may occasionally radiate into the ipsilateral shoulder and arm. The pain is described as a throbbing, boring, pulsatile, or stabbing sensation that ranges in severity from moderate to excruciating. In 28 previous reports, mild discomfort was noted interictally at the usual site of pain.[4] During headaches, sufferers usually prefer to sit quietly or lie in bed in the fetal position; rarely, however, some sufferers assume the pacing activity usually seen in CH.

In CPH, attacks recur from 1 to 40 times daily. However, there is a marked variability in attack frequency; the frequency of mild attacks ranges from 2 to 14 daily, and severe attacks recur 6 to 40 times daily. Most patients report 15 or more attacks per day. Headaches usually last between 2 and 25 minutes each (range, 2 to 120 minutes).

In EPH, the daily attack frequency ranges from 2 to 30, with attacks lasting 3 to 30 minutes each. The headache phase lasts from 2 weeks to 4.5 months, whereas remission periods range from 1 to 36 months.

Both EPH and CPH are characterized by excruciatingly severe throbbing or piercing headaches localized in the temple and orbital regions and accompanied by the ipsilateral autonomic features typical of CH. Both EPH and CPH have clinically similar features; multiple short-duration daily headaches, nocturnal attacks, precipitation by alcoholic beverages, and absolute response to treatment with indomethacin.

EPH differs from CPH by temporal profile. EPH is characterized by discrete attack and remission phases, whereas CPH occurs chronically without remissions. EPH is therefore frequently mistaken for episodic CH (ECH), as both EPH and ECH occur as active periods consisting of brief excruciating headaches recurring numerous times daily with associated ipsilateral autonomic disturbances, separated by pain-free remissions. Both EPH and CPH may occur nocturnally, and both may be triggered by alcohol. EPH is differentiated from ECH by the increased frequency and shorter duration of individual headaches, and by its absolute response to indomethacin therapy. CPH must be differentiated from chronic CH.

SHORT-LASTING UNILATERAL NEURALGIFORM PAIN WITH CONJUNCTIVAL INJECTION AND TEARING

Short-lasting unilateral neuralgiform pain with conjunctival injection and tearing (SUNCT) is a curious benign, short-lasting headache with autonomic features.[5] SUNCT is distinguished from the paroxysmal hemicranias and CH by the ultrashort attack duration (average 61 seconds) and high frequency of attacks (average 28/day).

Most attacks occurred during the day, with a bimodal distribution (i.e., morning and afternoon/evening peaks).[6] Nocturnal attacks are rare. Pain is confined to the first division. A status-like pattern has been reported in SUNCT syndrome.[7] SUNCT syndrome is characterized by less severe pain but marked autonomic activation during attacks. SUNCT syndrome usually does not respond to indomethacin and in general is resistant to therapy. SUNCT syndrome "transformed" from trigeminal neuralgia has been reported.[8]

HEMICRANIA CONTINUA

Hemicrania continua (HC), also known as alarm clock headache, is another rare unilateral continuous disorder that responds to indomethacin.[9] Remitting and unremitting forms have been described.[10]

HC remains a rare disorder, with less than 50 reported cases found in the literature. Recent clinical experience suggests that the disorder may be more common than previously recognized. HC is one of the causes of refractory, unilateral, chronic daily headache. The disorder demonstrates a marked female preponderance, with a female-to-male ratio of 1.9:1. The age of onset of the disorder ranges from 11 to 58 years (mean, 34 years). Responsiveness to indomethacin is diagnostic.

HYPNIC HEADACHE

The hypnic headache syndrome is a rare, benign headache disorder (also see Chapter 9). Although it is not truly a CH variant, the short-lived attacks of nocturnal headache resemble CH. This syndrome is characterized by recurrent attacks of a generalized or unilateral nocturnal headache that awakens the patient from sleep at a consistent time each night.[10,11] The diffuse and pulsatile pain is of moderate intensity. The pain lasts from 15 minutes to 6 hours and is unassociated with any autonomic features. Attacks may occur from one to three times nightly. These headaches are distinguished from CH by a number of important features. They begin after age 40 years, whereas CH tends to begin between ages 20 and 40 years. With hypnic headaches, the pain is usually generalized, pulsating, or steady. In CH, the pain is usually unilateral and boring. Unilateral hypnic headache has been reported.[12,13] In hypnic headache, the pain is of moderate severity. In CH, pain is excruciating. Hypnic headache is notable for the absence of autonomic features; cluster variants invariably have autonomic features. The recognition of this uncommon disorder is particularly important because of its unique response to lithium treatment at bedtime. A case of hypnic headache that responded well to indomethacin was reported.[14] Caffeine tablets or beverages were helpful in four patients.[15]

CLUSTER-MIGRAINE AND CLUSTER-TIC SYNDROMES

Occasionally, elements of both CH and another primary headache disorder appear together in the same patient. Recognition of these syndromes is important because therapeutic options are different from those available for treating each disorder separately.

Cluster-Migraine Syndrome

This syndrome is diagnosed when elements of migraine occur simultaneously in patients suffering with CH. Solomon et al.[16]

instituted an arbitrary diagnostic scheme to establish the diagnosis of cluster-migraine headache syndrome. They proposed that symptoms of one headache were prominent, but if four or five features of the other headache were also present, the designation of cluster-migraine headache syndrome was appropriate. For example, patients suffering from CH who also experienced nausea, vomiting, photophobia or phonophobia, or patients with migraine who experienced ipsilateral conjunctival injection, tearing, ptosis, and rhinorrhea would be candidates for this diagnosis. The criteria employed by these authors were not precise, and the number of associated features was arbitrarily selected. Similarly, if a patient met the International Headache Society (IHS) criteria for migraine but attacks occurred daily for weeks or months at a time in conjunction with ipsilateral autonomic features, the designation of cluster-migraine might also be appropriate.

The recognition of this mixed syndrome is important because of unique treatment strategies. Patients suffering from cluster-migraine syndrome have responded to oxygen to abort acute attacks of headache, and lithium is useful as a preventive agent. This combination of medications would not be expected to be helpful in patients suffering from typical migraine. Alternatively, beta-blockers may occasionally help in this syndrome, whereas patients suffering from CH do not typically remit with beta-blocker therapy.

Cluster-Tic Syndrome

The designation *cluster-tic syndrome* is used to describe patients who suffer from CH and trigeminal neuralgia.[17] This uncommon disorder is characterized by volleys of severe lancinating pains characteristic of trigeminal neuralgia but superimposed on other features common in CH sufferers. These ticlike pains are commonly triggered by light cutaneous or mucous membrane stimulation, as in typical tic douloureux. Concurrently, the patient suffers from the typical features of CH. Often the two pain syndromes may occur independently of each other for months to years prior to their actual melding together.

This disorder may be difficult to treat and may require more than one therapeutic modality. Recent reports have documented that carbamazepine is useful for treating ticlike pains, whereas standard CH therapy may successfully treat that portion of the syndrome. Solomon et al.[16] described four patients with the syndrome who underwent microvascular decompression of the trigeminal nerve. During the surgical exploration, compression of the root entry zone of the trigeminal nerve root by a blood vessel was found in all cases. In two of three cases in which there was facial nerve exploration, an arterial loop was found at the root entry zone of the facial nerve. Postoperatively, all patients experienced relief of the ticlike pains for up to 9 years. The features of CH, however, were unchanged by the surgery.

ICEPICK HEADACHE

Robert Schwartz and Raskin characterized the epidemiologic features of icepick headache (idiopathic stabbing headache) among 100 randomly selected control subjects and among 100 migraineurs.[18] Three of the control subjects reported sharp, jabbing pain about the head, and in all three it occurred at least once a year. One person noted that the jabs occurred only after strenuous running for several miles. Out of the 100 migraineurs, 42 had experienced sharp, jabbing pain, and more than half experienced it more often than monthly. Most described the pain as icepicklike; others described their repetitive pain as needle-, nail-, or pinpricklike. The majority noted single isolated jabs of pain, whereas 12 experienced volleys of jabs.

Icepick pains usually occurred focally at the temple or orbit but occasionally occurred at the occipital and parietal areas. Nearly half of the patients noted jabbing pain at the mirror locus in the opposite hemicranium.

Seven of the patients reported precipitants for their pain. Sudden postural change was reported by five; physical exertion, by three; dark/light transition and head motion during migraine attacks, by one each. Unprovoked pain was the most common presenting mode of sharp pain in these seven patients, as it was in the entire group.

Twenty-nine of the 42 patients with sharp pain experienced it concurrent with migrainous attacks as well as other times. Fourteen of the 29 patients noted it regularly with each headache attack. For seven patients, icepicklike pain heralded the onset of a migrainous episode. In a few patients, scintillating scotomas, acro- or facial paresthesia, or syncope had occurred on several occasions in association with jabbing pain.

Lansche described a benign jabbing unilateral eye pain that he termed *ophthalmodynia periodica*.[19] He also noted that more than 60% of such patients were migraine sufferers. Ekbom described what appears to be an identical phenomenon in patients with cluster headaches.[20] Eleven of 33 patients noted that during headache attacks paroxysms of "stabbing or pricking" pain sensations occurred, superimposed on the usual pain, lasting for a few seconds and usually indicating that the cluster attack was terminating. These sharp pains occurred around the eye, forehead, or upper jaw, homolateral to the pain of the cluster attack. The only other disorder in which this variety of pain is frequently encountered is giant cell arteritis. The dominant symptom of this disorder, headache, is invariably described as intense and boring, with superimposed icepicklike, lancinating pains.[21] Whereas the pain in giant cell arteritis is almost certainly generated by the arterial disease per se, it is probably mediated within the central nervous system in cluster headache, so that clear, common denominator is lacking.

Patients reporting icepick head pains are sometimes erroneously believed to have a neuralgic disorder. The tempo of icepick pains is, when occurring repetitively, at the rate of one per second; trigeminal neuralgia appears in machine gun–like volleys, with each jolt of pain occurring in a fraction of a second. Icepick pain status has been reported.[22]

SYMPTOMATIC CLUSTER HEADACHES

Symptomatic cluster headaches[23] are CH-like attacks that occur as a result of underlying intracranial lesion. Parasellar meningioma, adenoma of the pituitary, calcified lesion in the regional third ventricle, anterior carotid artery aneurysm, epidermoid tumor of the clivus expanding into the suprasellar cistern, vertebral artery aneurysms, nasopharyngeal carcinoma, ipsilateral large hemispheric arteriovenous malformation, and upper cervical meningiomas have been reported to produce symptomatic CH, which should be suspected when clinical features are atypical. Atypical features include (a) absence of typical periodicity, which is seen in episodic CH (in other words, the headaches behave more like chronic CH); (b) a certain degree of background headache that does not subside between attacks; (c) inadequate or unsatisfactory response to treatments that are effective in idiopathic CH, such as oxygen inhalation or ergotamine; and (d) presence of neurologic signs other than miosis and ptosis.

A careful neurologic examination is essential. Diminished corneal reflex and other signs of involvement of the fifth nerve and signs of involvement of other cranial nerves must be looked for. Most cases of symptomatic CH reported have had some parasellar abnormality, especially around the distal portions of the carotid artery in the cavernous sinus area, where nociceptive fibers of the trigeminal nerve and sympathetic and parasympathetic nerves come together.

Clusterlike headaches have been reported following head and facial trauma involving the trigeminal nerve territory.[24,25]

HEAD AND FACIAL NEURALGIAS

Definition and Classification

Neuralgia. A paroxysmal pain that extends along the course of a nerve.

Trigeminal neuralgia. A paroxysmal pain occurring repetitively, strictly confined to one or more branches of the trigeminal nerve.

Idiopathic trigeminal neuralgia. Structural causes have been excluded by imaging studies. (Note: current techniques rarely reveal a microvascular compression of the fifth nerve.)

Symptomatic trigeminal neuralgia. Pain is indistinguishable from the idiopathic pain. Imaging studies reveal a structural cause.

The International Headache Society (IHS) Classification[26] is as follows:

i. Idiopathic trigeminal neuralgia
ii. Symptomatic trigeminal neuralgia

The previously used term for trigeminal neuralgia was *tic douloureux* ("painful spasm").

Description

Trigeminal neuralgia is a painful unilateral affliction of the face, characterized by brief electric shock–like (lancinating) pains limited to the distribution of one or more divisions of the trigeminal nerve. Pain is commonly evoked by trivial stimuli—including washing, shaving, smoking, talking, and brushing the teeth—but may occur spontaneously. The pain is abrupt in onset and termination, and may remit for varying periods. A phase of "pretrigeminal neuralgia" is characterized by brief, milder episodes of pain often suspected of arising from the teeth.

Diagnostic Criteria

The following are diagnostic criteria:[26]

A. Paroxysmal attacks of facial pain lasting a few seconds to less than 2 minutes
B. Pain with at least four of the following criteria:
    1. Pain confined to one or more divisions of the nerve
    2. Pain that is sudden, intense, sharp, superficial, stabbing, or burning in quality
    3. Pain with severe intensity
    4. Pain that is precipitated by stimulation of trigger areas
    5. Symptomatic patient between spasms
C. No neurologic deficit
D. Attacks that are stereotyped in the individual
E. Other causes of facial pain are excluded

Epidemiology

Trigeminal neuralgia is more common in women (approximately 2:1) and begins after 40 years of age in 90% of cases.[27] It has been described in childhood, however. The annual incidence rate is about 4 per 100,000 of the population. A familial occurrence has been reported.

Pathogenesis

Degenerative changes in the gasserian ganglion have been described, but increasingly posterior fossa exploration has revealed focal demyelination of the main sensory root by compression with a loop of artery or vein.[28] This observation was originally made by Dandy in 1934 but was popularized and confirmed by Jannetta more recently. The microvascular compression produces demyelination, which in turn permits ephaptic impulse transmission.[28] (Ephapse is a point of lateral contact between nerve fibers across which impulses are conducted directly from one nerve fiber to another.)

Symptomatic causes, other than the vascular compression, include neuromas of the fifth nerve, meningiomas, metastases, malignant infiltration of the nerve and ganglion, and lesions within the root entry zone in the pons.

Diagnosis

The temporal profile, trigger mechanisms, and the strictly trigeminal distribution of the pain rapidly lead to the diagnosis. Imaging studies are used to exclude other conditions that may mimic the trigeminal pain. Computer-assisted tomography is especially useful for detecting bony destructive lesions of the skull base, such as nasopharyngeal carcinoma. The intracranial portions of the nerve and the gasserian ganglion are best seen by MRI. Angiography and MR angiography rarely demonstrate the vessel compressing the nerve (often the anterior superior cerebellar artery, persistent trigeminal artery, or simply an aberrant vessel, either arterial or venous).

Clinical Features

The intense pain is usually described as an "electric shock" or "lightninglike." The sufferer is protective of the face and will back away from the examiner and will be reluctant to touch the trigger region (if any) to even demonstrate the area. The pain rarely occurs during sleep.

After a series of attacks, there may be a period of refractoriness during which the subject can eat without triggering the pain.[29]

Distribution

Most frequently felt in a combination of V2 and V3, this neuralgia is rarely confined to V1.[29] When attacks are confined to the ophthalmic branch, one should suspect a symptomatic neuralgia.

Trigger zones are present in 90% of subjects. The trigger area is not always in the painful region.

When tic douloureux occurs bilaterally, not necessarily on both sides at the same time, a lesion in the pons is likely and is usually due to multiple sclerosis.

Course

Once it has developed, tic tends to persist but with an exacerbating and remitting course over many years. After some weeks or months of episodic pain, the disorder may remit for weeks, months, or years. Recurrence or initial onset after a dental procedure is a common history.

Treatment

Medical Management

Anticonvulsants, clonazepam, baclofen, tocainide, and pimozide are among the agents used for control of tic pain. The most effective agent is clearly carbamazepine.[29]

Carbamazepine (Tegretol) results in pain relief in 70% of patients but is unfortunately not always well tolerated in the elderly. At all ages, it should be started slowly—50 to 100 mg BID or TID with progressive upward titration of the dose. Relief may occur within 48 hours. The average effective dose range is 600 to 1,200 mg/day.

Drowsiness, dizziness, and ataxia occur in almost half of all subjects initially but are usually transient.

The complication of carbamazepine most feared is bone marrow suppression; therefore prior to starting treatment, a full blood count is obtained and the white cell count should be monitored as advised by the manufacturers. Liver and renal function should also be checked. Allergic reactions, such as a rash, are not uncommon. Inappropriate antidiuretic hormone secretion is a rare complication.

If pain control is complete, the medication can be discontinued after several months to see if a remission has developed. Long-term use of carbamazepine in this condition is appropriate if needed and if tolerated.

Phenytoin (Dilantin) is given in full anticonvulsant doses after an oral loading dose. It is far less effective than carbamazepine in the control of pain. The two agents can be combined.

Baclofen (Lioresal), either alone or in combination with an anticonvulsant, is an effective treatment. Initiated with 5 to 10 mg TID, the dose can be significantly higher as tolerated. Drowsiness, dryness of the mouth, and dizziness are not uncommon but may subside with time. Baclofen should be withdrawn slowly over 10 to 14 days if it has been used for more than a few days. Seizures and hallucinations can occur if withdrawal is abrupt.

Sodium valproate (Depakote) is given in antiseizure doses and has proven somewhat effective in the control of trigeminal neuralgia. It is not well tolerated by the elderly.

Clonazepam (Klonopin) in doses of 3 to 8 mg/day may be helpful but is excessively sedating.

Pimozide (Orap), a neuroleptic, is also effective for tic but is prone to produce unacceptable side effects, including tremor, sedation, and an extrapyramidal syndrome.

Surgical Treatment[29,30]

If medical management is ineffective, not tolerated, or refused, a series of procedures on the trigeminal pathway can be considered.

Factors that lead to a particular procedure include the age of the patient, the patient's general condition, personal preferences, and the availability of the procedures.

MICROVASCULAR COMPRESSION. All the procedures, with one exception, result in some sensory loss of the face for a variable period. The one exception is the *microvascular decompression* of the trigeminal root, known popularly as the Jannetta procedure. This posterior fossa exploration procedure is usually considered for those under 60 to 65 years of age, as it can result in permanent pain relief, without sensory loss, but is a major craniotomy (actually craniectomy) with some risk of complications, such as air embolism, damage to adjacent cranial nerves, and other structures. Even at exploration, vascular compression may not be located. When vascular decompression is achieved, there is a greater than 80% likelihood of long-term relief.

For older patients and those who do not wish to consider a posterior fossa exploration, there is a logical sequence in the choice of procedures.

PERIPHERAL BRANCH ALCOHOL INJECTION. Each of the three branches is suitable for blocking with alcohol. The supraorbital, the infraorbital, and the inferior alveolar (mandibular) nerves can be blocked with alcohol. Numbness lasts 3 to 9 months, during which period the pain may not be triggered or may occur spontaneously. As the sensory loss subsides, pain is likely to recur. The procedure can be repeated several times, but if the sensory loss is not considered unpleasant, a more permanent procedure may be used when pain returns. Alcohol can also be used to block the trigeminal nerve at the base of the skull in the region of the foramen ovale.

RADIOFREQUENCY THERMOCOAGULATION OF THE GASSERIAN GANGLION (GANGLIOLYSIS). Under a light anesthetic or narcosis, a needle can be placed percutaneously through the foramen ovale and a controlled thermal lesion can be achieved in the ganglion. Great skill is needed to place the lesion to achieve sensory loss in the appropriate portion of the face. Pain relief results in 93% to 100% of subjects in whom an adequate lesion is produced. The 2-year recurrence rate is about 10% to 15%. The procedure can be repeated as needed. Meningitis and damage to adjacent cranial nerves and structures can occur but are rare in the hands of an experienced neurosurgeon.

RETROGASSERIAN GLYCEROL INJECTION. Introduced by Hakanson, retrogasserian glycerol injection, a percutaneous injection into Meckel's cave, can be done without general anesthesia. Pain relief may be delayed for several days. Hakanson reported 86% of 75 patients were pain-free at 17 months. Painful dysesthesias are reported to be less common after this procedure than after a radiofrequency procedure or root section.

OTHER PROCEDURES. Balloon compression (percutaneously) of the gasserian ganglion, selective or total sensory root section, and brain stem tractotomy are rarely performed procedures.

RISKS OF ANY DENERVATING PROCEDURE ON THE TRIGEMINAL NERVES. Painful dysesthesias are common (but only rarely so severe as to justify the term *anesthesia dolorosa)*; corneal anesthesia leading to keratitis; difficulty chewing due to loss of proprioception, and trigeminal motor weakness.

GLOSSOPHARYNGEAL NEURALGIA

Description

Glossopharyngeal neuralgia is a severe transient stabbing pain experienced in the ear, at the base of the tongue, in the tonsillar fossa, or beneath the angle of the jaw. The pain is therefore felt in the distribution of the auricular and pharyngeal branches of the vagus nerve as well as that of the glossopharyngeal nerve. It is commonly provoked by swallowing, talking, and coughing, and may remit and relapse in the fashion of the trigeminal neuralgia.

Diagnostic Criteria

A. Paroxysmal attacks of facial pain that last a few seconds to less than 2 minutes
B. Pain that has at least four of the following characteristics:
   1. Unilateral location
   2. Distribution within the posterior part of the tongue, in the tonsillar fossa, in the pharynx, beneath the angle of the lower jaw, or in the ear
   3. Sudden, sharp, stabbing, or burning pain
   4. Pain intensity severe
   5. Precipitation from trigger areas or by swallowing, chewing, talking, coughing, or yawning
C. No neurologic deficit
D. Attacks that are stereotyped in the individual patient
E. Other causes of pain ruled out by history, physical, and special investigations
F. Pharmacotherapy is the same as that described for trigeminal neuralgia.

OCCIPITAL NEURALGIA

Description

Occipital neuralgia is a paroxysmal jabbing pain in the distribution of the greater or lesser occipital nerves, accompanied by diminished sensation or dysasthesias in the affected area. It is commonly associated with tenderness over the nerve concerned.

Diagnostic Criteria

A. Pain is felt in the distribution of greater or lesser occipital nerves.
B. Pain is stabbing in quality, although aching may persist between paroxysms.
C. The affected nerve is tender to palpation.
D. The condition is eased temporarily by local anaesthetic block of the appropriate nerve.

Comment

Occipital neuralgia must be distinguished from the occipital referral of pain from the atlantoaxial or upper zygapophyseal joints or from tender trigger points in neck muscles or their insertion. Occipital neuralgia and treatment are further discussed in Chapter 6.

REFERENCES

 1. Sjaastad O, Dale I. Evidence for a new (?) treatable headache entity. *Headache* 1974;14:105–108.
 2. Sjaastad O, Dale I. A new (?) clinical headache entity "chronic paroxysmal hemicrania" 2. *Acta Neurol Scand* 1976;54:140–159.
 3. Kudro WL, Esperanz AP, Vijaya NN. Episodic paroxysmal hemicrania? *Cephalalgia* 1987;7:197–201.
 4. Antonac IF, Sjaasta DO. Chronic paroxysmal hemicrania (CPH): a review of the clinical manifestations. *Headache* 1989;29:648–656.
 5. Sjaasta DO, Saunt EC, Salvese NR, et al. Short-lasting, unilateral neuralgiform headache attacks with conjunctival injection, tearing, sweating, and rhinorrhea. *Cephalalgia* 1989;9:147–156.
 6. Pareja JA, Shen JM, Kruszewski P, et al. SUNCT syndrome: duration, frequency, and temporal distribution of attacks. *Headache* 1996;36:161–165.
 7. Pareja JS, Caballero V, Sjaastad O. SUNCT syndrome: status-like pattern. *Headache* 1996;36:622–624.
 8. Sjaastad O, Spierings ELH. "Hemicrania Continua": another headache absolutely responsive to indomethacin. *Cephalalgia* 1984;4:65–70.
 9. Newman LC, Lipton RB, Solomon S. Hemicrania continua: ten new cases and a review of the literature. *Neurology* 1994;44: 2111–2114.
10. Raskin NH. The hypnic headache syndrome. *Headache* 1988; 28:534–536.
11. Newman LC, Lipton RB, Solomon S. The hypnic headache syndrome: a benign headache disorder of the elderly. *Neurology* 1990;40:1904–1905.
12. Morales-Asin F, Mauri JA, Iniguez C, et al. The hypnic headache syndrome: report of three new cases. *Cephalalgia* 1998;18: 157–158.

13. Gould JD, Silberstein SD. Unilateral hypnic headache: a case study. *Neurology* 1997;49:1749–1751.
14. Ivanez V, Soler R, Barreiro P. Hypnic headache syndrome: a case with good response to indomethacin. *Cephalalgia* 1998;18: 225–226.
15. Dodick DW, Mosek AC, Campbell JK. The hypnic ("alarm clock") headache syndrome. *Cephalalgia* 1998;18:152–156.
16. Solomon S, Karfunkel P, Guglielmo KM. Migraine-cluster headache syndrome. *Headache* 1995;25:236–239.
17. Solomon S, Apfelbaum R, Guglielmo KM. The cluster-tic syndrome and its surgical treatment. *Cephalalgia* 1985;5:83–89.
18. Raskin NH, Schwartz RJ. Icepick-like pain. *Neurology* 1980;203.
19. Lansche RK. Ophthalmodynia periodica. *Headache* 1964;4:247.
20. Ekbom K. Some observations on pain in cluster headache. *Headache* 1975;14:219.
21. Russell RWR. Giant cell arteritis: a review of 35 cases. *Q J Med* 1959;28:471.
22. Martins IP, Parreira E, Costa I. Extratrigeminal ice-pick status. *Headache* 1995;35:107.
23. Mathew NT. Symptomatic cluster. *Neurology* 1993;43:1270.
24. Reik L. Cluster headache after head injury. *Headache* 1987;27: 509–511.
25. Mathew NT, Rueveni U. Cluster-like headache following head trauma. *Headache* 1988;28:297.
26. Headache Classification Committee of the International Headache Society. Classification and diagnostic criteria for headache disorders, cranial neuralgias and facial pain. *Cephalalgia* 1988; 8[Suppl 7]:10–17.
27. Terrence CF, Jensen TS. Trigeminal neuralgia and other facial neuralgias. In: Olesen J, Tfelt-Hansen P, Welch KMA, eds. *The headaches,* 2nd edition. Philadelphia: Lippincott Williams & Wilkins, 2000:929–938.
28. Fromm GH, Sessle BJ, eds. *Trigeminal neuralgia current concepts regarding pathogenesis and treatment.* Boston: Butterworth-Heinemann, 1991.
29. Campbell JK. Cranial and facial neuralgias. In: Bradley WG, Daroff RB, Fenichel GM, Marsden CE, eds. *Neurology in clinical practice.* Boston: Butterworth-Heinemann, 1995:1683–1719.
30. From GH. Neuralgias of the face and the oral cavity. *Pain Digest* 1991;1:67–77.

Vascular Disorders and Headaches

Randolph W. Evans

Vascular disorders are commonly associated with headaches. Topics covered in this chapter are migraine and stroke, stroke, carotid endarterectomy, unruptured arteriovenous malformations and migraine, carotid and vertebral dissections, cerebral venous thrombosis, hypertension, carotidynia, and anginal headache. Vascular disorders reviewed in other chapters are subarachnoid hemorrhage (Chapter 5), subdural and epidural hematomas (Chapter 6), preeclampsia and eclampsia (Chapter 8), and temporal arteritis (Chapter 9).

MIGRAINE AND STROKE

Relationships

Between 1% and 17% of cerebral infarctions in young persons, especially females, have been attributed to migrainous infarction in various studies (also see Chapter 8). Migraineurs with aura have a greater stroke risk than those without aura. The strokes are often in the distribution of the posterior cerebral artery.[1] Welch et al. consider four relationships.[2]

1. Migraineurs can have a stroke due to another mechanism that occurs remotely in time from a typical attack of migraine.
2. A structural lesion (such as an arteriovenous malformation [AVM] or carotid dissection) unrelated to migraine can present with clinical features typical of migraine with neurologic aura. A nonstructural mimic is pseudomigraine with temporary neurologic symptoms and lymphocytic pleocytosis (PMP syndrome).[3] This condition usually affects those under 40 years of age who often have a history of migraine. Twenty-five percent report a viruslike illness up to 3 weeks prior to symptoms. Patients may have one to 12 episodes of changing variable neurologic deficits (including sensory and motor symptoms and dysphasia) associated with a throbbing, bilateral moderate to severe headache. Patients are asymptomatic between episodes and following the symptomatic period, which can last up to 49 days. The cerebrospinal fluid (CSF) typically reveals a CSF lymphocytic pleocytosis and elevated protein without evidence of oligoclonal bands. Studies for infectious causes are negative. Computed tomography (CT) and magnetic resonance imaging (MRI) scans of the brain are normal.
3. A migraine-induced stroke should meet the following criteria: the neurologic deficit must be identical to the migrainous symptoms of previous attacks; the stroke must occur during the course of a typical migraine attack; and all other causes of stroke must be excluded, although stroke risk factors may be present. Migrainous cerebral infarction is defined by the

International Headache Society (IHS) classification as one or more symptoms and signs of migrainous aura that are not fully reversible within 7 days and associated with neuroimaging confirmation of ischemic stroke. Possible causes of migraine-induced stroke are decreased regional cerebral blood flow and platelet dysfunction.

There are types of migraine that can mimic other disorders that cause cerebral ischemia. Examples include hemiplegic migraine, basilar migraine, and rare genetic disorders such as mitochondrial encephalomyopathy, lactic acidosis, and stroke-like episodes (MELAS) (Chapter 7) and cerebral autosomal dominant arteriopathy with subcortical infarcts and leukoencephalopathy (CADASIL). CADASIL[4] is a rare inherited arterial disease of the brain that has been mapped to chromosome 19. Clinical presentations include recurrent subcortical ischemic events, dementia (90% before death), migraine with aura (in 22% of cases), and depression.

4. Many migraine-related strokes cannot be categorized with certainty. Complex or multiple factors can interact with migraine and lead to stroke. Examples include medications (ergots, triptans, oral contraceptives, and beta-blocker use in basilar migraine); smoking; antiphospholipid antibody syndrome; stroke occurring when cerebral angiography is performed during a migraine episode; and late-life migrainous accompaniments (Chapter 9).

White-Matter Abnormalities

White-matter abnormalities (WMA) are foci of hyperintensity on both proton density and T2-weighted images in the deep and periventricular white matter due to either interstitial edema or perivascular demyelination. WMA are easily detected on MRI but are not seen on CT scan. WMA have been reported in 12% to 46% of migraineurs, compared with 2% to 14% of controls.[5] Although the cause of WMA in migraine is uncertain, various hypotheses have been advanced, including increased platelet aggregability with microemboli, abnormal cerebrovascular regulation, and repeated attacks of hypoperfusion during the aura. The presence of antiphospholipid antibodies might be a risk factor for WMAs in migraine, but the antibodies may not be an additional risk factor for stroke in migraineurs.[6]

Retinal Migraine

Retinal migraine[7] is a rare disorder defined by the following IHS criteria: fully reversible monocular scotoma or blindness lasting less than 60 minutes; headache preceding or following visual symptoms with a free interval of less than 60 minutes; and a normal ophthalmologic examination outside of an attack and embolism ruled out by appropriate investigations. (Because the retinal and ciliary circulations may be affected, the terms *ocular* or *anterior visual pathway migraine* have been proposed as more accurate.) The symptoms include unilateral quadrantic; altitudinal; or total gray-out, white-out, or blackout visual loss. Some patients report a concentric constriction of the monocular visual field proceeding from the periphery to the center, with spots and splatches of darkness that look like ink spots running together. There may be total loss of vision or a small piece of normal central vision remaining. Retinal migraine can also cause posterior ischemic optic neuropathy, mimicking retrobulbar optic neuritis. The retinal vessels appear to be in spasm during an attack. Permanent visual loss can occasionally occur with altitudinal field loss (especially nasal inferior loss), small blind spot extensions, and total visual loss.[8]

Persistent Positive Visual Phenomena

Persistent positive visual phenomena in migraine are visual disturbances such as dots or flashes in both visual fields that persist indefinitely without evidence of infarction.[9] Persistent migraine aura may respond to divalproex sodium.[10]

Management

Preventive treatment that may be beneficial for patients with prolonged migraine aura or migrainous infarction include antiplatelet agents (aspirin, ticlopidine, and clopidogrel) and verapamil. Beta-blockers should be avoided because they may worsen intracranial vasoconstriction.[11] Ergots and triptans should not be used for treatment of headache associated with prolonged migraine aura because of the potential for increased vasoconstriction.

STROKE

Epidemiology

Headaches due to stroke may be due to electrochemical or mechanical stimulation of the trigeminovascular afferent system. Headaches commonly accompany stroke.[12] In a prospective study of 163 patients with stroke, headache occurred in 29% with bland infarcts, 57% with parenchymal hemorrhage, 36% with transient ischemic attacks, and 17% with lacunar infarcts.[13] Patients with a history of prior recurrent throbbing headaches and women were more likely to have headaches associated with stroke. The headache began prior to the event in 60% and at its onset in 25%. The quality, onset, and duration of the headaches varied widely. The headaches are equally likely to be abrupt or gradual in onset.

Clinical Manifestations

Various studies report a usually unilateral and focal headache of mild to moderate severity, although up to 46% of patients may have an incapacitating headache. The headache may be throbbing or nonthrobbing and may rarely be stabbing. The headache is more often ipsilateral than contralateral to the side of the cerebral ischemia. Headache is more common in ischemia of the posterior than the anterior circulation and in cortical than subcortical events. The duration of the headache is longest in cardioembolic infarcts and thrombotic infarcts, of medium duration in lacunar infarction, and shortest in transient ischemic attacks.[14] Associated symptoms in one study include nausea in 44%, vomiting in 23%, and light and noise sensitivity in 25%.[15] Bending, straining, and jarring the head usually increase the intensity. A sentinel or warning headache has been reported in 10% to 43% of patients before ischemic strokes, especially before cardioembolic stroke. The headache is usually unilateral and focal and lasts more than 24 hours.[16] The occurrence may be hours to days before the stroke. Sentinel and other headaches due to subarachnoid hemorrhage (SAH) are reviewed in Chapter 5.

CAROTID ENDARTERECTOMY

A benign ipsilateral frontotemporal intense headache may follow endarterectomy with a latency of 36 to 72 hours. The headache may recur intermittently for up to 6 months. Headache can also develop postoperatively due to intracerebral hemorrhage, which is a complication of 0.75% of operations.[17] The hemorrhage occurs at a median of 3 days after surgery with a range of 0 to 18 days.

UNRUPTURED AVM AND MIGRAINE

The prevalence of AVMs is about 0.5% in postmortem studies. In contrast to saccular aneurysms, up to 50% present with symptoms or signs other than hemorrhage. Migrainelike headaches with and without visual symptoms can be associated with arteriovenous malformations, especially those in the occipital lobe, which is the predominant location of about 20% of parenchymal AVMs.[18] Although headaches always occurring on the same side (side-locked) are present in 95% of those with AVMs, 17% of those with migraine without aura and 15% of patients with migraine with aura have side-locked headaches.[19] Typical migraine due to an AVM is the exception, as there are usually distinguishing features. Bruyn reported the following features in patients with migrainelike symptoms and AVM: unusual associated signs (papilledema, field cut, bruit), 65%; short duration of headache attacks, 20%; brief scintillating scotoma, 10%, absent family history, 15%; atypical sequence of aura, headache, and vomiting, 10%; and seizures, 25%.[20]

CAROTID AND VERTEBRAL ARTERY DISSECTIONS[21-23]

Epidemiology

Two and a half percent of all patients with a first stroke have an internal carotid artery (ICA) dissection, with 90% involving the cervical carotid and 10% the intracranial. The frequency of vertebral artery (VA) dissections is about one-third that of carotid. Twenty percent of spontaneous ICA dissections and almost half of VA dissections are bilateral. Combined ICA and VA dissections occasionally occur. Rarely, headache can be the initial manifestation of aortic dissection type A extending into the cervical arteries.

Dissections occur due to penetration of circulating blood through an intimal tear into the subintimal, medial, and, less commonly, adventitial layers of the vascular wall that extends for varying distances along the vessel. Risk and predisposing factors for spontaneous dissections include migraine, hypertension, oral contraceptives, fibromuscular dysplasia (found in about 15% of cases), temporal arteritis, polyarteritis nodosa, meningovascular syphilis, Ehlers-Danlos syndrome, Marfan syndrome, cystic medial necrosis, and moyamoya disease. Traumatic dissections due to penetrating or nonpenetrating injuries have even been associated with minor or trivial trauma, including coughing, blowing the nose, turning the head, sleeping in the wrong position, sports activities, chiropractic manipulation, yoga exercises, sexual activity, and whiplash injuries. More than 70% of the patients are younger than 50 years of age, with a mean age of approximately 45. Dissections occur slightly more often in women.

Clinical Manifestations

Head, face, orbital, or neck pain, usually ipsilateral to the site of the dissection, is the initial manifestation in about 80% of patients with extracranial ICA dissection. Focal cerebral ischemic symptoms occur in about 60% of patients and may follow the headache by up to 4 weeks, or may precede it. The presence of deficits is as follows: neurologically normal, 50%; mild deficits only, 21%; moderate to severe deficits, 25%; and death, 4%. An incomplete ipsilateral Horner's syndrome with ptosis and miosis but not anhidrosis is present in about 50% of cases due to damage of the sympathetic fibers. Either subjective or objective bruits or both are present in about 45% of patients.

Uncommon symptoms and signs of extracranial ICA dissection include syncope, amaurosis fugax, scalp tenderness, neck swelling, positive visual phenomena (e.g., scintillations), sixth cranial nerve palsies, lower cranial nerve palsies (e.g., ipsilateral tongue paresis and dysgeusia from involvement of the hypoglossal nerve and chorda tympani), and a sensation of pulsation in the neck. Transient symptoms resembling migraine with aura[24] and cluster headache[25] have been reported.

Intracranial ICA dissection typically presents with a severe ipsilateral headache and a major stroke. SAH can occur in 20% of cases. Rarely, prolonged isolated orbital pain can be the only symptom of intrapetrous ICA dissection.[26]

The most common symptom of VA dissection is headache and neck pain (present in 88%) followed by vertebrobasilar distribution stroke or transient ischemic attacks (TIAs)—especially lateral medullary syndrome—from within hours to 2 weeks. Less frequently, the patients may present with vertebrobasilar stroke or TIAs only or with only headache and/or neck pain. The presence of deficits is as follows: neurologically normal or mild deficits only, 83%; moderate to severe deficits, 11%; and death, 6%. SAH can occur with dissection of the intracranial portion of the VA. Rare symptoms and signs of VA dissection include vertigo and upside-down vision, hemifacial spasm, upper-extremity pain that can mimic myocardial ischemia, acute cervical epidural hemorrhage, bilateral distal upper-limb amyotrophy, respiratory arrest, and transient amnesia.

The onset of headache is gradual in about 75% of patients with ICA and VA dissections. More than 10% of those with ICA and more than 20% of those with VA dissections report a thunderclap headache, a severe sudden headache usually without associated SAH. The headaches in both dissections are usually described as constant, steady aching or steady sharp pain and, less commonly, as throbbing. Facial pain, including ear pain, is reported by about one-third, and orbital and eye pain occurs in about 40% of patients with ICA dissection. This pain is always ipsilateral to the dissection. Neck pain (usually anterolateral) is reported by about 25% of those with ICA dissection. About half of those with VA dissection report posterolateral neck pain, which is bilateral in one-third of patients.

Diagnostic Evaluation

Arteriograms are the standard study for evaluating ICA and VA dissections and may reveal stenosis, often irregular and tapered, dissecting aneurysms, intimal flaps, and occlusion of distal branches. ICA dissections usually begin 2 cm or more distal to the origin and extend rostrally for a variable distance. Irregular narrowing may give a "wavy ribbon" appearance, and severe narrowing may produce a "string sign."

Axial MRI may demonstrate the abnormal lumen and the intramural clot. Magnetic resonance angiography (MRA) increases the yield of MRI studies. Table 11-1 gives the sensitivity and specificity of MRI and MRA compared with conventional angiography according to the study of Levy et al.[27] The sensitivity for detection of VA dissections is less than that for ICA dissections because of technical artifacts due to the smaller size and the broad variation in the normal caliber of the vertebral arteries. MRA is particularly useful for followup of patients. Occasionally, MRI and MRA may detect dissections not seen on conventional angiography due to undetectable narrowing of the lumen by intraluminal hematomas. Helical (spiral) CT angiography may have a similar sensitivity and specificity to MRA.

Carotid duplex ultrasound may show a tapering luminal stenosis and a double lumen. Extracranial Doppler may show reduced or absent distal carotid artery flow at the level of the bifurcation. Limitations of duplex ultrasound include anatomic factors (e.g., a short or fat neck and a high bifurcation) and not detecting intracranial ICA involvement. Extracranial vertebral duplex ultrasound has only fair sensitivity and specificity and does not image the intracranial portions.

Management

In the absence of SAH, intracranial hemorrhage, or a massive stroke, the standard treatment for dissection is anticoagulation with heparin followed by warfarin to prevent thrombus propagation and embolic stroke. The optimal time for treatment is unknown. Since most arteries will heal within 3 months, a follow-up study such as MRA is typically done. Then a decision is made on whether to continue warfarin or not. Many patients do

Table 11-1. Sensitivity and specificity of MRI and MRA for the evaluation of internal carotid and vertebral artery dissections compared to conventional angiography

Artery	Study	Sensitivity (%)	Specificity (%)
Carotid	MRI	84	99
	MRA	95	99
Vertebral	MRI	60	98
	MRA	20	100

well with or without treatment: a complete or excellent recovery occurs in about 85% of those with ICA and VA dissections. Antiplatelet agents are being studied as an alternative to anti-coagulation. The recurrence rate for second dissections is 2% for the first month and then about 1% per year. Occasionally, resection of a residual dissecting aneurysm that has been a source of embolization or the source of SAH is performed. Another occasional surgical option is superficial temporal artery-middle cerebral artery bypass for those with tight ICA stenosis and hemodynamic ischemic symptoms.

CEREBRAL VENOUS THROMBOSIS

Introduction and Epidemiology

Cerebral venous thrombosis (CVT)[28,29] is commonly associated with headaches. There are numerous causes and predisposing conditions. Local infectious causes include direct septic trauma, intracranial infection (e.g., abscess or meningitis), and regional infections (such as otitis, tonsillitis, and sinusitis). Systemic infections that can be causative include bacterial infections (e.g., septicemia and endocarditis), viral infections (e.g., herpes, HIV, CMV), parasitic infections (malaria, trichinosis), and aspergillosis. There are many noninfectious causes. Local pathology includes head injury, neurosurgical operations, cerebral infarcts and hemorrhages, tumors, porencephaly, arachnoid cysts, dural AVMs, and internal jugular vein infusions. Any type of surgery with or without deep venous thrombosis has been associated. Pregnancy and the puerperium as a cause is discussed in Chapter 8. Oral contraceptives are also a risk factor.

There are numerous medical associations, including cardiac disease, malignancies, red blood cell disorders (e.g., polycythemia, sickle cell disease), thrombocythemia, coagulation disorders (protein C and protein S deficiency and antiphospholipid antibody deficiency), severe dehydration, ulcerative colitis and Crohn's disease, connective-tissue disorders, venous thromboembolic disease, Behçet's disease, sarcoidosis, nephrotic syndrome, androgen therapy, homocystinuria, and thyrotoxicosis. Increased resistance to activated protein C with factor V Leiden mutation may be found in up to 20% of cases. Despite this extensive list of associations and causes, up to 35% of causes are idiopathic.

The incidence of CVT is not known. All age groups may be affected. Postpartum women appear to have the greatest risk of this disease. Neonates or young infants with severe dehydration are also a high-risk group.

Clinical Manifestations

In 75% of cases, multiple veins or sinuses are involved. The superior sagittal sinus (SSS), which drains the major part of the cerebral cortices and reabsorbs CSF, is involved in about 70% of cases of cerebral venous thrombosis (CVT). Thrombotic obstruction of the SSS elevates intracranial pressure by increasing intravenous and CSF pressure. The presentation of raised intracranial pressure is often headaches and papilledema. Extension of the thrombus into the superficial cortical veins can result in cerebral edema, infarction, hemorrhage, and seizures.

The lateral sinus, which drains blood from the sagittal sinus, cerebellum, brain stem, and posterior part of the cerebral hemispheres, is involved in about 70% of cases. Patients usually present with symptoms and signs of raised intracranial pressure.

The deep cerebral veins and sinuses, which drain the deep white matter of the cerebral hemispheres and the basal ganglia, are involved in more than 10% of cases. Headache and alterations in the level of consciousness are present with extensive thrombosis of these structures. More severe cases may result findings such as hemorrhagic infarction of the thalami and basal ganglia, dysphasia, and hemiparesis. The cavernous sinuses, which drain blood from the orbits and the anterior part of the base of the brain, are involved in less than 5% of cases. Headache, chemosis, proptosis, and painful ophthalmoplegia (initially unilateral but often becomes bilateral) are the usual presentations of cavernous sinus thrombosis.

Headache is present in 80% and is the earlier symptom in two-thirds of cases. The headaches, usually due to raised intracranial pressure, are typically diffuse, progressive, and rather constant. However, a sudden severe thunderclap headache can result if CVT leads to SAH. The headache of CVT is almost always associated with the following signs: papilledema in up to 80% of cases, which can cause transient visual obscurations (visual clouding in one or both eyes lasting seconds) when severe; focal deficits, which are present at some time during the course of the disease in 50% of patients; and partial and/or generalized seizures, which are present at some time during the disease in 40% of cases.

There are some important patterns of symptoms and signs that can simulate other disorders. Isolated intracranial hypertension, with headache, papilledema, and sixth cranial nerve palsy, occurs in up to 40% of patients. This presentation can exactly mimic pseudotumor cerebri (see later). Subacute encephalopathy, with an altered level of consciousness and no focal findings similar to a metabolic encephalopathy, often occurs in either very young or very old patients. During the postpartum period, some presentations of CVT can mimic other disorders as follows: headache alone can be mistaken for postpartum migraine; headache and seizures can be taken for eclampsia; and depression, irritability, anxiety, and lack of interest can be misdiagnosed as postpartum depression.

Diagnostic Evaluation

CT scan of the brain, which can exclude associated findings, such as cerebral infarction or hemorrhage, has limited sensitivity for the detection of CVT. The "empty delta sign" on an enhanced study, which is due to the opacification of collateral veins in the wall of the SSS surrounding the nonenhancing clot within the sinus, is present in only 35% of cases. In addition, false positives can occur because the posterior sagittal sinus divides into two channels in about 25% of normal.

MRI, especially when combined with MR venography, is the best way to detect CVT.[30] The studies can demonstrate flow void, the thrombus, and, later, recanalization. Cerebral angiography can certainly reveal partial or complete lack of filling of a sinus. However, false positives can occur due to normal variants such as absence of the anterior part of the sagittal sinus or partial or total agenesis of one lateral sinus.

Lumbar puncture, which should be avoided if there is a large cerebral infarction or hemorrhage, can document elevated intracranial pressure and help to exclude infectious or leptomeningeal malignancy as the cause of CVT. CSF findings include mild to moderate elevation of CSF protein in two-thirds of patients, more than 20 red cells in two-thirds, and a mild pleocytosis in one-third of cases. An abnormal CSF protein and cell count can help diagnose CVT in cases of isolated intracranial hypertension simulating pseudotumor cerebri where only a CT scan of the brain is obtained with normal findings.

Management

The treatment of CVT includes the following: the limitation or elimination of thrombus; treatment of an underlying cause, if present; control of seizures; treatment of raised intracranial pressure; and management of cerebral infarctions and hemorrhages.

Intravenous or subcutaneous heparin is the treatment of choice (except for neonates) with prolongation of the partial thromboplastic time (PTT) to 2 to 2.5 times normal. Some authorities recommend prolongation of the PTT to only 1.25 to 1.5 times normal in patients with associated hemorrhagic infarction. Heparin is continued until the patient improves or stabilizes. Warfarin then replaces heparin and is usually continued for at least 3 months. The dosage of warfarin is adjusted to obtain an international normalized ratio (INR) between 2.5 and 3.5. Serial MRI and magnetic resonance venography studies are useful in determining the duration of warfarin therapy.

Management of symptomatic raised intracranial pressure is controversial. Treatments sometimes used, depending on the clinical picture, include lumbar puncture before starting anticoagulation, steroids, mannitol, glycerol, acetazolamide, furosemide, shunting, optic nerve fenestration (in cases of progressive visual loss), intracranial pressure monitoring, and pentobarbital-induced coma. There is concern, however, that use of diuretics might lead to additional thrombus extension. If patients worsen despite optimal symptomatic and heparin treatment, some authorities recommend local urokinase infusion through the internal jugular route or tissue plasminogen activator via catheter at the site of the clot.[30a]

The mortality rate of CVT in recent series ranges from 6% to 30%. Full recovery occurs in more than 75% of survivors.

HYPERTENSION

Although mild or moderate hypertension does not usually cause headache, hypertension due to the following can cause headache: acute pressor response to exogenous agents; pheochromocytoma; malignant hypertension; and preeclampsia and eclampsia (Chapter 8). Headaches due to severe hypertension are usually a biooccipital throbbing but can be generalized or a frontal throbbing (especially in children). The headache is often present in the morning on awakening. The diastolic blood pressure is usually elevated to 120 mm Hg or higher.

Acute Pressor Responses

A sudden severe headache can occur due to a rapid increase in blood pressure when patients taking monoamine oxidase inhibitors drink red wine or eat foods such as cheese, chicken livers, or pickled herring, which have a high tyramine content, or also take sympathomimetic medications such as pseudoephedrine. Use of illicit drugs with sympathomimetic actions such as cocaine, methamphetamine, and methylenedioxymethamphetamine ("ecstasy") can also cause acute hypertension (sometimes leading to strokes) and headache.

Pheochromocytoma

Epidemiology

Pheochromocytoma,[31,32] a rare tumor, arises from the chromaffin cells of the adrenal medulla and is named for the color of its cut surface (from the Greek *phaios*, meaning "dusky"). The tumor usually secretes norepinephrine and epinephrine with a ratio of 4:1 or more. Ten percent to 20% are associated with genetic disorders such as multiple endocrine neoplasia syndromes, von Hippel-Lindau complex, neurofibromatosis type I, Sturge-Weber syndrome, tuberous sclerosis, and Zollinger-Ellison syndrome. Of the 80% to 90% of sporadic cases, 10% are malignant, 10% are bilateral, and 10% are found outside the adrenal gland. Ninety percent of the extraadrenal tumors are located within the abdomen, typically in the sympathetic ganglia between the diaphragm and the lower poles of the kidneys (paragangliomas), in the urinary bladder (where micturition can trigger attacks), and in the organ of Zuckerkandl (at the bifurcation of the aorta). Extraabdominal locations are the chest (pericardium, myocardium, and posterior mediastinum) and neck (in the carotid body, vagus nerve, or jugular bulb).

Clinical Manifestations

The most common symptom of pheochromocytoma is a rapid-onset headache that is reported by up to 92% of patients. The headache, which lasts less than 1 hour in 70%, is bilateral, severe, and throbbing, and may be associated with nausea in 50% of cases. Some patients may not get headaches even with blood pressures as high as 260/100 mm Hg. Hypertension, which is paroxysmal in 50% and sustained in 50%, is found in 90% of patients. The paroxysmal hypertension may show elevations to 300/160 mm Hg. Symptoms and signs of adrenergic stimulation are common with sweating, palpitations, and tachycardia with palpitations each reported by about 70% of patients. Anxiety, dizziness, abdominal pain, chest pain, weight loss, heat intolerance, nausea/vomiting, pallor (less often flushing), syncope, and orthostatic hypotension may also occur. Many patients have spells lasting between 15 and 60 minutes occurring from several times per day to once or twice a year. Paroxysms can begin spontaneously or be triggered by physical exertion, certain medications, emotional stress, changes in posture, and increases in intraabdominal pressure.

Diagnostic Evaluation

Laboratory and imaging studies are required to make the diagnosis. A 24-hour urine collection reveals elevations and sensitivity for diagnosis as follows: metanephrine and normetanephrine, up to 98%; vanillymandelic acid, 60% to 70%; and total catecholamines, 60% to 79%. MRI of the abdomen, pelvis, chest, and neck is almost 100% sensitive in detecting pheochromocytomas. CT scans have a sensitivity of 95% and specificity of 65% for detection of adrenal tumors. Scintigraphic imaging with I-131 metaiodobenzylguadnidine has a sensitivity of 88% and specificity of 99%. Indications include evaluation of extraadrenal, recurrent, or metastatic pheochromoctyomas or those with silent adrenal masses and borderline catecholamine levels.

Management

The hypertension due to pheochromocytoma is treated first with slow upward titration of an alpha-blocker (e.g., prazosin, terazosin, and phenoxybenzamine) and later addition of a beta-blocker for rate control after full alpha-blockade. A combination drug such as labetalol can sometimes be useful. Direct vasodilators, calcium channel blockers, and angiotensin-converting enzyme inhibits are sometimes used cautiously when the hypertension is resistant to initial therapy. Surgical removal can be curative, especially in benign tumors.

Malignant Hypertension

Hypertensive encephalopathy is an acute cerebral syndrome due to sudden, severe hypertension. The rate and extent of the rise of the blood pressure are the most important factors in the development of this condition. In those with chronic hypertension, hypertensive encephalopathy may not result unless the blood pressure is 250/150 mm Hg or higher. A previously normotensive person may develop the encephalopathy with a lower elevation. The presenting symptoms can be headache, nausea, and vomiting. Complaints of blurred or dim vision, scintillating scotoma, or visual loss may also be reported. Anxiety, agitation, and then decreased levels of consciousness and sometimes seizures can follow. Papilledema and focal neurologic deficits can be present.

CAROTIDYNIA

Carotidynia is neck pain associated with carotid artery tenderness, especially near the bifurcation.[33] Facial pain may also occur alone or with the neck pain. Symptomatic causes of carotidynia include disorders of the carotid artery, including dissection (see earlier), occlusion or stenosis, aneurysm, fibromuscular dysplasia, temporal arteritis (Chapter 9), and following endarterectomy. In the acute presentation, these disorders should be excluded with appropriate studies such as carotid ultrasound, MRI and MRA, angiography, and a sedimentation rate.

Acute monophasic carotidynia, which may have a viral basis, typically occurs in young or middle-aged adults and persists for an average of 11 days. Structural abnormalities and temporal arteritis are excluded by appropriate testing. Analgesics, nonsteroidal antiinflammatory drugs such as indomethacin, or a short course of corticosteroids may relieve the pain.[34]

Chronic or recurrent carotidynia, which occurs in adults, is characterized by recurring pain lasting minutes to hours with episodes occurring daily or weekly. This form, which may be related to migraine, may respond to treatment with indomethacin, a short course of corticosteroids, and migraine preventive medications. This is a diagnosis of exclusion. Evaluation by an ENT physician to exclude nonvascular abnormalities including thyroiditis and Eagle's syndrome (Chapter 12) may be useful.

ANGINAL HEADACHE

Cardiac ischemia can rarely cause a unilateral or bilateral headache brought on by exercise and relieved by rest.[35,36] The headache can occur alone or be accompanied by chest pain. The mechanism of the referral of cardiac pain to the head is obscure. Angina is generally believed to be due to afferent impulses that traverse cervicothoracic sympathetic ganglia, enter the spinal cord via the first and the fifth thoracic dorsal roots, and produce the characteristic pain in the chest or inner aspects of the arms. Cardiac vagal afferents, which mediate anginal pain in a minority of patients, join the tractus solitarius. A potential pathway for referral of cardiac pain to the head would be convergence with craniovascular afferents.[37]

REFERENCES

1. Suchurkova D, Moreau T, Lemesle M, et al. Migraine history and migraine-induced stroke in the Dijon Stroke Registry. *Neuroepidemiology* 1999;18:85–91.
2. Welch KMA, Tatemichi TK, Mohr JP. Migraine and stroke. In: Barnett HJM, Mohr JP, Stein BM, Yatsu FM, eds. *Stroke: pathophysiology, diagnosis, and management,* 3rd ed. New York: Churchill Livingstone, 1998:845–867.
3. Gomez-Aranda F, Canadillas F, Mrti -Masso JF, et al. Pseudomigraine with temporary neurological symptoms and lymphocytic pleocytosis: a report of 50 cases. *Brain* 1997;1270:1105–1113.
4. Mohr JP. CADASIL and white matter syndromes. *Ann Neurol* 1998;44:715–716.
5. Evans RW. Chapter 1. The evaluation of headaches. In: Evans RW, ed. *Diagnostic testing in neurology.* Philadelphia: WB Saunders, 1999.
6. Daras M, Koppel B, Leyfermann M, et al. Anticardiolipin antibodies in migraine patients: an additional risk factor for stroke? *Neurology* 1995;45[Suppl 4]:A367–A368.
7. Moore KL, Corbett JJ. Retinal migraine. In: Gilman S, Goldstein GW, Waxman SG, eds. *Neurobase.* San Diego: Arbor, 2000.
8. Beversdorf D, Stommel E, Allen C, et al. Recurrent branch retinal infarcts in association with migraine. *Headache* 1997;37:396–399.
9. Liu GT, Schatz NJ, Galetta SL, et al. Persistent positive visual phenomena in migraine. *Neurology* 1995;45:664–668.
10. Rothrock JF. Successful treatment of persistent migraine aura with divalproex sodium. *Neurology* 1997;48:261–262.
11. Alvarez SJ, Molins A, Turon A. et al. Migraine-infarct in patients treated with beta-blockers. *Rev Clin Esp* 1993;192:228–230.
12. Mitsias P, Welch KMA. Headache associated with ischemic cerebrovascular disease. In: Gilman S, Goldstein GW, Waxman SG, eds. *Neurobase.* San Diego: Arbor, 2000.

13. Portenoy RK, Abissi CJ, Lipton RB, et al. Headache in cerebrovascular disease. *Stroke* 1984;15:1009–1012.
14. Arboix A, Massons J, Oliveres M, et al. Headache in acute cerebrovascular disease: a prospective clinical study in 240 patients. *Cephalalgia* 1994;14:37–40.
15. Vestergaard K, Andersen G, Nielsen MI, et al. Headache in stroke. *Stroke* 1993;24:1621–1624.
16. Gorelick PB, Hier DB, Caplan LR, et al. Headache in acute cerebrovascular disease. *Neurology* 1986;36:144–150.
17. Ouriel K, Shortell CK, Illig KA, et al. Intracerebral hemorrhage after carotid endarterectomy: incidence, contribution to neurologic morbidity, and predictive factors. *J Vasc Endovasc Surg* 1999;29:82–87.
18. Kupersmith MJ, Vargas ME, Yashar A, et al. Occipital arteriovenous malformations: visual disturbances and presentation. *Neurology* 1996;46:953–957.
19. Leone M, D'Amico D, Frediani F, et al. Clinical considerations on side-locked unilaterality in long lasting primary headaches. *Headache* 1993;33:381–384.
20. Bruyn GW. Intracranial arteriovenous malformation and migraine. *Cephalalgia* 1984;4:191–207.
21. Mokri B. Chapter 20. Headache in spontaneous carotid and vertebral artery dissections. In: Goadsby PJ, Silberstein SD, eds. *Headache.* Boston: Butterworth-Heinemann, 1997:327–353.
22. Saver JL, Easton JD. Dissections and trauma of cervicocerebral arteries. In: Barnett HJM, Mohr JP, Stein BM, Yatsu FM, eds. *Stroke: pathophysiology, diagnosis, and management,* 3rd ed. New York: Churchill Livingstone, 1998:769–786.
23. Gomez CR. Spontaneous carotid artery dissection. In: Gilman S, Goldstein GW, Waxman SG, eds. *Neurobase.* San Diego: Arbor, 2000.
24. Silverman IE, Wityk RJ. Transient migraine-like symptoms with internal carotid artery dissection. *Clin Neurol Neurosurg* 1998;100:116–120.
25. Rosebraugh CJ, Griebel DJ, DiPette DJ. A case report of carotid artery dissection presenting as cluster headache. *Am J Med* 1997;102:418–419.
26. Guillon B, Biousse V, Massiou H, et al. Orbital pain as an isolated sign of internal carotid artery dissection: a diagnostic pitfall. *Cephalalgia* 1998;18:222–224.
27. Levy C, Laissy JP, Reveau V, et al. Carotid and vertebral dissections: three dimensional time-of-flight MR angiography and MR imaging versus conventional angiography. *Radiology* 1994; 190:97.
28. Bousser M-G, Barnett JHM. Cerebral venous thrombosis. In: Barnett HJM, Mohr JP, Stein BM, et al., eds. *Stroke: pathophysiology, diagnosis, and management,* 3rd ed. New York: Churchill Livingstone, 1998:623–647.
29. Broderick JP. Cerebral venous thrombosis. In: Gilman S, Goldstein GW, Waxman SG, eds. *Neurobase.* San Diego: Arbor, 2000.
30. Bianchi D, Maeder P, Bogousslavsky J, et al. Diagnosis of cerebral venous thrombosis with routine magnetic resonance: an update. *Eur Neurol* 1998;40:179–190.

30a. Frey JL, Muro GJ, McDougall CG, et al. Cerebral venous thrombosis: combined intrathrombus rtPA and intravenous heparin. *Stroke* 1999;30:489–494.

31. Pleet AB. Neuroendocrine disorders. In: Evans RW, ed. *Diagnostic testing in neurology*. Philadelphia: WB Saunders, 1999: 419–435.

32. Inzucchi SE, Brines ML. Pheochromocytoma. In: Gilman S, Goldstein GW, Waxman SG, eds. *Neurobase*. San Diego: Arbor, 2000.

33. Wesselmann U, Reich SG. The dynias. *Semin Neurol* 1996;16: 63–74.

34. Emmanuelli JL, Gutierrez JR, Chiossone JA, et al. Carotidynia: a frequently overlooked or misdiagnosed syndrome. *Ear Nose Throat J* 1998;77:462–469.

35. Lipton RB, Lowenkopf T, Bajwa ZH, et al. Cardiac cephalalgia: a treatable form of exertional headache. *Neurology* 1997;49: 813–816.

36. Grace A, Horgan J, Breathnach K, et al. Anginal headache and its basis. *Cephalalgia* 1997;17:195–196.

37. Lance JW, Lambros J. Unilateral exertional headache as a symptom of cardiac ischemia. *Headache* 1998;38:315–316.

Headaches and Neoplasms, High and Low Pressure, and HEENT Disorders

Randolph W. Evans

NEOPLASMS

Introduction and Epidemiology

Many patients with frequent or severe headaches are concerned that they may have a brain tumor. Fortunately, brain tumors are an uncommon cause of headaches. In the United States, about 18,000 primary brain tumors are diagnosed per year, including the following types: glioblastomas, 50%; astrocytomas, 10% (about 50% of these present with headache); meningiomas, 17%; pituitary adenomas, 4%; neurilemoma, 2%; ependymoma, 2%; and oligodendroglioma, 3%. About 170,000 new cases of metastatic brain tumors are diagnosed per year in the United States.[1] Eighty percent occur after the diagnosis of the primary and 70% have multiple cerebral lesions. The frequency by primary site in adults is as follows: lung, 64%; breast, 14%, unknown primary, 8%; melanoma, 4%; colorectal, 3%; hypernephroma, 2%; and other, 5%. The average interval between the diagnosis of the primary carcinoma and the development of brain metastasis is 4 months for lung carcinoma and 3 years for breast cancer. By contrast, slow-growing cancers of the ovary, uterus, or breast can result in cerebral metastasis up to 15 years after the diagnosis of the primary. Neoplasms in children and adolescents are discussed in Chapter 7.

The prevalence of adults with primary and metastatic brain tumors who complain of headaches at the time of diagnosis has been variably reported as 31%,[2] 48%,[3] 50%[3a] and 71%.[4] The median duration of headache at the time of diagnosis has been variably reported as from 3.5 weeks to 15.7 months. Headaches have been reported variably as equally frequent with primary and metastatic tumors and as more frequent with primary than with metastatic tumors.

Clinical Manifestations

Eight percent of patients with headaches and brain tumors have a normal neurologic examination. Papilledema, which is usually associated with headaches, is present in 40% of patients with brain tumors. The presence of headache is related to the size of the tumor and the amount of midline shift. Patients with previous headaches are more likely to have a headache with a brain tumor. The brain tumor headache may have an identical character to prior headaches but is more severe or frequent and is usually associated with other problems, such as seizure, confusion, prolonged nausea, hemiparesis, or other focal findings.

The most common location of headaches is bifrontal, although patients may complain of pain in other locations of the head as well as the neck. Unilateral headaches are usually on the same side as the neoplasm. Although the quality of the headache is usually similar to the tension type, occasional patients have headaches similar to migraine without aura and rarely migraine with aura and cluster headaches. Most of the headaches are intermittent with moderate to severe intensity, but a significant minority report only mild headaches relieved by simple analgesics. The "classic" brain tumor headache—severe, worse in the morning, and associated with nausea and vomiting—occurs in a minority of patients with brain tumors.

Pituitary Adenomas

The incidence of headaches in patients with pituitary adenomas has been reported as between 33% and 72%. The headache, which may be intermittent or continuous, is usually bilateral and occurs more frequently in the anterior half of the head.[5] In contrast, Sheehan's syndrome (the spontaneous ischemic necrosis of the pituitary gland in the postpartum period resulting in hypopituitarism) does not usually result in headache (Chapter 8).

Pain due to pituitary tumors can mimic seemingly benign disorders. Pituitary macroadenomas can present with trigeminal neuralgia, clusterlike headaches,[6] and Raeder's syndrome.[7] Raeder's syndrome is a rare disorder characterized by ptosis, miosis, impairment of sweating over the medial aspect of the forehead, and sudden onset of severe frontotemporal burning, aching pain often in a periorbital or trigeminal distribution. Episodic pain is usually due to cluster headaches (Chapter 4) and those with more constant pain can be due to lesions involving the internal carotid artery and impinging on the first division of the trigeminal nerve. In addition, other lesions than pituitary tumors include aneurysms, trauma, infections, and internal carotid artery dissection.[8]

Acute pituitary apoplexy is an uncommon syndrome due to hemorrhage of a pituitary macroadenoma with compression of neighboring neural and vascular structures. Signs and symptoms occur in the following percentages of patients: headache, 83%; visual disturbance, 59%; ocular palsies, 48%; nausea/vomiting, 38%; altered mentation, 22%; meningismus, 15%; and fever, 7%.[9] Rarely, entrapment of the internal carotid artery within the cavernous sinus can lead to hemiparesis.[10] The incidence of pituitary apoplexy in patients with known pituitary adenomas is reported as 2% to 5%, usually occurring in adenomas of more than 1 cm.

Pituitary hemorrhage can be clinically silent or present as a migrainelike headache without associated signs or as aseptic meningitis.[11] Pituitary hemorrhage even in a macroadenoma can be overlooked and underimaged on a routine computed tomography (CT) scan of the head for acute headache using 10-mm cuts. A magnetic resonance imaging (MRI) scan even without pituitary views will routinely identify the pathology.

Pituitary macroadenomas with hemorrhage can result in a migrainelike headache with a III nerve palsy[12] and a migrainelike headache without aura with a normal examination.[13] Although uncommon, pituitary hemorrhage with and without apoplexy should be considered in the differential diagnosis of acute headache (also see Chapter 5).

Meningeal Carcinomatosis

Meningeal involvement[14] occurs in about 5% of all patients with cancer. The primary in cases of meningeal carcinomatosis due to solid non–central nervous system (CNS) tumors are breast (39%), lung (34%), melanoma (8%), gastrointestinal (5%), genitourinary (4%), head and neck (2%), and miscellaneous and unknown primaries (8%). In addition, for every 100 patients with disease from these primaries, one can expect to see 76 patients with leukemia, 34 patients with lymphoma, and 15 patients with primary central nervous system (CNS) tumors. Symptoms and signs of meningeal carcinomatosis include cerebral involvement in 50% (headache, mental status alteration, seizures, nausea, and vomiting), cranial nerve dysfunction in 56% (most commonly involved are III, IV, and VI followed by VII and II), and spinal involvement in 82% (symptoms and signs due to spinal roots, spinal cord, and meningeal disease, including neck and back pain[15]). Headache, which is present in 33% to 62% of patients, is usually not severe.

A CT scan of the brain is usually normal in meningeal carcinomatosis, although meningeal enhancement with contrast administration is sometimes present. Hydrocephalus can be present in some cases. An MRI scan with contrast often demonstrated dural meningeal enhancement. Initial CSF examination demonstrates elevated white blood cells in 51%, elevated protein in 73%, and hypoglycorrhachia or decreased CSF glucose in 28%. CSF cytology is positive in 54% on the first lumbar puncture, in an additional 30% after the second, and in 1% more after the third. Sending a relatively large volume of 5 to 10 ml of CSF for cytology may increase the yield. CSF biochemical markers, such as beta-glucuronidase, carcinoembryonic antigen, and lactic dehydrogenase isoenzyeme 5, may be present in cases of meningeal involvement from breast and lung carcinoma and melanoma but are nonspecific.

Colloid Cysts of the Third Ventricle

Colloid cysts[16] account for up to 1% of primary intracranial mass lesions and are usually asymptomatic until between 20 and 50 years of age. Colloid cysts usually present with one of the following: headache, bilateral papilledema, and occasionally, false localizing focal, motor, and sensory signs; progressive or fluctuating dementia and raised intracranial pressure with or without headache; or paroxysmal severe headaches,[17] nausea, vomiting, syncope, stupor, or coma. Episodic positional headaches, which occur in a minority of cases, may be due to movement of the colloid cyst on its pedicle in and out of the foramen of Monro with intermittent obstruction of CSF. Acute neurologic deterioration, including coma in 15% and sudden death in 5%, is usually due to acute CSF obstruction by cysts 15 mm or greater in diameter.[18]

Because of the risk of sudden death, surgery is generally recommended even in asymptomatic persons. Options include shunting of CSF, stereotactic cyst aspiration, transcortical-transventricular microsurgery, transcollosal microsurgery, and endoscopic surgery.

PSEUDOTUMOR CEREBRI

Introduction and Epidemiology

Pseudotumor cerebri (PTC)[19,20] is also referred to as benign intracranial hypertension and as idiopathic intracranial hypertension (by those who do not believe that visual loss is so benign). PTC can be diagnosed using the following criteria: the neurologic examination is normal with the exceptions of papilledema, visual loss, and cranial nerve VI palsy; CSF pressure is increased (>20 cm H_2O in nonobese and >25 cm H_2O in obese patients); CSF analysis is normal with the exception of decreased protein; no hydrocephalus or mass lesions exist; and there are no other identifiable causes.

More than 90% of patients with PTC are young obese women. Obesity is present in 66% of adult men with PTC. The female-to-male ratio is 8:1, and the mean age at the time of diagnosis is 30 years. The average annual incidence per 100,000 population is as follows: 0.9 cases in the general population; 3.3 cases for females ages 15 to 44; and 19 cases for obese (20% above ideal body weight) women ages 20 to 44 years. In children, PTC affects boys and girls equally. Obesity occurs in 43% of patients with PTC ages 3 to 11, 81% in ages 12 to 14, and 91% in ages 15 to 17.[21] Associated conditions or secondary causes are common in children with PTC.[22]

PTC is usually primary or idiopathic. There are numerous secondary causes and associations (Table 12-1). Medications associated with PTC include nalidixic acid, vitamin A (over-supplementation with vitamins or use of isotretinoin [Accutane], for acne), minocycline,[23] anabolic steroids, and corticosteroid withdrawal. Oral contraceptives are probably not associated with this disorder. Other causes include head trauma, meningitis/encephalitis, intracranial and extracranial venous outflow obstruction and hypertension (cerebral venous thrombosis (Chapter 11), surgical ligation of extracranial veins, radical neck dissection, chronic otitis, hypercoaguable states, cerebral edema, cardiac failure, and chronic respiratory disease), systemic disease (renal disease and hypoparathyroidism), diseases with elevated CSF protein concentration (Guillain-Barré syndrome, systemic lupus erythematosis, and spinal tumors, especially oligodendrogliomas), hypertensive disorders (hypertensive encephalopathy, preeclampsia, and eclampsia) and large arteriovenous malformations. Other considerations in children include acute frontal sinusitis,[24] Lyme disease,[25] and parameningeal infections. Patients with optic drusen and a primary headache condition such as chronic daily headache might be confused with PTC. Optic neuritis and central retinal venous thrombosis are almost always unilateral.

Table 12-1.   Etiologies of papilledema and headache

Intracranial mass

Obstruction or deformity of the ventricular system

Cerebral venous thrombosis

Extracranial venous obstruction
    Radical neck dissection
    Cardiac failure
    Chronic respiratory disease

Hypertensive encephalopathy

Preeclampsia and eclampsia

Meningitis/encephalitis

Meningeal carcinomatosis

Elevated CSF protein concentration
    Guillain-Barré syndrome
    Systemic lupus erythematosus
    Spinal tumors, especially oligodendroglioma

Large arteriovenous malformations

Optic neuritis (usually unilateral)

Central retinal venous thrombosis (usually unilateral)

In children
    Lead toxicity
    Lyme disease
    Parameningeal infection

Head trauma

Medications
    Vitamin A
    Minocycline
    Anabolic steroids
    Steroid withdrawal
    Nalidixic acid

Other medical conditions
    Renal disease
    Hypoparathyroidism
    Hypercoaguable states

Clinical Manifestations

   Table 12-2 summarizes the features of idiopathic PTC. Headache is present in 75% or more of idiopathic cases of PTC. The headaches, which may be the patient's worst ever, are usually pulsatile, daily, and continuous. The headache can be unilateral, bilateral, frontal, or occipital, although a bifrontotemporal location is the most common. Nausea occurs in about 60%; vomiting, in 40%; and orbital pain, in about 40%. Pain on eye movement, retrobulbar and bilateral, is reported by up to 20% of patients.

   Papilledema is present in about 95%. Visual symptoms include transient visual obscuration (TVO, an episode of visual clouding in one or both eyes usually lasting seconds) in 70%, diplopia in 40%, and visual loss in 30%. Cranial nerve VI palsy, a nonlocalizing sign of raised intracranial pressure, is present in 25% of

Table 12-2. Features of idiopathic pseudotumor cerebri

Ninety percent of patients are young obese women

Headache present in 75% or more

Papilledema in 95%

Cranial nerve VI palsy in 25%

Transient visual obscurations in 70%

Visual loss in 30%

Secondary causes or associations are excluded

Diagnostic testing
  CT or MRI scan shown no evidence of intracranial mass,
    hydrocephalus, or cerebral venous thrombosis
  Lumbar puncture reveals an elevated opening pressure
  CSF analysis is normal except for decreased CSF protein
    concentration in some cases

patients. Visual field testing may show early enlargement of the blind spot and peripheral constriction, especially nasal inferior.

PTC without papilledema should be considered in patients with chronic daily headache with any of the following features: obesity, pulsatile tinnitus, an empty sella, a history of head trauma or meningitis, or a headache that is not relieved by standard therapy.[26] In patients with pseudopapilledema, headaches, and/or TVO (which can also be due to pseudopapilledema), a lumbar puncture is required to exclude PTC.[27]

Other symptoms and signs include back and shoulder pain, vomiting, tinnitus, and a cranial bruit over the mastoid or the temporalis (due to turbulence in the major venous sinuses). Uncommon manifestations include hearing loss, Lhermitte's sign, facial nerve paralysis in children, and facial pain. In infants and young children, PTC may present with nausea, vomiting, lethargy, and focal neurologic deficits. Papilledema may not occur when there is an open fontanelle.

Biologic Mechanisms

The cause of idiopathic PTC is unknown. Postulated mechanisms include an increased rate of CSF formation, an increased intracranial venous pressure, a decreased rate of CSF absorption, and an increase in brain interstitial fluid.

Diagnostic Evaluation

A number of causes of papilledema and headache need to be excluded (Table 12-1). A CT scan or MRI scan of the brain is first obtained to exclude a tumor or hydrocephalus. MRI is more sensitive than CT scans for the detection of some intracranial neoplasms and for the detection of cerebral venous thrombosis, especially with the addition of MR venography (Chapter 11). In some settings, MRI scans may be unavailable or impossible because the patient may be too obese, may be claustrophobic, or may have a contraindication. Elevation of intracranial pressure in PTC produced the following MRI findings in one study: empty sella, 70%; flattening of the posterior sclera, 80%; distension of the perioptic subarachnoid space, 45%; enhancement of the prelaminar optic nerve, 50%; vertical tortuosity of the orbital optic nerve, 40%; and intraocular protrusion of the prelaminar optic nerve, 30%.[28] The scan may also show small ventricles.

If the scan shows no other explanation for the papilledema, a lumbar puncture is mandatory. The opening pressure should be carefully measured in the lateral decubitus position with the legs partially extended. If the patient is not relaxed, increased intraabdominal pressure can raise the opening pressure. The CSF analysis should be normal except for a low protein level in some cases. An ophthalmologist usually sees the patient to evaluate the fundus, visual acuity, and visual fields, which are then followed periodically to help prevent visual loss.

Management

Symptomatic causes of PTC should be treated or eliminated as appropriate. The treatment of idiopathic PTC depends on the clinical presentation. Obese patients should be encouraged to lose weight. In a study comparing obese women with weight loss of more than or equal to 2.5 kg during any 3-month interval, those who lost weight recovered more rapidly from both papilledema and visual field dysfunction.[29]

Repeated lumbar punctures, withdrawing enough fluid to reduce the pressure to 12 to 17.5 cm H_2O, may benefit some patients. Many patients, especially obese ones where the lumbar puncture may be difficult or those who develop low back pain, do not want repeated lumbar punctures. Performance of the procedure using fluoroscopy can make the lumbar puncture easier. In some cases, the lumbar puncture may cause a low-CSF-pressure headache.

Medications may be of benefit.[30] Patients with persistent headache may benefit from preventive medications used for migraine. Frequent use of analgesics may complicate the picture if medication rebound headaches develop. Diuretics may be of benefit. Acetazolamide, which inhibits carbonic anhydrase and reduces CSF production, may be effective, starting with a dose of 500 mg twice daily and going up to 2 g or even more daily. Side effects include numbness and tingling of the hands and feet and periorally, nausea, and kidney stones. Furosemide, at a dose of 40 to 160 mg per day along with potassium supplementation, may also be effective. For some cases, there may be value in combining migraine-preventive drugs with a diuretic. Corticosteroids are typically used for emergent treatment of impending visual loss. Disadvantages of corticosteroids include a rebound rise in intracranial pressure when steroids are withdrawn and weight gain and fluid retention, especially in already obese patients.

There are surgical treatments for papilledema and headache. Optic nerve sheath fenestration usually improves or stabilizes visual fields and acuity,[31] and even improves headaches in up to 65%.[32] The operation might be effective due to improved optic nerve axoplasmic flow and continuous intraorbital CSF drainage. However, this procedure may fail any time postoperatively and has a small risk of visual loss. Lumboperitoneal shunting is often effective for treatment of patients with severe visual loss at presentation or with intractable headache (with or without visual loss).[33] Disadvantages include the need for frequent shunt revisions in a few patients, low-pressure headaches, lumbar radiculopathies, and headaches from an acquired Chiari I malformation (see later).

LOW-CEREBROSPINAL-FLUID-PRESSURE HEADACHES

Epidemiology

Low-CSF-pressure headaches are most often due to the following: post–lumbar puncture, the most common cause; spontaneous occurrence; and CSF shunt overdrainage.[34–36] Infrequent causes include those that are traumatic, postoperative (following craniotomy or spinal surgery), and associated with other medical conditions (e.g., severe dehydration, diabetic coma, uremia, hyperpnea, meningoencephalitis, and severe systemic infection). The features of low-CSF-pressure headaches of any cause are the same as those of post–lumbar puncture headaches (PLPH). Rarely, intracranial hypotension can present with a severe encephalopathy.[37]

Diagnostic Evaluation

A repeat lumbar puncture usually demonstrates an opening pressure from 0 to 70 cm H_2O, although the pressure can be in the normal range,[38] especially if the procedure is performed after a period of bedrest. The CSF analysis may be normal or can demonstrate a moderate, primarily lymphocytic pleocytosis, the presence of red blood cells, and elevated protein that can even be more than 500 mg/dl.

An MRI scan of the brain may reveal diffuse meningeal enhancement with gadolinium and, in some cases, subdural fluid collections, which return to normal with resolution of the headache. The diffuse meningeal enhancement on MRI may be explained by dural vasodilation and a greater concentration of gadolinium in the dural microvasculature and in the interstitial fluid of the dura. (Before the characteristic picture of the postural headache and diffuse meningeal enhancement on MRI was recognized, some patients underwent extensive testing, including meningeal biopsy to exclude other conditions, such as meningeal carcinomatosis and neurosarcoidosis.) The pleocytosis and elevated protein in the CSF and the subdural fluid collections are probably due to decreased CSF volume and hydrostatic pressure changes resulting in meningeal vasodilation and vascular leak.

A recent study showed color Doppler imaging of the superior ophthalmic vein to be a highly sensitive method for diagnosis.[38a] Patients with low-CSF-pressure headache all had a substantially large mean diameter of the vein and significantly higher mean maximum flow velocity.

Reversible descent of the cerebellar tonsils below the foramen magnum (acquired Chiari I malformation) can occur following lumbar puncture and due to overdraining CSF shunts and spontaneous intracranial hypertension.[39] Lumbar MRI may also be abnormal following lumbar puncture. In one study of 11 patients, all had evidence of CSF leakage ranging from 1 to 460 ml.[40]

POST–LUMBAR PUNCTURE HEADACHE

Epidemiology

Headache is the most common complication of lumbar puncture,[41] occurring in up to 40% of patients after diagnostic lumbar puncture. There are a variety of unmodifiable and modifiable risk factors (Table 12-3). The five following demographic features increase the risk of PLPH: female gender, age (greatest in those 18 to 30 years of age), lesser body mass index, prior chronic or recurrent headaches, and prior PLPH. PLPH occurs twice as often in women as in men. The highest incidence is in the 18- to 30-year-old age group. Younger women may be at greater risk because of increased dural fiber elasticity, which could maintain a patent dural defect better than a less elastic dura. Estrogens might also increase substance P receptor sensitivity. The incidence is much less in children younger than 13 years and adults older than 60. Decreased dural fiber elasticity, a smaller epidural space, and decreased sensitivity of pain structures in the dura and blood vessels may explain the lower incidence in those over age 60. The incidence is greater in patients with lesser body mass index (wt/ht^2). Younger female patients with a low body mass index may have the highest risk in developing PLPH.

Patients with a headache before the lumbar puncture are at greater risk for PLPHs, which are more severe and last longer than headaches of those with no preceding headache. Patients with chronic or recurrent headaches are three times more likely to develop PLPH as those without. Patients with a prior history of PLPH are also at increased risk. Risk factors related to the lumbar puncture needle are discussed later.

Clinical Manifestations

PLPH is a bilateral, frontal, occipital, or generalized pressure or throbbing occurring in the upright position and decreasing or resolving when supine. The headache is worse with head movement, coughing, straining, sneezing, and jugular venous compression. The headache begins within 48 hours in about 80% and within 72 hours in about 90% of patients. The onset can be immediately after the lumbar puncture or delayed for as long as 14

Table 12-3. Risk factors for developing post–lumbar puncture headache

Patient demographics
  Female gender
  Age (greatest in range of 18–30 years)
  Lesser body mass index
  Prior chronic or recurrent headache
  Prior post–lumbar puncture headache

Quincke lumbar puncture needle
  Larger-diameter needle
  Perpendicular orientation of the bevel

Sprotte lumbar puncture needle
  Not reinserting the stylet

days. The headache lasts for less than 5 days in about 80%, although it can persist for 12 months. In one study, the headaches were reported as mild in 11%, moderate in 22%, and severe in 69%.[42] Additional symptoms were present in the following percentages: neck stiffness, 43%; nausea, 66%; vomiting, 27%; cochlear symptoms, 15%; and ocular symptoms, 12%. In another series, nausea was present in 22% and vomiting occurred in 2%.

Dysfunction of cranial nerves III, IV, V, VI, VII, and VIII, usually transient, can also occur after lumbar puncture. Abducens paresis may follow as often as 1 in 400 lumbar punctures or spinal anesthetics and can be unilateral or bilateral. The paresis usually occurs 4 to 14 days after the procedure and usually resolves over 4 to 6 weeks. Reversible hearing loss may be symptomatic in up to 8% of patients.

Other complications of lumbar puncture include the following: uncal or tonsillar herniation; reversible tonsillar descent; spinal coning in patients with rostral subarachnoid block; nerve root irritation, herniation, and transection; low back pain; implantation of epidermoid tumors if a stylet is not used; infections; bleeding complications, including intracranial bleeding, traumatic lumbar puncture, and spinal hematomas; other complications include vasovagal syncope, cardiac arrest, seizures, and incorrect laboratory analysis of CSF.

Biologic Mechanisms

Although the cause of PLPH is not entirely certain, the best explanation is low CSF pressure due to CSF leakage through a dural and arachnoid tear produced by the puncture that exceeds the rate of CSF production. CSF hypotension can produce headache and cranial nerve symptoms through downward descent of the brain and stretching of pain-sensitive structures, including the dura, nerves (cranial nerves V, IX, and X and the upper three cervical nerves), and bridging veins. Traction on cranial nerves can also result in the cranial neuropathies. Intracranial venous dilatation and increased brain volume occur secondarily as the veins passively dilate in response to decreased extravascular pressure.

Prevention

Activity

Although many physicians recommend bedrest of varying durations for prevention, controlled prospective studies show no benefit for prevention of PLPH from bedrest for up to 24 hours in the supine, prone, or head-down position.[43–45] There may be an increased incidence of PLPH in those recumbent as compared with patients immediately mobilized.[46] An increased intake of oral fluids after the lumbar puncture does not prevent PLPH.[47]

Diameter of Quincke Needle

The incidence of PLPH decreases with a smaller diameter of the Quincke (standard) needle. A smaller-diameter needle produces a smaller tear in the dura and less potential for leakage. The incidence of PLPH decreases from up to 40% with use of a 20 gauge (G) needle down to 5% to 12% with use of a 24- to 27-G needle. Although smaller-diameter needles can be used for spinal anesthesia and myelography, they are not a practical choice for diagnostic lumbar puncture. The CSF flow rate is very slow with smaller-diameter needles. The flow rate in milliliters per hour for various needles is as follows: 20 G, 133; 22 G, 30.4 and 25 G, 10.5. In addition, the time needed to measure the CSF opening pressure with the manometer is increased from 43 seconds with a 20-G needle to 225 seconds with 22-G needle, and 336 seconds with one of 25 G.

Parallel Insertion of the Bevel

Insertion of the bevel parallel to the longitudinal dural fibers reduces the incidence of PLPH by about 50%.[48] Parallel insertion means that a plane passing through the flat part of the bevel, going through both edges of the bevel, is parallel to the long or vertical axis of the spine. This reduction of PLPH occurs because puncturing the dura with the bevel parallel to the fibers severs fewer fibers than when the bevel is perpendicular. The dural fibers run parallel to the long axis of the spine.

Atraumatic Needles

Atraumatic or pencil-point needles such as the Whitacre or Sprotte (Fig. 12-1) significantly reduce the incidence of PLPH when used for diagnostic lumbar puncture, myelography,[49] and spinal anesthesia.[50] This reduction is probably due to atraumatic needles spreading rather than cutting dural fibers. Based on one study using the Sprotte 21-G needle, the incidence is also reduced by replacing the stylet and rotating the needle 90 degrees before withdrawing it.[51] (This is thought to be beneficial because a strand of arachnoid may enter the needle with the CSF, and when the needle is removed, the strand may be threaded back through the dural defect and produce prolonged CSF leakage). Following diagnostic lumbar puncture with a Sprotte 21-G needle, for example, the incidence of PLPH is about 5%,[52,53] compared with about 30% with a Quincke 20-G (standard) needle. The physician should consider use of an atraumatic needle in patients with risk factors (Table 12-4) for PLPH.

A few lumbar punctures with the Sprotte needle are usually necessary for the physician to feel comfortable. Because the tip of the needle is relatively dull, a sharp, short introducer is provided with the Sprotte needle. The introducer should be inserted to two-thirds of its length before inserting the Sprotte needle. Unlike the Quincke needle, which can be wiggled and where the direction can be easily changed, the direction of the introducer has to be changed if the needle is not in the proper location. The procedure can be performed without the introducer by using the anesthetic needle to make a skin entry first, but use of the introducer is simpler for most physicians and may result in less damage to the needle tip. The feel of the atraumatic needle is different from that with the Quincke needle and the physician must push harder with the introduction of the needle. Occasionally, the LP cannot be performed with the Sprotte needle and the physician will have to change to the Quincke.

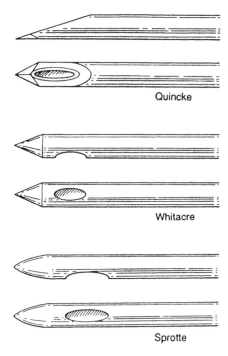

Quincke

Whitacre

Sprotte

Figure 12-1. Three types of spinal needle tips: the Quincke, Whitacre, and Sprotte. (From Peterman SB. Postmyelography headache rates with Whitacre versus Quincke 22-gauge spinal needles. *Radiology* 1996;200:771–778, with permission.)

Management

Table 12-4 lists the treatments available for PLPH. Recumbent position relieves the headache but is inconvenient. Relief usually occurs within 20 seconds but can be delayed for up to 15 minutes. The longer the patient is upright, the longer the headache takes to resolve when supine. For more severe or persistent

Table 12-4.   Treatments for post–lumbar puncture headaches

Initial or for mild headache
    Bedrest
    Caffeine 300 mg orally every 6–8 hours or
    Theophylline 300 mg orally every 8 hours
Moderate to severe headache present for more than 24 hours
    Bedrest
    Caffeine sodium benzoate 500 mg slow intravenous bolus
    Epidural blood patch

headaches, there are other effective treatments for PLPH.[54] Analgesics are usually not helpful.

Caffeine and Theophylline

The methylxanthines caffeine and theophylline may relieve PLPH. The mechanism may be blockade of cerebral adenosine receptors leading to intracerebral arterial constriction, resulting in a decrease of cerebral blood flow and intracranial pressure or increased CSF production by stimulating the sodium-potassium pump. Oral caffeine, 300 mg every 4 to 6 hours (in tablet form or in beverages), is worthwhile trying initially for PLPH,[55] although the relief may be transient. In a study of postpartum women with PLPH as a complication of epidural anesthetics, a single oral dose of 300 mg of caffeine reduced headache intensity within 4 hours in 90% of patients, with improvement persisting for 24 hours in 70%.[56] A slow intravenous bolus of 500 mg of caffeine sodium benzoate may initially relieve headache in 75%, but permanent relief occurs in only about 50%.[57] Intravenous caffeine should be used with caution in patients with coronary artery disease and seizure disorders. In a pilot study, sustained-release theophylline (281.7 mg of theophylline) given orally three times per day also reduced the intensity of PLPH.[58]

Epidural Blood Patch

The epidural blood patch (EBP) is the most effective treatment for PLPH and is indicated for patients with moderate to severe headache present for more than 24 hours. The success rate is about 85% after one injection and near 98% after a second.[59] The EBP is performed by slowly injecting 10 to 20 ml of the patient's blood into the lumbar epidural space at the same interspace or the interspace below the prior puncture. Following the procedure, the patient should stay in the decubitus position for at least 1 hour, and preferably for 2 hours, to obtain maximum benefit.

Based on a MRI study, the EBP has a mass effect that compresses the dural sac and displaces the conus medullaris and cauda equina.[60] The mass effect disappeared after 7 hours. The main bulk of the clot occupied four or five vertebral levels with a thinner spread cephalad and caudad. The presumed mechanism of action is an immediate gelatinous tamponade of the dural hole.[61] Alternative hypotheses include a sudden increase in CSF pressure that antagonizes adenosine receptors and compression of the dural sac, leading to activation of adrenergic, cholinergic, or peptidergic fibers.[62]

Side effects of EBP are usually mild and transient. In a retrospective study of 196 patients, the following percentages reported various side effects: 37%, pain at the site of injection; 12%, pain in the lower extremities; 10%, sensory disturbances in the lower extremities; 8%, walking disturbances; and 8%, weakness in the lower extremities.[63] The low back pain usually resolves from within 1 to 3 days. Potential complications include infection and arachnoiditis. Spinal subdural hematoma is a rare complication of EBP.

HEAD, EAR, NOSE, AND THROAT (HEENT) DISORDERS

Painful Ophthalmoplegias

With the exceptions of myasthenia gravis and chronic progressive external ophthalmoplegia, ophthalmoplegias[64,65] can cause unilateral orbitofrontal pain. The possible causes are extensive and include lesions from the midbrain to the orbit (Table 12-5). Ophthalmoplegic migraine is further discussed in Chapter 7.

Clinical Manifestations

Orbital pseudotumor and Tolosa-Hunt syndrome, which are inflammatory disorders of unknown etiology, have overlapping features. Orbital pseudotumor may be diffuse or localized to extraocular muscles, sclera, or the lacrimal gland and may cause uveitis or optic neuropathy. Unlike Tolosa-Hunt syndrome, orbital signs are often present in orbital pseudotumor, including

Table 12-5.   Conditions causing painful ophthalmoplegia*

Vascular
  Arterial: hypertension, diabetes, carotid dissection, internal carotid aneurysm, posterior communicating aneurysm,† pituitary apoplexy, midbrain infarction†
  Venous: cavernous sinus thrombosis, carotid-cavernous fistula, dural-cavernous shunt
Inflammatory
  Granulomatous: sarcoid, Wegener's granulomatosis, Tolosa-Hunt syndrome
  Dysimmune: systemic lupus erythematosus, rheumatoid arthritis,† mixed connective-tissue disorder, necrotizing vasculitis, temporal arteritis, multiple sclerosis,† segmental Guillain-Barré syndrome, chronic inflammatory demyelinating polyneuropathy†
  Parainfectious/postinfectious: Epstein-Barr virus,† mycoplasma,† herpes simplex,† herpes zoster, idiopathic cranial polyneuropathy
  Infectious: mucormycosis, aspergillosis, syphilis, tuberculosis, Lyme disease
Neoplastic
  Solid: epidermoid, meningioma, craniopharyngioma, chordoma,† chondrosarcoma, hemangioma, hemangiopericytoma, pituitary adenoma, metastases
  Hematologic: lymphoma, macroglobulinemia, lymphoid hyperplasia
  Meningeal carcinomatosis
Other
  Ophthalmoplegic migraine

From Averbuch-Heller L, Daroff RB. Painful ophthalmoplegias, Tolosa-Hunt syndrome, and ophthalmoplegic migraine. In: Goadsby PJ, Silberstein SD, eds. *Headache.* Boston: Butterworth-Heinemann, 1997:287, with permission.
*All may result in combined painful ophthalmoplegia
†This condition usually involves a single ocular motor nerve

unilateral lid swelling or ptosis, globe protrusion or displacement, and a palpable or visible orbital mass. Tolosa-Hunt syndrome is a recurrent granulomatous inflammation in the cavernous sinus and superior orbital fissure. The ipsilateral optic, oculomotor, trochlear, abducens, and first two divisions of the trigeminal nerve may be involved either singly or in different combinations. The pupil may be dilated or sluggish. The pain in both, which is ipsilateral to the involved side, is most intense in the orbit, brow, or directly in or behind the eye. The pain of Tolosa-Hunt may radiate to the ipsilateral frontal, temporal, or occipital areas. Both conditions respond to corticosteroids.

Diagnostic Evaluation

The diagnosis of both is one of exclusion using CT and MRI scans of the brain and orbit. Orbital pseudotumor may demonstrate infiltration of retrobulbar fat, enlargement of extraocular muscles, thickening of the optic nerve sheath complex, and proptosis. Imaging studies in Tolosa-Hunt syndrome may show soft-tissue infiltration in either the orbital apex or the cavernous sinus without bony changes.

Ophthalmologic Disorders

Refractive errors, imbalance of the extraocular muscles, diplopia, and a new refraction can cause tension-type headaches.[66,67] However, the eye is rarely responsible for headache localized to the eye and orbit without obvious signs, such as a red eye; symptoms, such as decreased vision; or a history of eye trauma. The exceptions to the maxim that a white eye is not the cause of a monosymptomatic painful eye or headache are the following: optic neuritis, where pain on eye movement may precede visual loss; the first 30 minutes of acute angle-closure glaucoma, where the eye may hurt before the cornea clouds; subacute angle-closure glaucoma; and posterior scleritis (Table 12-6).

Clinical Manifestations

Pain in or behind the eye or brow occurs in 77% of cases of optic neuritis and can precede visual loss. The pain can be present at rest, with voluntary movement, and with pressure on the globe. Eye movement worsens the pain because of traction of the superior and medial recti on the optic nerve sheath at the orbital apex.

Acute angle-closure glaucoma presents with the rapid onset of severe orbitofrontal pain, nausea, vomiting, photophobia, visual halos, and loss of vision. A decreased level of consciousness may be present. Examination reveals a red eye, hazy cornea, fixed and mid-dilated pupil, and markedly elevated intraocular pressure. Chronic angle-closure glaucoma does not cause headache

Table 12-6. Causes of a white eye and monosymptomatic ocular pain or headache

Optic neuritis when pain on eye movement precedes visual loss

The first 30 minutes of acute angle-closure glaucoma

Subacute angle-closure glaucoma

Posterior scleritis

or a red eye. The presentation is visual loss due to a gradual elevation of intraocular pressure.

Subacute angle-closure glaucoma (SACG) is uncommon. Episodes of nausea, vomiting, blurred vision, facial pain, or headache last 1 to 4 hours and may occur at any time of the day or night. The headache may be in or over the eye or temporal. The eye is usually normal in appearance. Intraocular pressure measurement is normal between attacks. Gonioscopy (use of a mirrored prism on the surface of the eye) makes the diagnosis and reveals peripheral anterior synechiae, pathologic adhesions between the iris and trabecular meshwork tissue, which close the outflow chamber of the eye and raise intraocular pressure. The symptoms of SACG can be misdiagnosed as due to migraine, cluster headache, or temporal arteritis.

In addition to acute angle-closure glaucoma, there are many other causes of a red eye (Table 12-7). The uveal tract is the pigmented middle ocular tissue, the iris, ciliary body, and choroid. About 50% of patients with uveitis have pure anterior involvement, iritis. The presentation of acute disease includes ocular pain, photophobia, miosis, and decreased vision. A subacute onset is often asymptomatic. Causes include rheumatologic disorders (psoriatic arthritis, Reiter's syndrome, juvenile chronic arthritis), sarcoidosis, postoperative trauma, Kawasaki disease, Behcet's syndrome, syphilis, and herpesvirus.

About 50% of patients with uveitis will have posterior involvement, chorioretinitis, with inflammation of the ciliary body and/or choroid. Posterior uveitis is more likely to cause visual loss than anterior disease and produces blurred vision, scotomas, and floaters. Toxoplasmosis is the most common cause. There are numerous infectious causes of panuveitis. Pars planitis is associated with multiple sclerosis.

Inflammation of the sclera (scleritis) produces a violaceous hue of the sclera, a tender globe to touch, and fixed blood vessels to the globe. Severe and piercing referred pain to the jaw and forehead is usually present. About 50% of cases are idiopathic with other causes, including herpes simplex virus, herpes zoster, and collagen vascular disease. Posterior scleritis, a rare disorder, usually presents with pain, proptosis, ptosis, lid edema, and

Table 12-7. Differential diagnosis of red eye

Conjunctivitis, the most common cause
  Infectious (bacterial and viral), allergic, and sicca syndromes
Trauma
Iritis
Keratopathy, including corneal ulcer
Scleritis
Episcleritis
Subconjunctival hemorrhage
Periocular or orbital cellulitis
Angle-closure glaucoma
Blepharitis, inflammation of the lid margins

decreased vision but can present with only ocular pain. Episcleritis presents more acutely and with milder pain than scleritis.

Preseptal cellulitis involves the lids and structures anterior to the orbital septum. Orbital cellulitis, which is an infection of tissues posterior to the septum, can cause conjunctival infection and chemosis; proptosis with restricted ocular motility and pain; and optic nerve findings with decreased acuity and color vision and an afferent pupillary defect.

Ophthalmodynia

More than 60% of patients with ophthalmodynia (benign, brief, jabbing, unilateral eye pain) are migraineurs. Similar pain can occur with cluster headaches and temporal arteritis.

Nose and Paranasal Sinus Disorders

Introduction and Epidemiology

Nose and paranasal sinus disorders[68-70] are often misdiagnosed as the cause of headaches by lay persons and some physicians, perhaps the result of the ubiquitous sinus medication commercials and ads. Many of the 60% of persons with unrecognized migraines attribute their symptoms to sinusitis. However, disorders of the nose and paranasal sinuses are common and can cause headaches. The term *rhinosinusitis* may be more accurate than *sinusitis* because rhinitis usually precedes sinusitis, the mucosa of the nose and sinuses are contiguous, symptoms of nasal obstruction and discharge are common in sinusitis, and sinusitis without rhinitis is rare.

The lifetime prevalence of headaches associated with disorders of the nose and sinuses is 15%. About 50% of patients presenting to ear, nose, and throat (ENT) physicians with symptoms of sinusitis complain of severe headaches. About 70% of patients with chronic sinusitis requiring surgery have headaches. Sinusitis affects more than 30 million people per year in the United States. It is a complication of about 0.5% of upper-respiratory infections in adults. Sinusitis is more common in children than in adults. It rarely involves the frontal and sphenoid sinuses in children because of the late development of these sinuses (the sphenoid sinus starts to pneumatize at 8 years of age and the frontal sinuses develop from the anterior ethmoid sinus at about 6 years of age) but is involved in teenagers. Radiographic evidence of sinusitis is present in about 40% of adults without symptoms as an incidental finding.

Clinical Manifestations

Acute sinusitis lasts from 1 day to 4 weeks; subacute sinusitis, from 4 to 12 weeks; and chronic sinusitis, for more than 12 weeks. The headaches associated with sinusitis are usually continuous.

The location of the pain and the position that improves the headache vary, depending on the sinus involved (Table 12-8). Nasal congestion, purulent nasal drainage, and facial tenderness and pain are commonly present in acute sinusitis. Fever is present in 50% of adults and 60% of children. Anosmia, pain on mastication, and halitosis may also be present.

The pain of acute maxillary sinusitis is usually in the cheek, the gums, and the maxillary teeth. Less often, the pain is in the

Table 12-8. Possible locations of pain and position that improves pain in acute sinusitis

Paranasal sinus	Possible locations of pain	Position which improves pain
Maxillary	Cheek, gums, maxillary teeth	Lying supine
	Periorbital, supraorbital, temporal	
Frontal	Frontal	Head upright
Ethmoid	Periorbital, retroorbital, temporal, inner canthal area, midline behind the nose	Head upright
Sphenoid	Retroorbital, occipital, frontal, temporal, vertex	Head upright

periorbital, supraorbital, or temporal areas. The pain is improved when supine and worse when the head is upright. The maxillary sinus is tender to palpation. Maxillary sinusitis is usually accompanied by rhinitis.

Acute frontal sinusitis causes severe frontal headaches with tenderness over the frontal sinus on percussion or palpation. The pain is less when the head is upright and worse when it is supine. Frontal sinusitis can result in brain abscess, meningitis, subdural or epidural abscess, osteomyelitis, subperiosteal abscess, orbital edema, orbital cellulitis, and orbital abscess.

Acute sphenoid sinusitis is responsible for 3% of all cases of acute sinusitis and is usually associated with pansinusitis. Headache is always present and may be frontal, occipital, temporal, or a combination and periorbital. Vertex headache is rare. The pain is less when upright and worse when the head is supine. The headache may be aggravated by standing, walking, bending, or coughing; is frequently associated with nausea and vomiting; and may interfere with sleep. Nasal discharge and drainage are present in only about 30% of patients. Fever occurs in more than 50% of patients. Photophobia and eye tearing may be present. The headache and associated symptoms may lead to a misdiagnosis of migraine, meningitis, trigeminal neuralgia, or brain tumor. Complications of sphenoid sinusitis include bacterial meningitis, cavernous sinus thrombosis, subdural abscess, cortical vein thrombosis, ophthalmoplegia, and pituitary insufficiency. A parameningeal focus may cause an aseptic meningitis.

Acute ethmoid sinusitis typically produces pain in the periorbital, retroorbital, temporal, inner canthal area or between the eyes. Coughing, straining, or lying supine can worsen the pain, whereas keeping the head upright lessens it. Ethmoid sinusitis is usually associated with rhinitis. Complications of ethmoid sinusitis include meningitis, orbital cellulitis, cavernous sinus thrombosis, and cortical vein thrombosis.

Headaches associated with chronic sinusitis are usually low grade and diffuse and are often accompanied by nasal obstruction, congestion, and fullness. Symptoms often increase during the day. A nighttime cough can be present.

Numerous anatomic variants in the nose and paranasal sinuses can be seen on endoscopic examination, CT scan, or both and are reported as causing headaches that improve with surgery (Table 12-9).[71] For example, the headache associated with a septal spur is reported as mild to moderate, frontal or facial, and dull or deep with fullness or heaviness. Anatomic variants as a cause of headaches are controversial. Because both anatomic variants and primary headaches are common, a primary headache can be misattributed as due to an anatomic variant. In addition, daily headaches can develop from overuse of decongestants or analgesics. Surgery can also have a placebo effect.

A mucocele or mucous retention cyst is a mucus-containing cyst in the sinus. Those in the frontal, sphenoid, and ethmoid sinuses can enlarge and erode into surrounding structures. Mucoceles are most common in the maxillary sinus, where they are usually benign.

Biologic Mechanisms

Normal sinuses contain anaerobic bacteria, and more than one-third have a mix of anaerobes and aerobes. Aerobes present include Gram-positive streptococci (alpha, beta, and *Streptococcus pneumoniae*) and *Staphylococcus aureus*, and Gram-negative *Moraxella catarrhalis, Hemophilus influenzae*, and *Escherichia coli*. Anaerobes include Gram-positive peptococci and *Propionibac-*

Table 12-9.   Anatomic variations in the nose and paranasal sinuses reported as causes of headaches

Septal deviation/spurs

Agger nasi cells

Uncinate process
  Medially or laterally bent
  Curved anteriorly
  Contacting middle turbinate
  Pneumatized

Middle turbinate
  Concha bullosa (pneumatized middle turbinate)
  Paradoxically bent
  Bulging into lateral nasal wall

Ethmoid bulla
  Large, filling middle meatus
  Anterior growth, overlapping hiatus semilunaris or protruding
    from middle meatus

Sphenoid sinus lesions
  Cysts, polyps, or mucoceles
  Mycotic infection

Maxillary sinus disease
  Cysts, polyps or mucosal disease in contact with infraorbital
    nerve

From Close LG, Aviv J. Headaches and disease of the nose and paranasal sinuses. *Semin Neurol* 1997;17:351–354.

terium species. The *Bacteroides* and *Fusobacterium* species can cause chronic sinusitis. Obstruction of the ostia can result in ciliary dysfunction and retention of secretions, bacterial proliferation, and sinusitis.

Risk factors for sinusitis include systemic diseases (cystic fibrosis, immune deficiency, bronchiectasis, and the immobile cilia syndrome) and local factors (upper-respiratory infection, allergic rhinitis, overuse of topical decongestants, hypertrophied adenoids, deviated nasal septum, nasal polyps, tumors, and cigarette smoke). The sinuses are involved in nearly 90% of viral upper-respiratory infections and usually clear spontaneously.

Diagnostic Evaluation

Plain sinus radiographs can diagnose acute maxillary or frontal sinusitis but are often inadequate for ethmoid or sphenoid sinusitis. CT scans of the sinuses without contrast in the coronal plain are highly sensitive for the detection of nasal and paranasal sinus disease, including the ethmoid and sphenoid sinuses. Routine CT scan of the head may inadequately cover these structures. Because a MRI scan of the brain will also visualize nasal and paranasal sinus structures, MRI is the study of choice for the evaluation of headaches.

MRI is more sensitive than CT scan for the detection of fungal infection and the evaluation of nasal or paranasal sinus neoplasms. MRI is highly sensitive on T2-weighted images for the detection of retained fluid and inflamed tissue of the sinuses and may lead to an exaggeration of the significance of minimal sinus disease such as mild inflammation, small polyps, and retention cysts. In some cases on MRI, chronic sinusitis can mimic a tumor or an air-filled sinus. CT scan is the preferred examination when inflammatory sinus disease is suspected.

Transillumination and ultrasonography of the sinuses have low sensitivity and specificity. Diagnostic endoscopy with the flexible fiberoptic rhinoscope permits direct visualization of the nasal passages and sinus drainage areas. This procedure is complementary to a CT or MRI scan.

Management

Treatment of acute sinusitis includes a decongestant (phenylpropanolamine), mucoevacuant (guiafenesine), steam, saline, and appropriate antibiotics for at least 10 to 14 days. Intranasal steroids may improve the symptoms of nasal obstruction, but antihistamines are not helpful. Acute frontal and sphenoid sinusitis require immediate referral to an otolaryngologist for appropriate treatment to avoid intracranial complications.

The initial treatment of chronic sinusitis is the same as that for acute sinusitis. Otolaryngology consultation should be considered when the symptoms are not relieved with at least two consecutive 2-week courses of treatment.

Temporomandibular Disorders

Introduction and Epidemiology

The pain of migraine, cluster headache, chronic paroxysmal hemicrania, trigeminal neuralgia, and cough headache can be referred to oromandibular structures, including the teeth.[72,73]

Conversely, pain from the temporomandibular joint (TMJ) and associated musculature and ligaments—temporomandibular disorders (TMD)—can be referred to the head. TMD are common in the general population, with at least one sign present in 75% and at least one symptom in 33%. The lifetime prevalence of TMD is up to 69%. Women report symptoms of TMD 2.1 times more often than men. Only 5% of patients with signs of TMD require treatment, and fewer than 5% have associated headache.

Clinical Manifestations

Pain—usually localized in the muscles of mastication, the preauricular area, or the TMJ—is the most common presenting symptom of TMD. It is usually aggravated by jaw function. Because both the ear and TMJ have sensory innervation from the auriculotemporal nerve, otalgia is a common initial symptom of TMD. Signs include limited or asymmetric jaw movements, joint noise on movement, and locking on opening. Joint noises, such as clicking and crepitus on movement (caused by poor lubrication in the joint associated with inflammation, arthritis, or a slipped disc), are also very common in asymptomatic subjects. TMJ joint displacement also occurs in up to 38% of asymptomatic people. Because TMD and headache are both so common, it can be easy to misattribute headache as due to TMD.

The extraoral examination includes palpation of the TMJ both laterally (the lateral capsule of the TMJ) and endaurally (the posterior recess and capsule of the TMJ) for tenderness. Mandibular range of motion can be measured vertically and laterally. The maximum vertical opening, measured with a ruler from the incisal edge of the upper and lower central incisors, normally ranges from 35 to 55 mm. Deviation of the mandibular midline to one side is usually due to a failure of the condyle to slide forward on the side to which the chin is deviating. Lateral excursion distance to the right and left, measured from the midline of the maxillary central incisors to the midline of the mandibular central incisor teeth, usually ranges from 8 to 15 mm. Protrusive or forward mandibular movements can also be measured.

Biologic Mechanisms

The TMJ is a diarthrodial synovial joint with two compartments separated by a fibrous disc. Rotation of the condyle within the fossa occurs with the first 25 mm of mouth opening. Then translation of the disc condyle complex along the articular complex allows for the second 25 mm of mouth opening.

There are numerous disorders which can cause TMD, including the following: synovitis, which can be due to excessive loading of the joint; myofascial pain, which can be associated with stress, grinding the teeth, and bruxism; osteoarthritis with roughened articular surfaces and worn-away cartilage; anterior disc displacement; adhesions, which can be due to trauma, synovitis, and lack of mobility; bony ankylosis, which can be due to trauma, infection, previous placement of TMJ implants or arthropathies; systemic arthropathies, including rheumatoid arthritis, Lyme disease, systemic lupus erythematosis, psoriatic arthritis, and gouty arthritis; and other conditions, such as tumors of the mandibular condyle, trigeminal neuropathy, parotid tumors, carcinoma with invasion of the pterygoid muscles, and traumatic condylar or subcondylar fractures.

Myofascial pain is the most common cause of pain arising from the TMJ. Malocclusion as a cause of TMD and headache is a controversial topic, with proponents arguing for and against an etiologic role.

Diagnostic Evaluation

Tomograms of the maxilla and mandible, including open and closed position views of bilateral TMJs, and a panoramic radiograph are useful for diagnosing bony pathology. CT scan of the TMJs is useful for further defining bony pathology, such as tumors, bony/fibrous ankylosis, and osteoarthritis. MRI can diagnose soft-tissue and other pathology, including synovial joint effusion, osteoarthritis, and disc displacement.

Management

TMD usually responds to conservative reversible therapies. An oral appliance or bite plate, which fits between the upper and lower teeth, relieves pressure or unloads the TMJ by creating a space between the upper and lower teeth. Forces are distributed throughout the dental arch. The appliance is placed in the mouth at night and sometimes during the day. A soft diet and the application of moist heat help to relieve exacerbations of TMD. Physical therapy may be worthwhile initially; then the patient can continue passive jaw motion exercises and apply moist heat, ice, or both at home. Clenching or grinding habits may be reversed in some cases with patient education. Other patients may benefit from stress reduction techniques, such as biofeedback. Medications such as nonsteroidal antiinflammatory drugs, muscle relaxants, tricyclic antidepressants, and the judicious use of narcotics can also be helpful.

When conservative treatment fails and the patient's TMJ symptoms are significant, surgery is indicated for a small percentage of cases. TMJ arthroscopy can be used for removal of fibrous adhesions and osteoarthritic cartilage, in cases of an anterior displaced disc without reduction (closed lock), and for steroid injection of inflamed synovial membranes. TMJ arthrotomy or open-joint surgery may be indicated for more advanced cases with obliteration of the joint space with adhesions and/or bone and for neoplasia.

Dental Disease

Dental disease uncommonly causes headache. Pericoronitis, infection or traumatic irritation around a partially erupted tooth, usually a molar, is the most common periodontal inflammation causing headache. Less often, pulpitis causes headache. Apical root infection or dental caries can cause a neuralgic pain in the second or third trigeminal divisions, with a constant aching and paroxysmal, jabbing pains. Hot or cold liquids in the mouth worsen the pain. Maxillary pain can be due to dental disease and maxillary sinusitis. Atypical odontalgia is pain in a tooth or tooth site in the absence of a detectable organic cause.

Atypical Facial Pain

Atypical facial pain[74] often affects patients in their fourth and fifth decades and is more common in women than in men. The pain has a steady, diffuse quality—described as deep, aching, pulling, boring, or gnawing—and can last hours or days. The pain is usually not limited to the distribution of the fifth or ninth cranial nerves and can spread over the areas supplied by the cervical root. The most common locations are the nasolabial fold or the chin overlying the lower gum. Atypical facial pain often begins after a dental procedure or insignificant facial trauma. Trigger zones are rare. The attacks are not precipitated by swallowing, cold water in the mouth, talking, or chewing. The pain is often refractive to analgesics, nerve blocks, and surgical intervention.

The diagnosis is made after excluding disorders of the eyes, nose, teeth, sinuses, and pharynx, including nasopharyngeal cancer as well as neuralgias and facial migraine. Depending on the symptoms, evaluation may include examinations by ophthalmologists, ENT physicians, dentists, and neurologists, and imaging studies, such as panorama radiographs and MRI scans of the head. A variety of medications can be used, such as antidepressants and baclofen, as well as behavioral and pain clinic approaches.

Gradenigo's Syndrome

Lesions of the apex of the petrous temporal bone, such as middle ear infections and tumors, can cause pain referred to the frontotemporal region and ear associated with a sixth cranial nerve palsy.

Eagle's Syndrome

Eagle's syndrome[75] is an uncommon disorder due to an elongated styloid process. (Either the styloid process alone or the combined lengths of the process and stylohyoid or stylomandibular ligaments exceed 40 mm.) Symptoms include dysphagia and unilateral pharyngeal pain radiating to the ear, which is worse with swallowing. Digital palpation (either through the pharynx or externally in the region of the mandibular angle) of an elongated styloid process can precipitate or increase pain.

There are numerous conditions in the differential diagnosis, including the following: neuralgias (glossopharyngeal, superior laryngeal, occipital, and nervus intermedius), migraine, cervicogenic headache, carotidynia, oromandibular disorders (TMJ disorders, unerupted or distorted third molar, faulty dental prostheses, and sialolithiasis), and ENT disorders (chronic tonsillitis, tonsillar calculi, otitis, mastoiditis, fracture of the hyoid bone, spasm of the pharyngeal constrictor muscle, Ernest syndrome, pterygoid hamulus bursitis, elongated pterygoid uncinus), and others (psychosomatic, foreign bodies, inflammatory and neoplastic diseases, nuchal cellulitis and fibrositis, and neck-tongue syndrome).

Some patients with Eagle's syndrome may respond to transpharyngeal injection of steroid and local anesthetic at the hyoid bone's inferior cornu or into the inferior tonsillar fossa. Surgical excision (there are advocates for both an intraoral and extraoral approach) often relieves the pain. In some cases, the styloid process may regenerate.

Neck-Tongue Syndrome

Neck-tongue syndrome is an uncommon disorder character-ized by acute unilateral occipital pain and numbness of the ipsi-lateral tongue precipitated by sudden movement, usually rota-tion, of the head.[76,77] The symptoms are due to transient subluxation of the atlantoaxial joint that stretches the joint cap-sule and the C2 ventral ramus (which contains proprioceptive fibers from the tongue originating from the lingual nerve to the hypoglossal nerve to the C2 root). Although neck-tongue syn-drome can occur without obvious abnormalities, associated dis-orders include degenerative spondylosis, ankylosing spondylitis, psoriatic arthritis, and genetically determined laxity of liga-ments of joint capsules.

The Red Ear Syndrome

Some patients with TMD, glossopharyngeal neuralgia, or irrita-tion of the third cervical root may have episodic burning pain in one ear lobe, with associated reddening of the ear.[78] Touch or heat can cause a similar problem in some people without any apparent structural disorders. The cause is uncertain. ABC (angry backfir-ing C-nociceptor) syndrome is a hypothesized cause with pain and increased ear temperature due to antidromic release of vasodila-tor peptides.

Ice Cream Headache

Ice cream headache (cold stimulus headache) can result from swallowing or holding in the mouth a cold food, beverage, or ice. This can cause shortlasting moderate to severe pain in the palate and throat that can be referred to the forehead, temple, or ears. The pain is usually bilateral but can be unilateral. The average onset of the pain is 12.5 seconds after the cold stimulus, and the average duration is 21 seconds.[79] Occasionally, later-onset and longer-duration pain can occur.

ACKNOWLEDGMENT

Larry P. Conrad is appreciated for reviewing the section on nose and paranasal sinus disease.

REFERENCES

1. Patchell RA. Metastatic brain tumors. *Neurol Clin* 1995;13: 915–925.
2. Vasquez-Barquero A, Ibanez FJ, Herrera S, et al. Isolated head-ache as the presenting clinical manifestation of intracranial tumors: a prospective study. *Cephalalgia* 1994;14:270–272.
3. Forsyth PA, Posner JB. Headaches in patients with brain tumors: a study of 111 patients. *Neurology* 1993;43:1678–1683.
3a. Pfund Z, Szapary L, Jaszbernyi O, et al. Headache in intracra-nial tumors. *Cephalalgia* 1999;19:787–790.
4. Suwanwela N, Phanthumchinda K, Kaoropthum S. Headache in brain tumor: a cross-sectional study. *Headache* 1994;34:435–438.
5. Abe T, Matsumoto K, Kuwazawa J, et al. Headache associated with pituitary adenomas. *Headache* 1998;38:782–786.
6. Milos P, Havelius U, Hindfelt B. Clusterlike headache in a patient with a pituitary adenoma. With a review of the litera-ture. *Headache* 1996;35:184–188.

7. Friedman AH, Wilkins RH, Kenan PD, et al. Pituitary adenoma presenting as facial pain: report of two cases and review of the literature. *Neurosurgery* 1982;10:742–745.

8. Selky AK, Pascuzzi R. Raeder's paratrigeminal syndrome due to spontaneous dissection of the cervical and petrous internal carotid artery. *Headache* 1995;35:432–435.

9. Brines ML. Pituitary apoplexy. In: Gilman S, Goldstein GW, Waxman SG, eds. *Neurobase*. San Diego: Arbor, 2000.

10. Rolih CA, Ober KP. Pituitary apoplexy. *Endocrinol Metab Clin North Am* 1993;22:291–302.

11. Haviv YS, Goldschmidt N, Safadi R. Pituitary apoplexy manifested by sterile meningitis. *Eur J Med Res* 1998;12:263–264.

12. Silvestrini M, Matteis M, Cupini LM, et al. Ophthalmoplegic migraine-like syndrome due to pituitary apoplexy. *Headache* 1994;34:484–486.

13. Evans RW. Migraine-like headaches associated with pituitary hemorrhage. *Headache* 1997;37:455–456.

14. Junck L. Leptomeningeal metastasis. In: Gilman S, Goldstein GW, Waxman SG, eds. *Neurobase*. San Diego: Arbor, 2000.

15. Wasserstrom W, Glass J, Posner J. Diagnosis and treatment of leptomeningeal metastases from solid tumors: experience with 90 patients. *Cancer* 1982;49:759–772.

16. Recht LD. Colloid cysts. In: Gilman S, Goldstein GW, Waxman SG, eds. *Neurobase*. San Diego: Arbor, 2000.

17. Young WB, Silberstein SD. Paroxysmal headache caused by colloid cyst of the third ventricle: case report and review of the literature. *Headache* 1997;37:15–20.

18. Mathiesen T, Grane P, Lindgren L, Lindquist C. Third ventricular colloid cysts: a consecutive 12-year series. *J Neurosurg* 1997;86:5–12.

19. Friedman DI. Pseudotumor cerebri. In: Gilman S, Goldstein GW, Waxman SG, eds. *Neurobase*. San Diego: Arbor, 2000.

20. Silberstein SD, Lipton RB, Goadsby PJ. Headache associated with non-vascular intracranial disease. In: *Headache in clinical practice*. Oxford: Isis, 1998:143–164.

21. Balcer LJ, Liu GT, Forman S, et al. Idiopathic intracranial hypertension: relation of age and obesity in children. *Neurology* 1999;52:870–872.

22. Scott IU, Siatkowsky RM, Eneyni M, et al. Idiopathic intracranial hypertension in children and adolescents. *Am J Ophthalmol* 1997;124:253–255.

23. Chiu AM, Chuenkongkaew WL, Cornblath WT, et al. Minocycline treatment and pseudotumor cerebri syndrome. *Am J Ophthalmol* 1998;126:116–121.

24. Keren T, Lahat E. Pseudotumor cerebri as a presenting symptom of acute sinusitis in a child. *Pediatr Neurol* 1998;19:153–154.

25. Kan L, Sood KS, Maytal J. Pseudotumor cerebri in Lyme disease: a case report and literature review. *Pediatr Neurol* 1998;18:439–441.

26. Wang SJ, Silberstein SD, Patterson S, et al. Idiopathic intracranial hypertension without papilledema: a case-control study in a headache center. *Neurology* 1998;51:245–249.

27. Jacome DE. Headaches, idiopathic intracranial hypertension, and pseudopapilledema. *Am J Med Sci* 1998;316:408–410.

28. Brodsky MC, Vaphiades M. Magnetic resonance imaging in pseudotumor cerebri. *Ophthalmology* 1998;105:1686–1693.
29. Kupersmith MJ, Garnell L, Turbin R, et al. Effects of weight loss on the course of idiopathic intracranial hypertension in women. *Neurology* 1998;50:1094–1098.
30. Corbett JJ. Headache due to idiopathic intracranial hypertension. In: Goadsby PJ, Silberstein SD, eds. *Headache.* Boston: Butterworth-Heinemann, 1997:279–283.
31. Kelman SE, Heaps R, Wolf A, et al. Optic nerve decompression surgery improves visual function in patients with pseudotumor cerebri. *Neurosurgery* 1992;30:391–395.
32. Corbett JJ, Nerad JA, Tse DT, et al. Results of optic nerve sheath fenestration for pseudotumor cerebri: the lateral orbitotomy approach. *Arch Ophthalmol* 1988;106:1391.
33. Burgett RA, Purvin VA, Kawasaki A. Lumboperitoneal shunting for pseudotumor cerebri. *Neurology* 1997;49:734–739.
34. Lay CL, Campbell JK, Mokri B. Low cerebrospinal fluid pressure headache. In: Goadsby PJ, Silberstein SD, eds. *Headache.* Boston: Butterworth-Heinemann, 1997:355–367.
35. Mokri B, Piepgras DG, Miller GM. Syndrome of orthostatic headaches and diffuse pachymeningeal gadolinium enhancement. *Mayo Clin Proc* 1997;72:400–413.
36. Ferrante E, Riva M, Gatti A, et al. Intracranial hypotension syndrome: neuroimaging in five spontaneous cases and etiopathogenetic correlations. *Clin Neurol Neurosurg* 1998;100:33–39.
37. Beck CE, Rizk NW, Kiger LT, et al. Intracranial hypotension presenting with severe encephalopathy: case report. *J Neurosurg* 1998;89:470–473.
38. Mokri B, Hunter SF, Atkinson JL, et al. Orthostatic headaches caused by CSF leak but with normal CSF pressures. *Neurology* 1998;51:786–790.
38a. Chen CC, Luo CL, Wang SJ, at al. Colour Doppler imaging for diagnosis of intracranial hypotension. *Lancet* 1999;354:826–829.
39. Atkinson JLD, Weinshenker BG, Miller GM, et al. Acquired Chiari I malformation secondary to spontaneous cerebrospinal fluid leakage and chronic intracranial hypotension syndrome in seven cases. *J Neurosurg* 88:237–242, 1998.
40. Iqbal J, Davis LE, Orrison WW. An MRI study of lumbar puncture headaches. *Headache* 1995;35:420–422.
41. Evans RW. Complications of lumbar puncture. *Neurol Clin* 1998;16:83–105.
42. Kuntz KM, Kokmen E, Stevens JC, et al. Post-lumbar puncture headaches: experience in 501 consecutive patients. *Neurology* 1992;42:1884–1887.
43. Hilton-Jones D, Harrad RA, Gill MW, et al. Failure of postural maneuvers to prevent lumbar puncture headache. *J Neurol Neurosurg Psychiatry* 1982;45:743–746.
44. Cook PT, Davies MJ, Beavis RE. Bed rest and postlumbar puncture headache. The effectiveness of 24 hours' recumbency in reducing the incidence of postlumbar puncture headache. *Anaesthesia* 1989;44:389–391.
45. Spriggs DA, Burn DJ, French J, et al. Is bed rest useful after diagnostic lumbar puncture? *Postgrad Med J* 1992;68:518–583.

46. Vilming ST, Schrader H, Monstad I. Post-lumbar puncture headache: the significance of body posture. A controlled study of 300 patients. *Cephalalgia* 1988;8:75–78.
47. Dieterich M, Brandt T. Incidence of post lumbar puncture headache is independent of daily fluid intake. *Eur Arch Psychiatry Neurol Sci* 1988;237:194–195.
48. Fishman RA. Cerebrospinal fluid in diseases of the nervous system, 2nd ed. Philadelphia: WB Saunders, 1992.
49. Prager JM, Roychowdhury S, Gorey MT, et al. Spinal headaches after myelograms: comparison of needle types. *AJR* 1996;196:1289–1292.
50. Jeanjean P, Montpellier D, Carnec J, et al. Post-spinal headache: a prospective, multicentre study in young adults. *Ann Fr Anesth Reanim* 1997;16:350–353.
51. Strupp M, Brandt T. Should one reinsert the stylet during lumbar puncture? *N Engl J Med* 1997;336:1190.
52. Engelhardt A, Oheim S, Neundörfer B. Post-lumbar puncture headache: experiences with Sprotte's atraumatic needle. *Cephalalgia* 1992;12:259.
53. Jager H, Krane M, Schimrigk K. [Lumbar puncture: the post-puncture syndrome. Prevention with an "atraumatic" puncture needle, clinical observations.] *Schweiz Med Wochenschr* 1993;123:1985–1990.
54. Choi A, Launto CE, Cunningham FE. Pharmacologic management of postdural puncture headache. *Ann Pharmacother* 1996;30:832–839.
55. Leibold RA, Yealy DM, Coppola M, et al. Post-dural-puncture headache: characteristics, management, and prevention. *Ann Emerg Med* 1993;22:1863–1870.
56. Camann WR, Murray RS, Mushlin PS, et al. Effects of oral caffeine on postdural puncture headache: a double-blind, placebo-controlled trial. *Anesth Analg* 1990;70:181–184.
57. Sechzer PH, Abel L. Post-spinal anesthesia headache treated with caffeine: evaluation with demand method. Part 1. *Curr Ther Res* 1978;24:307–312.
58. Feuerstein TJ, Zeides A. Theophylline relieves headache following lumbar puncture: placebo-controlled, double-blind pilot study. *Klin Wochenschr* 1986;64:216–218.
59. Tarkkila PJ, Miralles JA, Palomaki EA. The subjective complications and efficiency of the epidural blood patch in the treatment of postdural puncture headache. *Reg Anesth Pain Med* 1989;14:247–250.
60. Beards SCD, Jackson A, Griffiths AG, et al. Magnetic resonance imaging of extradural blood patches: appearances from 30 min to 18 h. *Br J Anaesth* 1993;71:182–188.
61. Olsen KS. Epidural blood patch in the treatment of post-lumbar puncture headache. *Pain* 1987;30:293–301.
62. Raskin NH. Lumbar puncture headache: a review. *Headache* 1990;30:197–200.
63. Tarkkila PJ, Miralles JA, Palomaki EA. The subjective complications and efficiency of the epidural blood patch in the treatment of postdural puncture headache. *Reg Anesth Pain Med* 1989;14:247–250.
64. Averbuch-Heller L, Daroff RB. Painful ophthalmoplegias, Tolosa-Hunt syndrome, and ophthalmoplegic migraine. In:

Goadsby PJ, Silberstein SD, eds. *Headache,* Boston: Butterworth-Heinemann, 1997:285–297.

65. Goodwin J. Orbital pseudotumor and Tolosa-Hunt syndrome. In: Gilman S, Goldstein GW, Waxman SG, eds. *Neurobase.* San Diego: Arbor, 2000.

66. Lewis J, Fourman S. Subacute angle-closure glaucoma as a cause of headache in the presence of a white eye. *Headache* 1998;38:684–686.

67. Daroff RB. Ocular causes of headache. *Headache* 1998;38:661.

68. Close LG, Aviv J. Headaches and disease of the nose and paranasal sinuses. *Semin Neurol* 1997;17:351–354.

69. Evans KL. Recognition and management of sinusitis. *Drugs* 1998;56:59–71.

70. Silberstein SD. Sinus-related headache. In: Gilman S, Goldstein GW, Waxman SG, eds. *Neurobase.* San Diego: Arbor, 2000.

71. Clerico DM. Sinus headaches reconsidered: referred cephalgia of rhinologic origin masquerading as refractory primary headaches. *Headache* 1995;35:185–192.

72. Israel HA. Temporomandibular disorders: what the neurologist needs to know. *Semin Neurol* 1997;17:355–366.

73. Graff-Radford SB. Head pain relating to oromandibular structures. In: Gilman S, Goldstein GW, Waxman SG, eds. *Neurobase.* San Diego: Arbor, 2000.

74. Davidoff RA. Cranial neuralgias and atypical facial pain. In: Gilman S, Goldstein GW, Waxman SG, eds. *Neurobase.* San Diego: Arbor, 2000.

75. Montalbetti L, Ferrandi D, Pergami P, et al. Elongated styloid process and Eagle's syndrome. *Cephalalgia* 1995;15:80–93.

76. Lance JW, Anthony W. Neck-tongue syndrome on sudden turning of the head. *J Neurol Neurosurg Psychiatry* 1980;43:97–101.

77. Orrell RW, Marsden CD. The neck-tongue syndrome. *J Neurol Neurosurg Psychiatry* 1994;57:348–352.

78. Lance JW. The red ear syndrome. *Neurology* 1996;47:617–620.

79. Bird N, MacGregor EA, Wilkinson MI. Ice cream headache-site, duration, and relationship to migraine. *Headache* 1992;32:35–38.

Other Secondary Headaches and Associated Disorders

Randolph W. Evans

This chapter covers other secondary headaches and associated disorders, including the following: cough, exertional, and sexual headaches; Chiari I malformation; infection and inflammation; metabolic disorders; sleep disorders; seizures; multiple sclerosis; and central pain syndrome.[1,2]

COUGH, EXERTIONAL, AND SEXUAL HEADACHES

Introduction and Epidemiology

Headaches can be triggered by coughing, exertion, and sexual activity.[3,4] The definitions of the International Headache Society (IHS) follow. The lifetime prevalence of benign cough headache, benign exertional headache, and headache associated with sexual activity is 1% for each.[5] All three headache types occur most often in men.

Clinical Manifestations

Benign cough headache is a bilateral headache of sudden onset lasting less than 1 minute and precipitated by coughing. It may be prevented by avoiding coughing and may be diagnosed only after structural lesions such as posterior fossa tumor, Arnold-Chiari malformation (discussed later), platybasia, and basilar impression have been excluded by neuroimaging. In some cases, the onset can be after a respiratory infection with cough. Internal carotid stenosis can rarely cause unilateral cough headache. The term *cough headache* also includes headache brought on by sneezing, weightlifting, bending, stooping, or straining with a bowel movement. Weightlifting can also cause an acute bilateral nuchal-occipital or nuchal-occipital-parietal headache that can persist as a residual ache for days or weeks.

Benign exertional headache is specifically brought on by physical exercise and lasts from 5 minutes to 24 hours. It is bilateral, is throbbing at onset, and may develop migrainous features in patients susceptible to migraine. Reported causes include running, rowing, tennis, and swimming. One particular activity may precipitate the headache in some individuals but not others. This headache type is prevented by avoiding excessive exertion, particularly in hot weather or at high altitude, and is unassociated with any systemic or intracranial disorder. Subarachnoid hemorrhage (SAH) (Chapter 5), pheochromocytomas, cardiac ischemia, middle cerebral artery dissection (see Chapter 11 for the last three topics), and hypoplasia of the aortic arch after successful coarctation repair are rare secondary causes of exertional headaches.

Three types of headache are precipitated by sexual excitement (masturbation or coitus); all are bilateral at onset, prevented or eased by ceasing sexual activity before orgasm, and unassociated with any intracranial disorder, such as aneurysm. The dull type is a dull ache in the head and neck that intensifies as sexual excitement increases. The explosive type is a sudden severe headache occurring at orgasm. The postural type is a postural headache resembling that of low cerebrospinal fluid (CSF) pressure developing after coitus.

In one study of patients with the explosive type, those who stop sexual activity with headache onset before orgasm had a duration of 5 minutes to 2 hours.[6] Those who proceeded to orgasm had a severe headache for 3 minutes to 4 hours and a milder headache for 1 to 48 hours afterward. Forty percent of patients with the explosive type also have exertional headache.[7] A personal or family history of migraine is common in sexual headaches, which occur more frequently when the person tries to have more than one orgasm after a brief interval. Caution is necessary in diagnosing the first sex headache because sexual activity is the precipitant of up to 12% of ruptured saccular aneurysms and of up to 4% of patients with SAH resulting from bleeding arteriovenous malformations. Rarely, pheochromocytomas (Chapter 11) can present with paroxysmal hypertension precipitated by sexual activity. Viagra can cause headaches in 10% of users. Extracephalic pain can be due to masturbation. Severe paroxysmal icepicklike pain has been described referred to the neck in a patient with compressive spondylitic cervical myelopathy and the groin and genitalia in another patient with a tethered cord.[8]

In 1991, Sands et al. reviewed 219 previously reported cases of cough and exertional headaches, most from the era before computed tomography (CT) scans.[9] From the two combined headache types, 78% were benign. The following were found in the 22% with structural lesions: posterior fossa space–occupying lesions, 37.5%; after trauma or after craniotomy, 27%; supratentorial space–occupying lesions, 18.7%; basilar impression/platybasia, 12.5%; and syrinx, 4.2%.

In 1996, Pascual et al. reported 72 benign and symptomatic cases of cough, exertional, and sexual headaches they had evaluated over a 15-year period.[10] The findings are summarized in Table 13-1. The sexual headache reported is the explosive type. The one patient with a SAH had only a single headache; those with the benign type had multiple sexual headaches. Pascual et al. state that neuroradiologic studies could be avoided in cases with clinically typical benign sexual or exertional headaches (men around the third decade of life, with short-duration, multiple episodes of pulsating pain, response to ergotamine or to preventive beta-blockers), the remaining patients must have brain CT scan and CSF examination if the CT scan is normal (see Chapter 5 on evaluation of SAH). They recommend magnetic resonance imaging (MRI) in all patients with cough headache and mandate the scan when there is no response to indomethacin, in those with posterior fossa signs, or in those under 50 years of age.

Management

Benign cough headaches may respond to indomethacin 25 to 50 mg three times a day,[11] lumbar puncture,[12] or methysergide.[13] Some patients may have an abrupt recovery after extraction of abscessed teeth. In some cases, exertional headache may be pre-

Table 13-1. Cough, exertional, and sexual headaches

Parameter	Cough headache		Exertional headache		Sexual headache	
	Benign	Symptomatic	Benign	Symptomatic	Benign	Symptomatic
Patients (n)	13	17	16	12	13	1
Age, range (years)	67 ± 11, 44–81	39 ± 14, 15–63	24 ± 11, 10–48	42 ± 14, 18–61	41 ± 9, 24–57	60
Sex (% men)	77	59	88	43	85	100
Duration	Secs to 30 min	Secs to days	Min to 2 days	1 day to 1 month	1 min to 3 hours	10 days
Bilateral localization	92%	94%	56%	100%	77%	Yes
Quality	Sharp, stabbing, pulsating	Bursting, stabbing	Pulsating, stabbing	Explosive,	Explosive + pulsating	Explosive + pulsating
Other manifestations	No	Posterior fossa signs	Nausea, photophobia	Nausea, vomiting, double vision, rigidity neck	None	Vomiting, neck rigidity
Diagnosis	Idiopathic	Chiari Type I malformation	Idiopathic	SAH, sinusitis, brain metastases	Idiopathic	SAH

From Pascual J, Iglesias F, Oterino A, et al. Cough, exertional, and sexual headaches: an analysis of 72 benign and symptomatic cases. *Neurology* 1996;46:1520–1524, modified with permission.

vented by a warm-up period. Some patients may choose to avoid the particular activity. Indomethacin may be preventive. Prophylactic drugs used for migraine such as beta-blockers may be effective for some patients.

The natural history of the benign explosive type of sexual headaches is variable. In one study of 26 patients, the headaches went away in 50% after 6 weeks to 6 months but recurred in 50% after remissions of up to 6 years.[14] Headaches may be prevented in some patients by weight loss, an exercise program, a more passive role during intercourse, variation in posture, limitation of additional sexual activity on the same day, and medications.[15] Again, indomethacin may be useful. Ergotamine tartrate or methylsergide given before sexual activity may also be preventive. Propranolol (40 to 200 mg/day) and diltiazem (60 mg three times daily)[16] can be given as a daily preventive if this headache type occurs frequently.

CHIARI TYPE I MALFORMATION AND HEADACHE

Epidemiology

Chiari type I malformation describes herniation of the cerebellar tonsils below the level of the foramen magnum. Although Chiari I malformation is usually congenital, reversible descent of the cerebellar tonsils below the foramen magnum (acquired Chiari I malformation) can occur due to lumbar puncture, overdraining CSF shunts, and spontaneous intracranial hypertension. In one study, Chiari I was more common in women (3:2) and was associated with syringomyelia in 40%, most commonly between the levels of C4 and C6.[17] All patients with tonsillar herniations greater than 12 mm and 70% of those with herniations of 5 to 10 mm were symptomatic. Information is unavailable about the prevalence of this disorder. With the advent of MRI, minimal tonsillar herniation is frequently detected as an incidental finding.

Clinical Manifestations

Presentations include foramen magnum compression, central cord syndrome, cerebellar dysfunction, bulbar palsy, and paroxysmal intracranial hypertension.[17a] Syncope can occasionally occur with headache similar to basilar migraine or with Valsalva-like maneuvers or exercise.

In a study of 35 patients with Chiari I who subsequently underwent surgery (decompression of the foramen magnum, opening of the fourth ventricular outlet, and plugging of the obex), the frequency of clinical presentations in Chiari I were as follows: headache and neck pain, 73%; sensory dysesthesias/numbness, 56%; gait problems, 43%; upper-extremity weakness, 25%; cranial nerve dysfunction, 23%; blurred vision, 17%; and lower-extremity weakness, 15%.[18] Significant improvement following surgery was described in 45% with syringomyelia and in 87% without syringomyelia.

Headaches have been reported in 15% to 75% of those with Chiari I. Stovner et al. described 20 patients with headaches out of 34 Chiari I patients seen with tonsillar herniation of ≥5 mm. Many patients had several headache types. Fifty percent had short-lasting cough headache types (see earlier) of less than 5 minutes; 70% had headaches lasting 3 hours to several days; and 40% had continuous headaches. Associated symptoms present in some patients included intermittent dizziness, visual symptoms (visual field defects, oscilloscopia, diplopia, blurred vision, and skew vision), and tinnitus. Long-lasting headaches were similar to cervicogenic headaches with occipital and neck pain, pain in the arm, and restriction of neck movement. Long-lasting headaches were unilateral in 50% and could shift sides. Those with long-lasting headaches averaged 6.25 attacks/month. The headaches, which were present in various locations—including below the eyes, eye(s), forehead, vertex, temple, and occiput—often were severe. The degree of tonsillar herniation was not correlated with the presence or absence of headaches or the presence of short-duration headaches. The headaches were improved in the five out of eight patients who had surgery.

Pascual et al. reported 26 patients with headaches out of 50 with Chiari I. Suboccipital-occipital headaches were present in 28%, with a duration that ranged from seconds to weeks and variable quality, including throbbing, dull, and lancinating pain.[19] The pain was aggravated by Valsalva-like maneuvers in all the patients. This headache correlated with the degree of tonsillar herniation.

Thus a variety of headaches have been associated with Chiari I, including those that are similar to migraine with and without aura, are tension type, are cervicogenic, and result from high and low CSF pressure.[20] Migraine and tension-type headaches can also occur unrelated to the Chiari I. If the tonsillar herniation is less than 5 mm, the physician should be wary of attributing the headache to Chiari I.

Biologic Basis

Intermittent or persistent intracranial hypertension can be due to obstruction of CSF flow from the fourth ventricle to the cisterna magna or within the subarachnoid space at the level of the foramen magnum. The short-lasting cough headaches are due to a transient pressure dissociation between the intracranial and intraspinal compartments that causes further impaction of the cerebellar tonsils in the foramen magnum and produces pain by traction and pressure on pain-sensitive structures, such as the C1 and C2 nerve roots, cranial nerves, meninges, and vessels. The mechanism of recurrent, long-lasting headaches not induced by Valsalva-like maneuvers is not understood.[21]

HEADACHES DUE TO INFECTION AND INFLAMMATION

HIV and Headaches

A variety of headaches result from HIV infection.[22] Primary headaches can also occur in those infected with HIV. Medication rebound should also be considered as a cause in those patients with chronic headaches or pain syndromes who frequently use pain medications.

HIV-Related Headaches

Two to 4 weeks after HIV-1 infection, up to 93% of patients develop an acute illness, often associated with headache, that lasts 1 to 2 weeks. Acute headaches with fever, meningeal signs,

**Table 13-2.   Frequency of headache based
on diagnosis in the HIV-infected individual**

Diagnosis	Percentage with headache
Cryptococcal meningitis	88
Neurosyphillis	88
Tuberculous meningitis	59
Toxoplasmosis encephalitis	55
Cytomegalovirus encephalitis	30
Progressive multifocal leukoencephalopathy	23
HIV-associated dementia	14

From Holloway RG, Kieburtz KD. Headache associated with AIDS. In: Gilman S, Goldstein GW, Waxman SG, eds. *Neurobase*. San Diego: Arbor, 2000, modified with permission.

cranial nerve palsies, and CSF lymphocytic pleocytosis (20 to 300 cells/mm^3) can develop at any stage of the disease. In the late stages of the disease, the CSF may show no white blood cells because of lymphocyte depletion. Because CSF pleocytosis and elevated protein concentration can be seen in asymptomatic HIV-seropositive patients, this finding in a patient with headache does not exclude other etiologies. Up to 30% of HIV-seropositive people develop chronic headache and persistent pleocytosis.

Opportunistic infections and tumors can also cause headaches in HIV-1 disease. Meningitides include cryptococcal meningitis, tuberculous meningitis, syphilitic meningitis, and lymphomatous meningitis. Focal brain lesions that can cause headache include toxoplasmosis encephalitis, primary central nervous system lymphoma, progressive multifocal leukoencephalopathy, cryptococcomas, tuberculomas, and *Candida* abscess. Diffuse brain lesions that can cause headache include cytomegalovirus encephalitis, herpes simplex virus encephalitis, toxoplasmosis encephalitis, and HIV-associated dementia. Table 13-2 lists the frequency of headache with these various causes. Sinusitis, which is common in patients with AIDS, should also be considered as the cause of headaches.

A variety of medications taken by HIV-seropositive patients may be associated with headaches, including zidovudine, trimethoprim-sulfamethoxazole, fluoxetine, rifampin, ethambutol, methotrexate, and acyclovir. The protease inhibitors do not appear to cause or worsen headaches.

Primary Headaches

Early in the AIDS epidemic in the United States, opportunistic infections such as cryptococcal meningitis were the commonest cause of headaches. With better opportunistic and antiretroviral treatments, primary headaches have become more common. Stress and depression associated with HIV infection can certainly contribute to primary headaches.

In a prospective study of patients with headaches seen in a neuro-AIDS clinic performed by Mirsattari et al., primary headaches were present in 66% and secondary headaches occurred in 34%.[23] Primary headaches have the following features: They are not uncommon in this population and are distinguished by the late age of onset, usual absence of family or personal history of headaches, and exacerbation following HIV infection; may present first in patients with severe immunosuppression; are unrelated to antiretroviral drug therapy; frequently do not respond to conventional treatments; and have a poor prognosis.

Diagnostic Evaluation

Diagnostic testing is often necessary to exclude secondary causes of headaches especially in those patients with headache and a CD4+ cell count of less than 500 cells/mm^3 (also see Chapter 1). An MRI scan is preferable to a CT scan because of greater sensitivity in detecting lesions associated with HIV infection. If the findings of the scan do not explain the headache, then a lumbar puncture is necessary, including routine CSF studies as well as bacterial, fungal, mycobacterial stains and cultures; sometimes viral studies and cytology; and cryptococcal antigen titers and venereal disease research laboratory (VDRL) titers. The CSF VDRL is nonreactive in 30% of cases of neurosyphillis. A nonreactive CSF-FTA-ABS or CSF-MHA-TP excludes neurosyphillis.

The diagnosis of tuberculous meningitis can be difficult. The sensitivity of acid-fast bacilli (AFB) stains is no more than 24%, and cultures may take 2 to 6 weeks for growth to occur. However, CSF polymerase chain reaction (PCR) for *Mycobacterium* tuberculosis has high sensitivity (variably reported as 32% to 100%) and specificity (about 8% false positives) for diagnosis.

In undiagnosed patients, HIV infection should be considered as the cause in patients with risk factors presenting with aseptic meningitis, cranial herpes zoster, facial pain associated with Bell's palsy, and new-onset or chronic progressive headaches. An enzyme-linked immunosorbent assay (ELISA) test, which is 99% specific and 98% sensitive when properly performed, is the initial test for HIV infection. Because false positives can occur, the diagnosis must be confirmed with more specific PCR or Western blot techniques. If the ELISA is negative, testing should be repeated in 6 months if there is sufficient concern because of the possible delay in the development of detectable serum antibodies.

Brain Abscess

Epidemiology

The annual incidence of brain abscess[24,25] is about four in 1 million. The most common age is the third decade of life. Abscesses due to paranasal sinus infection are most common between the ages of 10 and 30, whereas otogenic abscesses are most common in childhood and after 40 years of age. In children, the peak incidence is between 4 and 7 years of age, and 25% have cyanotic congenital heart disease.

Brain abscesses are usually the result of hematogenous spread of organisms from distant sites (e.g., bronchiectasis, lung abscess, and acute bacterial endocarditis) or spread from sinusitis (especially frontal, ethmoid, or sphenoid sinusitis), otitis, or mastoiditis through emissary veins. Less common causes include penetrating trauma, neurosurgical procedures, facial infections, and dental sepsis. In 20% to 30% of cases, no predisposing condition is identified. The microbiologic profile, which includes a variety of aerobes and anaerobes, often reflects the origin of the infection. Multiple organisms may be present, especially when due to sinusitis or otitis. Infection in immunocompromised patients may be due to *Enterobacteriaceae, Pseudomonas aeruginosa,* and *Nocardia asteroides.* Brain abscesses in diabetics may be associated with *Cryptococcus neoformans, Candida, Mucor,* and *Aspergillus* species. Focal infections in AIDS are listed in the prior section.

Clinical Manifestations

Headaches, unilateral or bilateral, are present in about 75% of patients, and nausea and vomiting occur in about 50%. Fever is present in less than 50% of patients. Focal neurologic signs are also present in less than 50%. About one-third of patients present with seizures, which are usually generalized. Nuchal rigidity and papilledema are present in about 25% of cases.

Diagnostic Evaluation

CT and MRI scans are the key to diagnosis. CT scan classically shows a ring-enhancing lesion with a variable appearance, depending on the age and cause of the abscess. Early lesions may not show enhancement. Metastatic neoplasms may be difficult to distinguish from multiple brain abscesses. MRI is more sensitive than CT scans. T1-weighted images show hypodense areas with ring enhancement after gadolinium injection. T2-weighted images show a hyperdense central area surrounded by a capsule. Better imaging of the abscess allows more accurate estimates of its age and amenability to aspiration or drainage. Single photon emission computed tomography (SPECT) with thallium 201 is useful in distinguishing central nervous system lymphoma from toxoplasmosis. Lumbar puncture is contraindicated in the presence of a mass lesion because of the risk of herniation.

Meningitis and Encephalitis

Epidemiology

The annual incidence of meningitis and encephalitis[25,26] per 100,000 in the United States for various infections is as follows: bacterial meningitis, 5 to 10; viral meningitis, 10.9; and viral encephalitis, 7.4. Bacterial meningitis occurs more often in winter than during other seasons. Because of the *Hemophilus influenzae* type B vaccine, the median age of patients with meningitis due to *Hemophilus influenzae, Streptococcus pneumoniae, Neisseria meningitidis,* group B streptococcus, and *Listeria monocytogenes* has increased in the last 15 years from 15 months of age to 25 years. Pneumococcal meningitis is the most common cause of bacterial meningitis in the United States.Viral meningitis usually occurs during the summer and typically occurs in children and young adults. The most common organisms are enteroviruses (echo and coxsackie), mumps, and the arboviruses. Most cases of viral encephalitis occur in the summer and early fall. There are numerous causes of viral encephalitis, including mumps, arboviruses, enteroviruses, lymphocytic choriomeningitis, herpes

simplex virus, Epstein-Barr virus, measles, influenza virus, varicella zoster, and mycoplasma.

Clinical Manifestations

Bacterial meningitis in adults classically presents with fever,
headache, meningismus, pain with eye movement, and altered
mental status. The headache is usually generalized (but may be
bifrontal), severe, and unremitting. Bacterial meningitis can present with a thunderclap headache. Young children and the
elderly have headaches less often than young adults. Nausea,
vomiting, photophobia, and myalgias are also common. Kernig's
or Brudzinski's sign or both are present in about 50% of cases.
Cranial nerve findings are found in less than 20% of cases. Subacute or chronic headache may be present in tuberculous or
cryptococcal meningitis.

Viral meningitis typically presents with a severe, sudden-onset
headache, fever, malaise, anorexia, pain with eye movement,
phonophobia, photophobia, and nuchal rigidity. The features of
encephalitis include headache, fever, alteration of consciousness,
meningeal signs, focal neurologic deficits, and seizures. Thunderclap headaches can also occur in viral encephalitis.

Diagnostic Evaluation

Patients with focal neurologic findings, papilledema, or altered
mental status should have a CT scan or MRI scan before a lumbar puncture. If there is a significant delay before the lumbar
puncture or the patient is seriously ill, blood cultures should be
taken and antibiotics empirically started when bacterial meningitis is suspected.

On lumbar puncture and CSF examination, the usual findings
in bacterial meningitis are the following: an elevated opening pressure, increased white blood cells (WBCs) with neutrophilic predominance (1,000 to 5,000 cells/mm^3), increased protein level (100
to 500 mg/dl), and low glucose level (<40 mg/dl or a CSF/serum
ratio of <0.3). Approximately 90% of patients will have more than
100 WBCs/mm^3; 65% to 70% will have more than 1,000 WBCs/mm^3.

Although the WBCs are predominantly neutrophils, initially
10% of patients may show mononuclear predominance, generally
with cell counts of less than 1,000. CSF findings with a very high
predictive value for bacterial meningitis include the following:
glucose <34 mg/dl; CSF/serum glucose <0.23; WBCs >2,000/mm^3;
and neutrophils >1,180/mm^3. Gram's stain of the CSF is positive
in 60% to 90% of patients. Blood cultures may be positive in up
to 50% of cases. Counterimmunoelectrophoresis (CIE) and latex
agglutination tests of the CSF to test for bacterial antigens can
be sensitive adjuncts, especially in partially treated meningitis.

On lumbar puncture and CSF examination, the usual findings
in viral meningitis are the following: normal or slightly elevated
opening CSF pressure; a mild pleocytosis (usually <1,000
cells/mm^3); protein either normal or slightly elevated; and glucose either normal or slightly decreased. Early in the course of
the disease there may be neutrophil cell predominance, but this
rapidly shifts to a lymphocytic pleocytosis.

On CSF examination, the usual findings in viral encephalitis
include the following: a mild CSF pleocytosis (usually <200

cells/mm^3); protein concentration either normal or slightly elevated; and glucose level either normal or slightly decreased. The CSF typically shows a lymphocytic predominance, although a neutrophil predominance may be seen in the first 48 hours. MRI studies may show focal findings in focal encephalitides, such as herpes simplex or Eastern equine. Other useful studies include electroencephalogram, acute and convalescent sera, and CSF PCR. CSF PCR for herpes simplex virus encephalitis, with a sensitivity of 98% and a specificity of 94%, has supplanted the need for brain biopsy in these cases. The results may become negative once acyclovir has been started.

Drug-Induced Aseptic Meningitis

Numerous medications can cause an aseptic meningitis,[27] including the following: nonsteroidal antiinflammatory drugs (ibuprofen, naproxen, diclofenac, sulindac, tolmetin, and ketoprofen); antibiotics (trimethoprim/sulfamethoxazole, sulfasalazine, cephalosporins, ciprofloxacin, isoniazide, and penicillin), intrathecal drugs and diagnostics (antineoplastics such as methotrexate and cytarabine; gentamicin; corticosteroids; spinal anesthesia; baclofen; repeated iophendylate for myelography; and radiolabeled albumin); intraventricular chemotherapy; intravenous immunoglobulin; vaccines (polio, measles, mumps, and rubella, and hepatitis B); and other drugs (e.g., carbamazepine, muromonab CD-3, and ranitidine).

The clinical presentation is the same as that of viral meningitis. The CSF findings are similar to viral meningitis except for a neutrophil predominance in most cases. Aseptic meningitis due to intravenous immunoglobulin demonstrates eosinophils in the CSF. The prognosis in drug-induced aseptic meningitis is generally good.

Postmeningitis Headache

Following recovery from bacterial or viral meningitis, preexisting primary headaches can have an increased severity or new-onset headaches, including migraine, beginning within weeks after recovery.[28]

Lyme Disease

Epidemiology

Lyme disease[29] is a multisystem infectious disease caused by the spirochete *Borrelia burdorferi sensu stricto*. The disease is a zoonosis spread by hard-shelled *Ixodes* ticks with humans as the inadvertent host. Mature ticks usually attach to large mammals, such as bears or deer. Only 1% to 2% of humans with identified *Ixodes* tick bites become infected. About 10,000 cases are reported yearly to the Centers for Disease Control. Although cases have been reported from 47 states, most cases occur along the eastern seaboard from Maryland to Massachusetts, in the upper Midwest (primarily Wisconsin and Minnesota), and in northern California.

Clinical Manifestations

Up to 90% of infected people have a usually painless rash, erythema migrans, which starts as a red macule or papule and expands to form a large red ring with central clearing. During erythema migrans, headache is present in about 50% of patients.

About 15% of patients will develop nervous system involvement with all or part of the triad of lymphocytic meningitis, cranial neuritis, and painful radiculitis. Although any cranial nerve can be involved, cranial nerve VII is most common and can be bilateral. (Sarcoid and Guillain-Barré syndrome can also cause bilateral palsies.) Late or chronic neurologic manifestations include a chronic encephalomyelitis (which is rare) and a mild peripheral neuropathy, which can be a symmetric distal polyneuropathy, more focal mononeuropathy multiplex, or a polyradiculopathy. A significant number of patients with chronic infection will develop a mild encephalomyelitis with mild confusion and difficulty with memory and complex intellectual tasks. Headache occurs commonly with lymphocytic meningitis with or without cranial neuritis or painful radiculoneuritis or both and with encephalomyelitis.

Diagnostic Evaluation

Diagnostic testing is problematic for Lyme disease because of difficulties with the sensitivity and specificity of the tests. Patients with headache alone usually do not require testing. Serum antibody testing by ELISA, which can have both false positives and negatives, is the first step. Western blot tests confirm a positive ELISA or identify false positives. PCR, to detect bacterial DNA, has a sensitivity of about 60%. For neurologic presentations, demonstration of intrathecal antibody production (the ratio of CSF to serum antibody) is very sensitive and specific.

Neurosarcoid

Sarcoidosis can affect any part of the central or peripheral nervous system. Neurosarcoid occurs in about 5% of cases. Sarcoid granulomas in the basal meninges, brain, and cranial nerves—the most common neurologic manifestations—often cause headaches either directly or due to obstruction of CSF pathways and hydrocephalus.

METABOLIC DISORDERS AND HEADACHE

Fever

Generalized headaches often occur with nonneurologic disorders,[30] such as pyelonephritis. The fever that results from the disorder in turn causes increased cerebral blood flow and headache.

Hypoxia

The IHS criteria for hypoxic headache include headache occurring within 24 hours after the acute onset of hypoxia with PaO_2 of less than or equal to 70 mm Hg or in chronic hypoxic patients with PaO_2 persistently at or below this level. Hypoxic headache can occur during exposure to reduced ambient oxygen or in patients with carbon monoxide exposure, pulmonary disease, anemia, cardiac failure, and sleep apnea. Hypoxia can also be a trigger for migraine and cluster headaches. Hypoxemia, especially when combined with an increased level of carbon dioxide, can produce headache due to dilation of arteries and arterioles.

Hypercapnia

Severe headaches can occur in some patients with hypercapnia caused by marked dilatation of cerebral vasculature. Prolonged hypercapnia can be a secondary cause of pseudotumor cerebri.

Hypoglycemia

Missing a meal can be a trigger for migraineurs. Headache due to hypoglycemia can occur in diabetics, pancreatic islet cell tumors, hypopituitarism, adrenocortical insufficiency, hypothyroidism, and liver disease such as cirrhosis.

Dialysis

Tension- or migraine-type headaches can be precipitated during dialysis. A new type of headache can also occur a few hours after dialysis, starting as a bifrontal aching and then a throbbing, sometimes with nausea and vomiting.[31]

High Altitude

Epidemiology

Acute mountain sickness (AMS) develops in about 25% of visitors to moderate altitudes (6,300 to 9,700 feet). Symptoms usually occur within the first 12 hours of arrival but may be delayed 24 hours or more. Those who are younger than 60 years of age, less physically fit, live at sea level, have a history of AMS, or have underlying lung problems are most likely to be affected by AMS.[32] AMS leads to high-altitude cerebral edema (HACE) in perhaps 1.5% of cases. Alcohol use inhibits acute ventilatory adaptation to mild hypoxia at moderate altitude. High altitude can also be a trigger for migraines.

Clinical Manifestations

AMS, which usually occurs above 8,200 feet, is defined by the presence of a headache and at least one of the following symptoms: gastrointestinal symptoms (anorexia, nausea, or vomiting), fatigue or weakness, dizziness or lightheadedness, and difficulty sleeping.[33] The headache is usually bilateral but may be unilateral. HACE, which is uncommon below 12,000 feet, is defined by the presence of a change in mental status and/or ataxia in a person with AMS or the presence of both mental status change and ataxia in a person without AMS. HACE, which can lead to coma and death, may be associated with abnormalities in limb tone, urinary incontinence, papilledema, cranial nerve palsies, and tremor.

High-altitude pulmonary edema (HAPE), which can occur along with HACE, usually occurs above 9,840 feet. High-altitude retinal hemorrhage is common in people who go above 15,000 feet.

Biologic Mechanisms

As the partial pressure of oxygen decreases with increasing altitude, ventilation increases, leading to respiratory alkalosis. Although hypocapnia alone results in cerebral vasoconstriction, hypoxia produces a net decline of cerebral vascular resistance and increased cerebral blood flow. Hypoxia can result in cerebral edema, which may be due to cerebral vasodilation and elevated cerebral capillary hydrostatic pressure. An increase in sympathetic activity follows, causing an increased heart rate, pulmonary vasoconstriction, and an initial increase and later decrease of cerebral blood flow.[34]

Management

Altitude sickness may be prevented in those planning higher ascents by starting below 8,000 feet, resting the first day, and then ascending about 1,000 feet each day. Sleeping at a lower altitude at night may be helpful because hypoxia is worse with sleep. It is also important to keep well hydrated and avoid alcohol. Acetazolamide, at a dose of 250 to 1,000 mg/day starting 8 to 12 hours before ascent and continuing for 3 to 4 days, may prevent AMS and improve sleep. Dexamethasone may also reduce the incidence and symptoms of AMS. Aspirin may also prevent AMS. In one study, the incidence of headache was greatly reduced by giving aspirin 320 mg starting 1 hour before arrival at high altitude and then one every 4 hours for two doses (for a total of three doses).[35]

AMS may be treated symptomatically with rest, mild analgesics, alcohol avoidance, and adequate hydration. Depending on the severity of symptoms, it may be necessary to not go any higher, slow the rate of ascent, or descend. Acetazolamide may also help acute symptoms. In addition to descent, HACE may be treated with acetazolamide, dexamethasone, supplemental oxygen, and a portable hyperbaric bag. Nifedipine and inhalation of nitric oxide may be beneficial for HAPE.[36]

AMS usually resolves after 16 to 72 hours at altitude. When descent is impossible and when treatment is lacking, HACE and HAPE have a mortality rate of up to 50%.

Decompression Sickness

Decompression sickness (DCS), also referred to as the "bends" or caisson disease, usually affects divers and caisson workers but can occur in pilots during rapid ascent in a nonpressurized cabin. DCS, which can occur after diving to a depth of more than 25 feet, usually appears within a few minutes to a few hours after the end of a dive. Mild DCS (type I) is defined by pain usually in the joints (bends) and/or itching of the skin. Serious DCS (type II) is characterized by neurologic problems. Involvement of the thoracic spinal cord, the most commonly affected area, leads to low back or pelvic pain and dysesthesias, which may be accompanied by sensory loss, weakness, and incontinence. Less often, the brain may be involved, resulting in various symptoms and signs, such as headache, confusion, lethargy, vertigo, speech disturbance, hemiparesis, visual impairment, and seizures, depending on the site of the insult.[37]

Hyperventilation Syndrome

Introduction and Epidemiology

Hyperventilation syndrome,[38] according to one consensus definition, is a "syndrome characterized by a variety of somatic symptoms induced by physiologically inappropriate hyperventilation and usually reproduced in whole or in part by voluntary hyperventilation."[39] Acute hyperventilation with obvious tachypnea accounts for about 1% of all cases of hyperventilation. The other 99% of cases is due to chronic hyperventilation where there may be a modest increase in respiratory rate and/or tidal volume that may not even be apparent to the patient or a medical observer.

The hyperventilation syndrome occurs in about 6% to 11% of the general patient population. Most studies have reported hyperventilation syndrome occurring two to seven times more frequently in women than in men, with most patients ranging in age between 15 and 55 years. One large study reported that patients with acute hyperventilation syndrome ranged in age from 5 to 85 years and that this condition was particularly prevalent in women in their late teens.[40] The prevalence of chronic hyperventilation is the highest in middle-aged women. In studies of patients with neurologic symptoms of hyperventilation syndrome, the percentage of females ranged from 50% to 87%.

Hyperventilation syndrome is frequently associated with anxiety or stress, although some patients have no detectable psychiatric disorder and develop a habit of inappropriately increased ventilatory rate and/or depth. Common triggers of acute hyperventilation syndrome include anxiety, nausea and vomiting, and fever due to the common cold.

Clinical Manifestations

The manifestations of hyperventilation syndrome that include headaches are listed in Table 13-3. Patients with different symptoms may see different types of physicians. Primary-care physicians may see an assortment of presentations. Cardiologists may see those with complaints of chest pain, palpitations, and shortness of breath. Neurologists frequently see patients describing dizziness, paresthesias, and pressure in the head. Ear, nose, and throat physicians may see those with dizziness. The most common cause of distal symmetric paresthesias is hyperventilation syndrome. Although physicians generally recognize bilateral paresthesias of the face, hands, and feet as due to hyperventilation syndrome, many are unaware that hyperventilation can cause unilateral paresthesias. Unilateral paresthesias more often involve the left side. In a study of medical students, hyperventilation produced predominantly unilateral paresthesias in 16%, which involved the left side in more than 60% of control groups.[41] Of those with hand numbness, often only the fourth and fifth fingers are involved. Unusual patterns of numbness reported include one side of the forehead, the shoulders, and one side of the abdomen.

Patients may report a variety of psychologic complaints commonly, including anxiety, nervousness, unreality, disorientation, or feeling "spacey." Impairment of concentration and memory may be described as part of episodes or alternatively as symptoms of an underlying anxiety neurosis or depression. A patient's concern about the cause of the various symptoms of hyperventilation may result in feelings of impending death, fear, or panic, which may accentuate the hyperventilation. Patients with

**Table 13-3.   Symptoms and signs
of the hyperventilation syndrome**

General
 Fatiguability, exhaustion, weakness, sleep disturbance, nausea,
  sweating
Cardiovascular
 Chest pain, palpitations, tachycardia, Raynaud's phenomenon
Gastrointestinal
 Aerophagia, dry mouth, pressure in throat, dysphagia, globus
  hystericus, epigastric fullness or pain, belching, flatulence
Neurologic
 Headache, pressure in the head, fullness in the head, head
 warmth
  Blurred vision, tunnel vision, momentary flashing lights, diplopia
  Dizziness, faintness, vertigo, giddiness, unsteadiness
  Tinnitus
  Numbness, tingling, coldness of face, extremities, trunk
  Muscle spasms, muscle stiffness, carpopedal spasm, generalized
   tetany, tremor
  Ataxia, weakness
  Syncope and seizures
Psychologic
  Impairment of concentration and memory
  Feelings of unreality, disorientation, confused or dreamlike
   feeling, déjà vu
  Hallucinations
  Anxiety, apprehension, nervousness, tension, fits of crying,
   agoraphobia, neuroses, phobic, panic
Respiratory
  Shortness of breath, suffocating feeling, smothering spell,
   inability to get a good breath or breathe deeply enough,
   frequent sighing, yawning

hyperventilation syndrome have a mean group profile very similar to patients with pseudoseizures: a neurotic pattern where
patients respond to psychologic stress with somatic symptoms.
Other complaints such as déjà vu or auditory and visual hallucinations are rare.

Biologic Mechanisms

Acute hyperventilation produces a reduction in arterial pCO_2
resulting in alkalosis. Respiratory alkalosis produces the Bohr
effect, a left shift of the oxygen dissociation curve with increased
binding of oxygen to hemoglobin and reduced oxygen delivery to
the tissues. The alkalosis also causes a reduction in plasma Ca^{2+}
concentration. Hypophosphatemia may be due to intracellular
shifts of phosphorus caused by altered glucose metabolism. In
chronic hyperventilation, bicarbonate and potassium levels may
be decreased because of increased renal excretion. Finally, stress
can trigger a hyperadrenergic state that may cause hyperventilation through beta-adrenergic stimulation.

Central and peripheral mechanisms have been postulated for production of neurologic symptoms during hyperventilation.[42] Voluntary hyperventilation can reduce cerebral blood flow by 30% to 40%. Such symptoms and signs as headache, visual disturbance, dizziness, tinnitus, ataxia, syncope, and various psychologic symptoms may be produced by diminished cerebral perfusion. Muscle spasms and tetany may be due to respiratory alkalosis and hypocalcemia. The finding that there is no relationship between the rate of fall of pCO_2 and the onset of dizziness and paresthesias suggests that symptoms may be due to hypophosphatemia. Hypophosphatemia can result in symptoms such as tiredness, dizziness, poor concentration, disorientation, and paresthesias. A hyperadrenergic state may result in tremor, tachycardia, anxiety, and sweating. Hypokalemia can cause muscle weakness and lethargy. The cause of bilateral and unilateral paresthesias is not certain. Evidence exists for both a central and peripheral mechanism, including a reduction in the concentration of extracellular Ca^{2+} and decreased cerebral perfusion.

Diagnostic Evaluation

The acute form of hyperventilation syndrome is easily recognized, even by the general public. However, the chronic form is less easily recognized, even by physicians, because the breathing rate is not reported as rapid or does not appear rapid and because the symptoms may appear to be atypical. For example, a respiration rate of 18 combined with an increased tidal volume of 750 ml/minute may lead to overbreathing that is not easily detectable. Because the chronic disorder is intermittent, spot arterial pCO_2 or end tidal volume pCO_2 results can be normal.

The diagnosis depends on reproducing some or all of the symptoms with the hyperventilation provocation test and excluding other possible causes by either clinical reasoning or laboratory testing when indicated. The symptoms of panic attacks and hyperventilation syndrome overlap. In patients with prominent chest pain, cardiac disease should be considered.

The hyperventilation provocation test can be performed with either an increased ventilation rate of up to 60/minute or simply deep breathing for 3 minutes. Dizziness, unsteadiness, and blurred vision commonly develop within 20 to 30 seconds, especially with the patient in the standing position; paresthesias start later. Chest pain is reported by 50% of patients after 3 minutes of hyperventilation and by all by 20 minutes. For clinical purposes, measurement of end tidal volume pCO_2 is unnecessary. In addition, there is no clear correlation between $PaCO_2$ and neurologic signs. The hyperventilation provocation test should not be performed in patients with ischemic heart disease, cerebrovascular disease, pulmonary insufficiency, hyperviscosity states, significant anemia, sickle cell disease, or uncontrolled hypertension.

Not infrequently, patients report only one or two symptoms, but on performing the hyperventilation provocation test, they report other symptoms that appear during their typical episodes that they did not remember to mention. For some patients with hyperventilation syndrome, symptoms cannot be reliably reproduced during the hyperventilation provocation test or even on consecutive tests. For others, antecedent anxiety and stress, not present during the test, may predispose to symptom formation, perhaps because of a hyperadrenergic state. Different patterns of hyperventilation with different respiratory rates, tidal volumes, and durations may induce different symptoms. In the individual case, if the hyperventilation provocation test fails to reproduce the symptoms but clinical suspicion persists, treatment such as breath holding, slow breathing, or breathing into a paper bag can certainly be suggested on a trial basis.

Management

Treatments for hyperventilation include patient reassurance and education; instructions to hold the breath, breathe more slowly, or breathe into a paper bag; breathing exercises and diaphragmatic retraining; biofeedback; hypnosis; psychologic and psychiatric treatment; and such medications as beta-blockers, benzodiazepines, and antidepressants. Educational sessions, breathing techniques and retraining, and progressive relaxation may be helpful.

Most patients respond to reassurance, education (see patient information sheet in Chapter 16), and instructions to hold the breath, breathe more slowly, or breathe into a paper bag. If significant symptoms of stress, anxiety, or depression are present, use of appropriate medication and psychologic or psychiatric referral may be helpful.

SLEEP AND HEADACHES

Headaches Occurring During Sleep

Secondary causes of nocturnal headaches[43,44] include drug withdrawal, temporal arteritis, sleep apnea, oxygen desaturation, pheochromocytomas, primary and secondary neoplasms, communicating hydrocephalus, subdural hematomas, subacute angle-closure glaucoma, and vascular lesions.[45] Migraine, cluster, hypnic, and chronic paroxysmal hemicrania are other primary headaches that can cause awakening from sleep. Hypnic headaches only occur during sleep (see Chapter 9). Migraine typically has associated symptoms and very uncommonly only occurs during sleep. Cluster headaches have autonomic symptoms and may occur during the day as well as during sleep. Chronic paroxysmal hemicrania occurs both during the day and at night, lasts for less than 30 minutes, and occurs 10 to 30 times a day.

Obstructive Sleep Apnea

Snoring and excessive daytime sleepiness are the most common symptoms of obstructive sleep apnea (OSA). Morning headaches are three times more common in those with OSA than in the general population[46] and may occur in 36% of those with OSA.

Sleep Bruxism

Bruxism[47] (grinding or clenching of teeth) during sleep occurs in up to 20% of the population as determined by visible tooth wear. Sleep bruxism is most common in children between the ages of 3 and 12 years and in adults between the ages of 19 and 45 years. Individuals are unaware of this behavior, which produces audible sounds in about 20% of episodes. Some patients report morning jaw discomfort and tension-type headaches that improve as the day goes on. Causes include dental factors (malocclusion and rough cusp ends), psychologic and emotional factors, and systemic disorders (encephalopathies, hyperthyroidism, allergies, gastrointestinal disturbances, and nutritional deficiencies). Occlusal bite splints protect against damage. Medications that can be helpful at bedtime include propranolol, L-dopa, bromocriptine, and, for acute exacerbations, diazepam.

Sleep Deprivation and Sleeping In

Lack of sleep can trigger migraine and tension-type headaches. In one study, 38.8% of medical and dental students reported headaches due to sleep deprivation.[48] Some migraineurs find sleeping later than their usual time of awakening is a trigger.

Sleep to Relieve Migraine

Many migraineurs obtain relief from acute attacks by sleeping. In one study, 28% could terminate a migraine with sleep.[49]

Parasomnias and Migraine

Somnambulism (sleepwalking) occurs in 28% of children with migraine and 5% of controls.[50] Children with migraine also have a greater incidence of night terrors (71% versus 11% in controls) and enuresis (41% versus 16% in controls).[51]

Exploding Head Syndrome

Episodes of exploding head syndrome[52] awaken people from sleep with a sensation of a loud bang in the head, like an explosion. Ten percent of cases are associated with the perception of a flash of light. The episodes take place in healthy individuals during awakenings without evidence of epileptogenic discharges.

SEIZURES AND HEADACHES

Migraine and Seizures

The frequency of migraine in an epileptic population has been variably reported as 8.4% to 23%, and the reported frequency of epilepsy in a migraine population ranges from 1% to 17%.[53] MELAS, arteriovenous malformations (Chapter 11), head trauma, and systemic lupus erythematosus can result in seizures and migraines or migrainelike headaches. Migraine with typical or prolonged aura, basilar migraine, and catamenial epilepsy can be triggers for seizures.[54] Migraine can rarely cause a cerebral infarction that can cause seizures.

Benign occipital epilepsy, benign rolandic epilepsy, and temporal and occipital lobe epilepsy can cause seizures that mimic some features of migraine.[54a] A seizure is more likely if the aura lasts less than 5 minutes and is associated with alteration of consciousness, automatisms, and abnormal motor activity such as tonic-clonic movements. Migraine is more likely if the aura lasts more than 5 minutes and has positive (tingling, scintillations) and negative features (visual loss, numbness).

Ictal and Postictal Headaches

Hemicrania epileptica or synchronous ipsilateral ictal headache with migraine features is a cause of headaches resulting from a seizure. Most patients have both ictal headaches and some other seizure manifestations, although ictal headaches can be the only symptom. The seizure discharges, usually on the same side as the ipsilateral headache, begin and end simultaneously with the headache. The headaches usually last a few seconds to minutes. Unilateral or bilateral headaches can occur during a temporal lobe seizure.[55]

Postictal headaches are common after partial complex and generalized tonic-clonic seizures, reported by 51% of subjects in one study.[56] The headaches can resemble those of migraine or tension type.

MULTIPLE SCLEROSIS AND HEADACHES

Acute Attacks and Headaches

Tension- and migrainelike headaches can occur with a first or subsequent attacks in 1.4%[57] to 7%[58] of cases. Some attacks with hemiparesis may raise the possibility of hemiplegic migraine.

Trigeminal Neuralgia and Multiple Sclerosis

A plaque at the point of entry of the trigeminal root, in the main sensory nucleus, or the descending root of the trigeminal nerve can cause trigeminal neuralgia.[59] Perhaps 1% of patients with multiple sclerosis have trigeminal neuralgia, and 2% of those with trigeminal neuralgia have multiple sclerosis. The pain becomes bilateral in about 14% of those with multiple sclerosis, compared with 4% of those without. New-onset trigeminal neuralgia under the age of 40 with normal facial sensation strongly suggests multiple sclerosis as the cause.

Migraine and Multiple Sclerosis

Migraine is twice as common in multiple sclerosis patients as in controls.

CENTRAL PAIN SYNDROME

The condition resulting from central lesions that cause pain, originally termed *thalamic pain syndrome*, is now called *central pain syndrome*, since lesions in other locations can cause the same symptoms. Central lesions of the second-order trigeminal neurons, the quintothalamic tract, the ventrobasal nuclei of the thalamus, the parietal lobe, and even the cerebellum can cause diminished pain and burning sensations in the face and scalp. The ipsilateral extremities and trunk are usually also involved. Diminished pinprick and temperature sensation are usually present. Patients also report mechanical and thermal, especially cold, hyperalgesia. Central pain syndrome is a complication of 8% of strokes. The onset of the pain may be delayed for 1 or 2 months after the stroke. Multiple sclerosis can also cause central pain syndrome.

Treatment is often difficult. Medications that may be beneficial include tricyclic antidepressants (e.g., amitriptyline), antiepileptics (including carbamazepine, valproic acid, and gabapentin), narcotics, clonidine, and neuroleptics.[60]

REFERENCES

1. Lance JW, Goadsby PJ. Other headaches without any structural abnormality. In: *Mechanism and management of headache,* 6th ed. Oxford: Butterworth-Heinemann, 1998:206–225.
2. Silberstein SD, Lipton RB, Goadsby PJ. Headache associated with non-vascular intracranial disease. In: *Headache in clinical practice.* Oxford: Isis, 1998:143–164.
3. Raskin NH. Short-lived head pains. *Neurol Clin* 1997;15: 143–152.
4. Davidoff RA, Dalessio DJ. Activity-related headache. In: Gilman S, Goldstein GW, Waxman SG, eds. *Neurobase.* San Diego: Arbor, 2000.
5. Rasmussen BK, Olesen J. Symptomatic and nonsymptomatic headaches in a general population. *Neurology* 1992;42: 1225–1231.
6. Lance JW. Headaches related to sexual activity. *J Neurol Neurosurg Psychiatry* 1976;39:1226–1230.
7. Silbert PL, Edis RH, Stewart-Wynne EG, et al. Benign vascular sexual headache and exertional headache: interrelationships and long term prognosis. *J Neurol Neurosurg Psychiatry* 1991; 54:417–421.
8. Jacome DE. Masturbatory-orgasmic extracephalic pain. *Headache* 1998;38:138–141.
9. Sands GH, Newman L, Lipton R. Cough, exertional, and other miscellaneous headaches. *Med Clin North Am* 1991;75: 733–743.
10. Pascual J, Iglesias F, Oterino A, et al. Cough, exertional, and sexual headaches: an analysis of 72 benign and symptomatic cases. *Neurology* 1996;46:1520–1524.
11. Mathew NT. Indomethacin-responsive headache syndromes. *Headache* 1981;21:147–150.
12. Raskin NH. The cough headache syndrome: treatment. *Neurology* 1995;47:1784.
13. Bahra A, Goadsby PJ. Cough headache responsive to methysergide. *Cephalalgia* 1998;18:495–496.
14. Ostergaard JR, Kraft M. Natural history of benign coital headache. *BMJ* 1992;305:1129.
15. Davidoff RA. Headache associated with sexual activity. In: Gilman S, Goldstein GW, Waxman SG, eds. *Neurobase.* San Diego: Arbor, 2000.
16. Akpunona SE, Ahrens J. Sexual headaches: case report, review, and treatment with calcium blocker. *Headache* 1991;31:141–145.
17. Elster AD, Chen MY. Chiari I malformations: clinical and radiologic reappraisal. *Radiology* 1992;183:347–353.
17a. Milhorat TH, Chou MW, Trinidad EM, et al. Chiari I malformation redefined: clinical and radiographic findings for 364 symptomatic patients. *Neurosurgery* 1999;44:1005–1017.
18. Pillay PK, Awad IA, Little JR, et al. Symptomatic Chiari malformation in adults: a new classification based on magnetic resonance imaging with clinical and prognostic significance. *Neurosurgery* 1991;28:639–645.
19. Pascual J, Oterino A, Berciano J. Headache in type I Chiari malformation. *Neurology* 1992;42:42:1519–1521.
20. Khurana RK. Headache spectrum in Arnold-Chiari malformation. *Headache* 1991;31:151–155.

21. Ramadan NB. Unusual causes of headache. *Neurology* 1997;48: 1494–1499.
22. Holloway RG, Kieburtz KD. Headache associated with AIDS. In: Gilman S, Goldstein GW, Waxman SG, eds. *Neurobase*. San Diego: Arbor, 2000.
23. Mirsattari SM, Power C, Nath A. Primary headaches in HIV-infected patients. *Headache* 1999;39:3–10.
24. Greenlee JE. Brain abscess. In: Gilman S, Goldstein GW, Waxman SG, eds. *Neurobase*. San Diego: Arbor, 2000.
25. Carlini ME, Harris RL. Central nervous system infections. In: Evans RW, ed. *Diagnostic testing in neurology*. Philadelphia: WB Saunders, 1999:405–417.
26. Silberstein SD, Pollack DA. Headache associated with meningitis, encephalitis, and brain abscess. In: Gilman S, Goldstein GW, Waxman SG, eds. *Neurobase*. San Diego: Arbor, 2000.
27. Jain KK. Drug-induced aseptic meningitis. In: Gilman S, Goldstein GW, Waxman SG, eds. *Neurobase*. San Diego: Arbor, 1999.
28. Neufeld MY, Treves TA, Chistik V, et al. Postmeningitis headache. *Headache* 1999;39:132–134.
29. Halperin JL. Lyme disease. In: Gilman S, Goldstein GW, Waxman SG, eds. *Neurobase*. San Diego: Arbor, 2000.
30. Meyer JS, Terayama Y, Konno S, et al. Headache associated with metabolic disorders. In: Gilman S, Goldstein GW, Waxman SG, eds. *Neurobase*. San Diego: Arbor, 2000.
31. Bana DS, Yap AU, Graham JR. Headache during dialysis. *Headache* 1972;2:1–14.
32. Honigman B, Theis MK, Koziol-McLain J, et al. Acute mountain sickness in a general tourist population at moderate altitudes. *Ann Intern Med* 1993;118:587–592.
33. Sutton JR. High-altitude physiology and medicine. In: Evans RW, ed. *Neurology and trauma*. Philadelphia: WB Saunders, 1996.
34. Krasney JA. A neurogenic basis for acute altitude illness. *Med Sci Sports Exerc* 1994;26:195–208.
35. Burtscher M, Likar R, Nachbauer W, et al. Aspirin for prophylaxis against headache at high altitudes: randomized, double blind, placebo controlled trial. *BMJ* 1998;316:1057–1058.
36. Jerome EH, Severinghaus JW. High-altitude pulmonary edema. *N Engl J Med* 1996;334:662–663.
37. Greer HD, Massey EW. Neurological injury from undersea diving. In: Evans RW, ed. *Neurology and trauma*. Philadelphia: WB Saunders, 1996.
38. Evans RW. Neurologic aspects of hyperventilation syndrome. *Semin Neurol* 1995;15:115–125.
39. Lewis RA, Howell JBL. Definition of the hyperventilation syndrome. *Bull Eur Physiopathol Respir* 1986;22:201–204.
40. Hirokawa Y, Kondo T, Ohta Y, et al. Clinical characteristics and outcome of 508 patients with hyperventilation syndrome. *Nippon Kyobu Shikkan Gakkai Zasshi* 1995;33:940–946.
41. Evans RW. Neurologic aspects of hyperventilation syndrome. *Semin Neurol* 1995;15:115–125.
42. Beumer HM, Bruyn GW. Hyperventilation syndrome. In: Goetz CG, Tanner CM, Aminoff MJ, eds. *Handbook of clinical neurology,* vol 19. Amsterdam: Elsevier, 1993:429–448.
43. Sahota PK, Dexter JD. Sleep and headache syndromes: a clinical review. *Headache* 1990;30:80–84.

44. Culebras A. Sleep disorders associated with headaches. In: Gilman S, Goldstein GW, Waxman SG, eds. *Neurobase*. San Diego: Arbor, 1999.

45. Gould JD, Silberstein SD. Unilateral hypnic headache: a case study. *Neurology* 1997;49:1749–1750.

46. Ulfberg J, Carter N, Talback M, et al. Headache, snoring, and sleep apnoea. *J Neurol* 1996;243:621–625.

47. Aldrich MA. Sleep bruxism. In: Gilman S, Goldstein GW, Waxman SG, eds. *Neurobase*. San Diego: Arbor, 2000.

48. Blau JN. Sleep deprivation headache. *Cephalalgia* 1990;10: 157–160.

49. Blau J. Resolution of migraine attacks: sleep and the recovery phase. *J Neurol Neurosurg Psychiatry* 1982;45:223–226.

50. Giroud M, Nivelon JL, Dumas R. [Somnambulism and migraine in children: a non-fortuitous association]. *Arch Fr Pediatr* 1987;44:263–265.

51. Dexter JD. The relationship between disorders of arousal from sleep and migraine. *Headache* 1986;26:322.

52. Pearce JMS. Clinical features of the exploding head syndrome. *J Neurol Neurosurg Psychiatry* 1989;52:907–910.

53. Welch KMA, Lewis D. Migraine and epilepsy. *Neurol Clin* 1997; 15:107–123.

54. Marks DA, Ehrenberg BL. Migraine-related seizures in adults with epilepsy with EEG correlation. *Neurology* 1993;43: 2476–2483.

54a. Panayiotopoulos CP. Elementary visual hallucinations, blindness, and headache in idiopathic occiptial epilepsy: differentiation from migraine. *J Neurol Neurosurg Psychiatry* 1999;66:536–540.

55. Young GB, Blume WT. Painful epileptic seizures. *Brain* 1983; 106:537–554.

56. Schon F, Blau JN. Post-epileptic headache and migraine. *J Neurol Neurosurg Psychiatry* 1987;50:1148–1152.

57. Freedman MS, Gray TA. Vascular headache: a presenting symptom of multiple sclerosis. *Can J Neurol Sci* 1989;16:63–66.

58. Rolak LA, Brown S. Headaches and multiple sclerosis: a clinical study and review of the literature. *J Neurol* 1990;237:300–302.

59. Davidoff RA. Trigeminal neuralgia. In: Gilman S, Goldstein GW, Waxman SG, eds. *Neurobase*. San Diego: Arbor, 2000.

60. Beric A. Central pain and dysesthesia syndrome. *Neurol Clin* 1998;16:899–918.

What's My Headache?

Randolph W. Evans

Now it's time to play, "What's my headache?" the popular game enjoyed by millions of Americans yearly when they come to see their doctors. The focus is on diagnosis and management. A brief summary of a case based on patients I have seen is provided. Then you should decide on your diagnosis and management. What tests, if any, would you order, or can the diagnosis be made without testing? What treatment is appropriate? Final answer? You can then compare your answers with my diagnosis and management provided in the answers section at the end of the case presentations where the chapter dealing with the topic is also provided. The cases range from common to uncommon to rare causes and presentations of headaches.

CASE PRESENTATIONS

Case 1

This 24-year-old man came in with a 6-day history of a nuchal-occipital bad-aching headache associated with nausea and with sensitivity to light and noise. His concentration seemed off and he had intermittent blurred vision. One week earlier he had been in a motor vehicle accident in which he had bumped his forehead and briefly lost consciousness. That day he was seen in the emergency room and discharged on ibuprofen after a normal cervical spine series was obtained. Neurologic examination was normal.

What is the diagnosis? Would you order an imaging study?

Case 2

This 10-year-old boy was seen with a 1.5-year history of headaches that were all the same. He described a bifrontal pounding associated with a little nausea and with light and noise sensitivity. The headaches lasted about 1 hour and were helped by lying down and ibuprofen. The headaches usually occurred three or four times per month. During the prior 2 weeks, he had had five. The mother reported no increased stress or changes in schoolwork. There was a medical history of sinus symptoms and allergy treated with Bromfed. Family history is noncontributory. Neurologic exam was normal.

What is the diagnosis? Would you order an imaging study? What treatment would you suggest?

Case 3

An 84-year-old woman was referred with a 2.5-week history of intermittent daily severe headaches described as a right retroorbital, hemicranial, and nuchal occipital pounding and pressure. She also reported pressure in the right posterior neck. Tylenol was of mild help. She thought she might have low-grade fever. She also complained of soreness of the right temporomandibular joint with eating. She denied any shoulder or pelvic girdle aching and had no recent weight loss. On examination, the right superficial temporal artery pulse was not present and the area was very tender.

What is the diagnosis? What studies are indicated? What is your treatment?

Case 4

This 31-year-old male complained of an 8-month history of daily severe headaches that often occurred in the afternoon. The headaches usually began bifrontally and then become a generalized throbbing with increased intensity with bending over or coughing. The headaches lasted several hours and could be associated with frequent nausea and occasional vomiting and photophobia. There was a history of occasional mild headaches. Neurologic exam was normal.

What is the diagnosis? Would you recommend an imaging study? What treatment would you recommend?

Case 5

A 44-year-old woman is referred to the office with a 3-day history of a severe nuchal occipital and generalized throbbing ache associated with nausea and worse with movement. She had been seen in an emergency room the day before, where she was given a Stadol injection with only mild help. About 1 month earlier she had a similar but less severe headache that lasted 1 day. She otherwise had a history of occasional mild headaches. Neurologic examination was normal.

What is your diagnosis? Would you recommend testing? Would you try giving a triptan?

Case 6

This 38-year-old pediatrician described recurring headaches since high school: a left more often than right temporal or occasionally bitemporal pressure associated with nausea and occasionally vomiting lasting about 24 hours. There were no other associated symptoms. The headaches could awaken her from sleep. Over-the-counter medications helped just a little. At times, the headaches interfered with her activity and she would go to bed and try to sleep. Frequency had been variable from one to four each month; recently, headaches occurred at the rate of one a week. They were not triggered by menses, foods, or alcohol but could be triggered by heat or stress. There was no recent oral contraceptive use. Family history was noncontributory. Neurologic exam was normal.

What is the diagnosis? Would you recommend an imaging study? What treatment would you recommend?

Case 7

On the day before the consultation, this 47-year-old male attorney had sex after a several-week abstinence. One minute before a second orgasm, he developed a bad, pounding nuchal occipital headache that increased in intensity with orgasm. The headache was bad for 1 hour and persisted as a mild nuchal-occipital ache when he was seen. He had no nausea, vomiting, or other symptoms. He had rare mild headaches in the past. Neurologic exam was normal. The neck was supple.

What is your diagnosis? Would you recommend testing?

Case 8

This 33-year-old woman had a history of only occasional mild headaches. One year before presentation, she developed increasingly frequent headaches that were daily for the month before consultation. She described having daily mild to moderate bifrontal aching and throbbing headaches. About twice a week, the headache became a bifrontal and nuchal occipital pounding associated with nausea, light and noise sensitivity, and occasional vomiting. The mild to moderate headaches lasted about 2 hours if she took Excedrin Migraine. The severe headaches could last all day and she would go to bed. She was taking from two to six Excedrin Migraine tablets daily. In the year prior, she had seen an internist, a chiropractor, and another neurologist. A magnetic resonance imaging (MRI) scan of the brain was normal. No new medications were started. Neurologic exam was normal.

What is the your diagnosis? Would you recommend additional testing? How would you manage this patient?

Case 9

A 23-year-old woman in the middle of her menses presented with a 4-day history of a constant severe headache described as a generalized heaviness associated with noise sensitivity but no nausea, vomiting, light sensitivity, fever, or systemic symptoms. She reported occasional headaches in the past. She did have a history of two throbbing headaches on the top of her head followed by brief syncopal episodes at the ages of 8 and 18. With the last episode, testing, including an electroencephalogram and computed tomography (CT) scan were reportedly negative. Family history was remarkable for two maternal aunts with migraine. Neurologic exam was normal. Toradol 60 mg intramuscularly (IM) was given in the office. Within 30 minutes, the headache was reduced from an intensity rating of 10 to a level of 1.

What is your diagnosis? Would you recommend testing?

Case 10

This 18-year-old woman reported headaches every 2 weeks for the previous few years described as a bifrontal pressure relieved by Advil. For the prior 2 years, every 3 or 4 months around her menses she had episodes of blurred vision in the right field of vision lasting 15 to 30 minutes without an associated headache or other symptoms. She presented with a 4-day history of an intermittent bitemporal and retroorbital pounding with noise sensitivity but no other symptoms. The headache was behind the right eye the day before the office visit and behind the left eye the next morning but had resolved by the afternoon office visit. There was no history of similar headaches. She had no sinus or systemic symptoms. She had been on oral contraceptives for 4 months. Family history was noncontributory. Neurologic exam was normal.

What is the diagnosis? Would you recommend testing?

Case 11

This 33-year-old man presented with a 6-year history of episodic headaches that occurred about every 1 to 2 years, often in the spring, and that recurred over an 8-week period. The current headaches were present for 10 days. He described a severe stabbing around the left eye and forehead associated with conjunctival injection, ipsilateral tearing of the eye, and clear drainage from the nares. The headaches lasted about 45 minutes, during which time he paced about and sometimes banged his head. He typically had two headaches per day, one in the afternoon and the other awakening him from sleep around 2 A.M.

What is your diagnosis? Would you recommend an imaging study? What treatment would you provide?

Case 12

This 35-year-old woman reported occasional headaches in the past. For the last few months, she has had a daily and fairly constant generalized intense ache without associated symptoms. Over-the-counter medications have been of little help and she stopped taking any medication. She drank occasional caffeinated beverages. Her posterior neck has been tight for a long time. She reports increased financial stress recently. Family history: 7-year-old daughter with chronic headaches. Neurologic exam was normal.

What is your diagnosis? Would you recommend testing? What treatment would you suggest?

Case 13

This 27-year-old woman had occasional headaches in the past. She presented with a 3-month history of daily, intermittent nuchal occipital pressure-type headaches on the left more than the right that could occur any time of the day but did not awaken her from sleep. She reported being under increased stress. Her husband was being transferred out of state, her family was here, and she would prefer not moving. She has three small children. Exam showed left mid-superior nuchal line tenderness. Digital pressure produced pain similar to her headache. Neurologic exam was otherwise normal.

What is the diagnosis? Would you recommend testing? What treatment would you recommend?

Case 14

This 26-year-old woman, 12 weeks pregnant, was admitted to the hospital by her obstetrician with a severe right nuchal-occipital and parietal pressure headache with nausea and vomiting present for 7 days. During the preceding 3 months, she had daily headaches. She had no fever or systemic symptoms. She was given intravenous morphine and phenergan, which did not help. She had a history of recurring generalized throbbing headaches with nausea, vomiting, and light and noise sensitivity lasting 3 to 4 days for the last 8 years. She saw a neurologist 4 months before admission and was diagnosed with migraine. Before this pregnancy, she was having headaches three times per month for the last 2 years. Neurologic exam was normal.

What is the diagnosis? Would you recommend testing? What treatment would you recommend?

Case 15

A 46-year-old male reports severe stabbing headaches shooting up from the palate lasting perhaps 30 seconds. The headaches are triggered by ice cream or yogurt. Although the headache is a 10, medical attention has never been sought. Neurologic exam is normal.

What is the diagnosis? Would you recommend testing?

Case 16

A 42-year-old female attorney was seen with a 4-year history of bad headaches about once every 3 to 4 months that could be triggered by stress or lack of sleep. She described a severe right- or left-sided throbbing with nausea, light, and noise sensitivity, and occasional vomiting. She occasionally saw spots before her eyes for a few minutes before the headache. The headache could last 1 to 2 days without treatment. Her family physician placed her on Imitrex with improvement but not complete relief.

For the last 2 years, she had been having daily headaches. She would wake up almost nightly about 2 A.M. with a generalized pressure headache and take a Vanquish; the headache would improve in about 30 minutes. The headache also occurred about 2 P.M. and was relieved by Tylenol ES in about 30 minutes. She took about 14 Vanquish and about 14 Tylenol weekly and also drank about 2 cups of coffee daily. She had been on Inderal LA 80 mg daily for 1.5 years for mitral valve prolapse and palpitations with benefit. Neurologic exam was normal.

What is your diagnosis? Would you recommend any testing? What treatment do you recommend?

Case 17

This 30-year-old obese woman was seen with a 3-month history of rather constant, daily, generalized aching and throbbing headaches associated with intermittent brief graying out of vision. Neurologic examination was normal except for bilateral papilledema.

What is the diagnosis? What tests would you recommend?

Case 18

This 11-year-old girl reported a history of four or five spells with the first at 7 years of age and the last 3 days before the consultation. The prior headache occurred 1 week previously. The episodes occurred while playing catch or running around except for the last one, which happened after she was dancing, layed down for a few minutes, and then got up. The episodes were described as an intense feeling of the right side of the head going to sleep or vibrating and lasting about 30 seconds. With all the episodes except the last, which was mild, she would fall down because of the pain. However, she did not believe that there was any alteration in or loss of consciousness. Otherwise, her history was one of occasional mild headaches. There was no history of syncope, seizures, significant head trauma, or meningitis. Family history was negative for migraine and seizures. Neurologic examination was normal.

What is the diagnosis? What tests would you recommend?

Case 19

This 35-year-old female developed severe stabbing and throbbing pain in the left anterior neck and left side of the face, but not the head, lasting about 5 hours. For years she had experienced frequent right nuchal occipital pressure–type headaches associated with posterior neck tightness. She went to the emergency department, where the exam was normal and she was advised to see her doctor the next day. The next day her examination was normal.

What is the diagnosis? Would you recommend any testing?

Case 20

A 13-year-old female presented with a 6-month history of new-onset daily headaches with only occasional mild headaches previously. Bad headaches occurred about three times a week and were described as a generalized throbbing associated with nausea, light and noise sensitivity, but no aura. Advil, Aleve, or Tylenol would relieve the headache in 2.5 hours. She had no triggers. She also had mild headaches on a daily basis that could occur any time of the day and last about 1.5 hours; these were relieved by Advil. These headaches involved a bitemporal, frontal, and generalized pressure without associated symptoms. For both headaches, she was taking about four Advil and one Aleve daily and an occasional Tylenol. Her pediatrician tried Claritin without any help. The headaches did not subside during the summer. She reported being under increased stress during the prior few months, with some problems at home and in school. She drank occasional caffeinated beverages. Her mother has migraines. Neurologic exam was normal.

What is the diagnosis? Would you recommend any testing? What treatment would you suggest?

Case 21

This 49-year-old female was referred by her family physician for severe headaches. The patient reported an 11-day history of a right retroorbital and hemicranial throbbing headache that was worse with movement; she also experienced lightheadedness. She had nausea and vomiting for 2 days 4 days prior to the consultation. She had no fever, sinus symptoms, or systemic symptoms. She also complained of low-back soreness for 3 days. Her family physician gave her a cortisone shot for possible allergies, which did not help. A few days later she was given a Demerol injection, which also did not help. She then saw her allergist and was given Imitrex 50 mg orally and Medrol for 2 days without benefit. She was also prescribed Fiorinal #3 and Vicodin, which only dulled the headache, and Antivert, which did not help the dizziness. From her mid-20s until about 35 years of age, she had throbbing headaches on the top of her head associated with nausea and vomiting. Since then, she has had only occasional mild headaches. Neurologic exam was normal. Her neck was supple.

What is your diagnosis? Would you recommend any testing? What treatment would you recommend?

Case 22

This 17-year-old male presented with a 6-month history of bilateral throbbing headaches triggered by sneezing, coughing, weight lifting, or bowel movements lasting about 3 minutes. About half of the time, a slight headache would persist for an additional 5 minutes. Before the visit, he was having about 10 headaches each week. He saw his family physician, who obtained a CT scan of the head with and without contrast, which was negative. He was placed on Inderal LA 60 mg daily without help. His father has cluster headaches. Neurologic exam was normal.

What is your diagnosis? Would you recommend any additional evaluation or treatment?

Case 23

One evening I received a frantic telephone call from a friend who was in her Suburban en route to a pediatric emergency room. Her 9-year-old son was playing just a short time before at home when he accidentally bumped the back of his head on a table. There was no loss of consciousness. Within a couple of minutes, he developed a left frontal pain, nausea, vomiting, and sleepiness. There was no prior history of significant headaches or motion sickness. Family history was negative for migraine.

What would you tell the mother?

Case 24

This 45-year-old female presented with a 4-day history of a right-sided throbbing headache with nausea and vomiting for 2 days. The day of the consultation, she complained of a right nuchal occipital and right frontal aching without nausea, fever, or systemic symptoms. There was a 15-year history of recurring headaches. The bad headaches had occurred about once weekly for the prior 6 months but were occasional for many years. She described a usually right-sided and occasionally left-sided throbbing associated with nausea and occasionally vomiting with light and noise sensitivity but no aura. The headaches usually lasted 1 day but could last up to 4. There were no triggers. Imitrex SC on one occasion did not help. Neurologic exam was normal except for intensification of the headache with digital pressure over the right mid-superior nuchal line (over the greater occipital nerve).

What is your diagnosis? Would you recommend testing? What treatment would you suggest?

Case 25

This 53-year-old female hospital administrator and physician's wife was seen with a 5-week history of daily headaches that were left nuchal-occipital at first and then became a fairly constant bitemporal pain with posterior neck tightness. She had no sinus or systemic symptoms. The headache was worse with coughing and sneezing. She tried Tylenol and Sudafed without help. I had treated her for 10 years for migraine headaches without aura that started at 28 years of age. The headaches were usually a right and occasionally left hemicranial throbbing associated with nausea, sometimes vomiting, light and noise sensitivity relieved by Imitrex SC or NS. Neurologic examination was normal.

What is your diagnosis? Would you recommend any testing? What treatment would you try?

Case 26

A 32-year-old woman has a 3-year history of headaches that are a bilateral occipital and retroorbital throbbing associated with nausea but no aura, vomiting, or light or noise sensitivity and lasting up to 2 days. Fiorinal #3 decreased but did not relieve the pain. The headaches were occurred one or two times each week 1 year ago, but in the last year they have been infrequent, with the last occurring 4 months ago while she was taking amitriptyline and propranolol. She presented with a 4-day history of a severe bilateral occipital and retroorbital throbbing associated with light and noise sensitivity, nausea, but no aura or vomiting. She had not had any fever or systemic symptoms. Neurologic examination was normal. She was admitted by her gynecologist and placed on parenteral narcotics without help.

What is the diagnosis? Would you recommend any testing? What treatment is indicated?

Case 27

This 61-year-old woman was seen with a 10-year history of a right mandibular sharp pain lasting seconds and extending from the chin to the TMJ area along the mandible. The pain was sometimes triggered by drinking water, talking, and chewing. There were no trigger zones to touch. She also had an intermittent right mandibular distribution dull ache at times. The pain would occur intermittently for a few months with up to 10 paroxysms daily and then go away for a few months but was almost daily for the prior year. She saw a dentist who gave her a partial bridge without help and then a second dentist who gave her a night guard without benefit. Neurologic examination was normal.

What is the diagnosis? Would you recommend any testing? What treatment would you suggest?

Case 28

This 23-year-old woman was seen with a 5-day history of a severe bifrontal-temporal throbbing headache associated with nausea and photophobia, which was worse supine. She had no fever, sinus, or systemic symptoms. There was a history of occasional "sinus headaches" described as a hemicranial throbbing with nausea and light sensitivity occurring before her menses. She had been evaluated in the emergency department the night before the office visit. A CT scan of the brain and lumbar puncture and cerebrospinal fluid (CSF) evaluation were reported as normal. She was afebrile. Neurologic examination was normal.

What is the diagnosis? Would you recommend any testing? What treatment would you suggest?

Case 29

A 69-year-old woman presented with a 6-month history of a recurring right retroorbital and occasionally nuchal-occipital piercing pain that could last up to 1 hour and often occurred at night. There was a history, going back a number of years, of posterior neck symptoms without upper-extremity complaints. Exam was normal except for marked right mid-superior nuchal line tenderness reproducing the headache.

What is the diagnosis? Would you recommend testing? What treatment would you recommend?

Case 30

This 35-year-old woman reported bad headaches that occurred since she was a teenager and averaged about one or two each year. The last occurred about 1.5 years ago. She described a generalized throbbing associated with nausea, vomiting, light and noise sensitivity lasting 1 to 3 days. She would take Tylenol and try to sleep. She had never seen a doctor for the headaches. She also had frequent mild headaches for years that occurred about two or three times per week previously but almost daily for the prior few weeks. The headaches were a nuchal-occipital pressure often in the afternoon and could last a few hours. She was taking about four Tylenol ES daily. She also drank about two cups of coffee and four Dr. Peppers daily.

Ten days before I saw her, she had a stabbing sensation in the left temple lasting about 30 minutes. She then developed a left-sided throbbing with an intensity of 10/10 within seconds. There was no associated nausea or sensitivity to light or noise. The headache lasted about 6 hours. She was seen in the emergency room and was reported to have a normal CT scan of the head. The family history was remarkable for her mother, with a history of a ruptured aneurysm. My neurologic exam was normal.

What are your diagnoses of the headaches? Would you recommend any further testing? What treatment would you recommend?

Case 31

This 38-year-old G2 P2 had a C-section 6 days previously for failure to progress. The epidural catheter was removed 1 day post partum. She was breastfeeding. The day before I saw her, she developed a mild headache that within 30 minutes became a severe 10/10 generalized throbbing associated with nausea, light, and noise sensitivity and blurred vision. The headache was not better supine. She had no fever, back pain, or systemic complaints. This headache, the worst of her life, was still severe the next day, when she was evaluated. There was a history of throbbing generalized headaches with nausea, vomiting, and light and noise sensitivity occurring several times per year but none since the first trimester. She was afebrile and had a supple neck. Neurologic exam was normal.

What is your diagnosis? Would you recommend any testing? What treatment would you recommend?

Case 32

An 82-year-old man was seen with an 8-hour history of a mild dull right frontal headache that had been present since awakening. He had played golf that morning but did not feel quite right and shot a 92, about 10 strokes higher than his usual. (He had had a single-digit handicap when he was younger.) The headache was more intense when he bent over to pick up the ball or tee it up. There was no history of significant headaches. He was in good health except for hypertension controlled with medication. Neurologic exam was normal.

What is your diagnosis? Would you recommend any testing? What treatment would you recommend?

Case 33

A 52-year-old overweight male police officer presented with a 2-month history of a dull intense bifrontal and retroorbital, rather constant headache that was worse with coughing or bending over. He had had occasional mild headaches in the past. Neurologic exam was normal except for the presence of papilledema. A MRI scan of the brain was normal.

What is your diagnosis? Would you recommend further testing? What treatment would you recommend?

Case 34

This 73-year-old woman presented with a 3-week history of a daily, mild to moderate, aching, generalized headache. She had experienced migraines for the last 15 years. There was a history of a mastectomy for breast carcinoma 3 years previously. Neurologic exam was normal. A CT scan of the brain with and without contrast obtained by her primary-care physician was normal.

What is your diagnosis? Would you recommend further testing? What treatment would you recommend?

Case 35

A 28-year-old woman is seen for evaluation of left-sided numbness. The patient developed a pounding bifrontal headache lasting about 5 hours. She went to sleep and the headache was gone the next morning. That afternoon she had the sudden onset of tingling of the left face and a numb and weak feeling on her left side. There was a history of occasional mild headaches. Neurologic exam showed decreased sensation over the entire left face and left side of the body and decreased rapid alternating movements of the left side. A CT scan of the brain was normal.

What is your diagnosis? Would you recommend further testing?

Case 36

This 76-year-old woman underwent a left carotid endarterectomy for asymptomatic 95% internal carotid stenosis. There was no neurologic deficit postoperatively. The next morning, she complained of a severe left frontotemporal-hemicranial aching headache without associated symptoms. Neurologic exam was again normal.

What is your diagnosis? Would you recommend further testing?

Case 37

A previously healthy 42-year-old man was hospitalized with a 1-month history of right-sided headaches. Neurologic exam was normal. A MRI scan of the brain revealed diffuse enhancement of the meninges.

What is your diagnosis? What further testing would you recommend?

The patient became progressively encephalopathic the day after admission and, by 2 weeks after admission, was comatose. What is your diagnosis now?

Case 38

A 62-year-old man saw an orthopedist, complaining of a 4-month history of fairly constant neck pain, which he believed started after having his head propped at an angle for a long period of time. For the prior 2 months, he had had a constant dull ache behind the eyes, across the forehead, and sometimes on the top of the head. The neck pain, which frequently awakened him from sleep, was better with heat and ice and worse with bending the neck backward and to the left or right. Coughing or sneezing would cause a brief stabbing pain behind the left or right ear. His internist had tried him on naproxen with little help. On exam, the neck was nontender, with a decreased range of motion in all directions. Neurologic exam was normal. A cervical spine series showed multilevel spondylosis. An erythrocyte sedimentation rate (ESR) was 1.

What is your diagnosis? What treatment would you recommend? Would you recommend any further testing?

The patient returned to see the orthopedist 2 weeks later with a 1-week history of complaints of intermittent slurred speech and difficulty eating, with problems coordinating his tongue and jaw. His wife was concerned that he might have had a stroke.

What would you recommend now?

Case 39

This 32-year-old woman was seen with an acute throbbing behind the left eye and across the forehead that was associated with nausea, vomiting, and light and noise sensitivity that had awakened her from sleep 9 hours earlier. This was the worst headache of her life and different from prior headaches. For 2 days previously she had had a mild constant bifrontal pressure headache. There was a history of left-sided throbbing headaches associated with nausea and noise sensitivity but no aura since the 9 years of age. These headaches would begin 3 to 4 days before her menses started and last about 3 to 4 days. Imitrex 50 mg orally would help the headache, which would then recur. For the prior 5 years, she also had a left nuchal occipital parietal pressure headache about every other day that could last hours. She was taking 12 Tylenol per week and about 30 Fiorecet per month for the headaches. She had been on Prozac 20 mg daily for the prior year without reducing the headaches. Neurologic exam was normal. She was afebrile.

What is your diagnosis? Would you recommend any testing? What treatment would you recommend?

CASE STUDY ANSWERS

Case 1

This presentation is consistent with a postconcussion syndrome. Because there is a 1% to 2% chance of a subdural or epidural hematoma, a CT scan of the brain without contrast was obtained with normal findings. The patient was initially placed on Tylenol #3 and Phenergan. The symptoms gradually resolved over a 3-week period. (Chapter 6)

Case 2

This is a typical case of childhood migraine, which occurs in about 5% of boys. Migraines can be different in children from those in adults because the headaches have a shorter duration, often less than 2 hours, and are more often bilateral, frontal, and temporal (65% versus 40% in adults) than unilateral. After discussion with his ear, nose, and throat (ENT) physician, who had started the Bromfed for atopic allergies, Bromfed was discontinued and he was started on Periactin 4 mg at bedtime. This is a treatment "two for" because Periactin is an antihistamine and an effective preventive migraine drug in children. (Other "two fors" are tricyclic antidepressants, for the treatment of migraine and depression; beta-blockers, for migraine and hypertension; and Depakote, for migraine and epilepsy.) After 2 weeks, the dose of Periactin was increased to 8 mg at bedtime. Within a few weeks, the frequency of the headaches decreased to two or three per month. (Chapter 7)

Case 3

A MRI scan of the brain was negative. The erythrocyte sedimentation rate (ESR) was 97 mm/hour. A superficial temporal artery (STA) biopsy was negative. The headache resolved within 24 hours of starting Prednisone 60 mg daily. A repeat ESR 2 weeks later was 55. The dose of Prednisone was slowly tapered.

The diagnosis is temporal arteritis. Headaches are present in 60% to 90% of patients and jaw claudication is found in 38%. The false-negative rate of STA biopsy ranges from 5% to 44% in different series. Although other positive findings were present in this patient, the STA has a normal pulse and is nontender in about 50% of cases. The ESR has been reported as normal in 10% to 36% of cases. When abnormal, the ESR averages 70 to 80 and may be as high as 130 mm/h. The C-reactive protein can also be very useful, providing additional sensitivity and specificity for the diagnosis, especially when the ESR is normal or only mildly elevated. (Chapter 9)

Case 4

This was the first headache patient I saw after completing my residency. Although the headaches are migrainelike, the daily occurrence does not fit for migraine. Medication rebound is a consideration, but he had stopped taking medications because nothing worked. A CT scan of the head demonstrated a colloid cyst of the third ventricle. He underwent craniotomy and transcollosal removal of the cyst. The headaches were gone postoperatively.

Colloid cysts of the third ventricle account for only 1% of primary intracranial mass lesions. Sudden death occurs in 5% of patients. Although you may never see a patient with a colloid cyst (some 35,000 patients later, I have seen only one other case), remember that the diagnosis of primary or benign headaches is one of exclusion. (Chapter 12)

Case 5

Statistically, this patient would probably have new-onset migraine even though migraines usually start before 40 years of age. She had a throbbing headache with nausea that was worse with activity. However, the criteria for migraine are based on a history of at least five attacks. This was her worst headache and warranted a "first or worst" evaluation. A CT scan of the brain was normal. Her neck was supple on exam. Have we now diagnosed migraine?

No! The probability of demonstrating subarachnoid hemorrhage (SAH) on CT scan is 74% on day 3. A lumbar puncture *must* be performed to exclude SAH. The lumbar puncture revealed xanthochromic CSF. A cerebral arteriogram demonstrated a 12 mm right middle cerebral artery aneurysm, which was successfully clipped. (Chapter 5)

Case 6

This is a typical case of migraine without aura diagnosed by the unilateral location, moderate or severe intensity, and associated nausea and occasional vomiting. Midrin and Anaprox did not help. Fiorinal #3 and dihydroergotamine (DHE) nasal spray were of mild help. She started using the subcutaneous form of Imitrex when it was released and later the oral form with relief of her headaches. Nortriptyline 25 mg at bedtime reduced the headaches to about two monthly. (Chapter 2)

Case 7

When a "first or worst" headache is associated with orgasm, SAH should be ruled out because sexual activity is the precipitant of up to 12% of ruptured saccular aneurysms and of 4% of bleeding arteriovenous malformations. To help remember the significance of this presentation, you may want to think of this as a "coming but going headache."

A CT scan of the head and lumbar puncture with CSF examination were normal. The headache resolved after 2 days. The patient then developed a severe post–lumbar puncture headache that was present for 3 days and resolved with a lumbar epidural blood patch. This is an example of the benign explosive type of sexual headache or benign orgasmic cephalalgia. The patient had a single recurrence of this type of headache and then experienced no further problems for the last 5 years. (Chapter 13)

Case 8

The headaches sound like a combination of tension and migraine type. However, with the frequent use of Excedrin Migraine (containing acetaminophen 250 mg, aspirin 250 mg, and caffeine 65 mg), medication rebound was the first consideration. (She was only drinking occasional caffeinated beverages.) She was advised to taper off the Excedrin Migraine and was started on nortriptyline 25 mg at bedtime. On an office visit 3 weeks later, she reported three headaches during the first week and then none for the next 2 weeks. She stopped nortriptyline on her own after 2 weeks due to constipation. She was seen again 2 months later. She had one migraine completely relieved by Zomig 2.5 mg and six mild headaches for which she took no medication. When next seen 3 months later, she reported only three mild headaches.

In some cases, medication rebound headaches can dramatically and rapidly improve when the overused medication or beverages, foods, or medications containing caffeine are tapered off. (See the list of caffeine content in Chapter 16.) Medication rebound headaches can be due to overuse of over-the-counter medications containing acetaminophen, aspirin, nonsteroidal antiinflammatory drugs, and caffeine as well as prescription drugs with these ingredients as well as others such as butalbital, narcotics, and benzodiazepines.

This patient's increased frequency of headaches coincided with her use of daily Excedrin Migraine, which she started taking after seeing a television commercial. She first thought that she must have a brain tumor or aneurysm. She was very skeptical when advised to discontinue the Excedrin Migraine because she had never heard of medication rebound headaches. The medication warning label states: "Stop using this product and see a doctor if: migraine headache pain worsens or continues for more than 48 hours." There is no warning about the potential for rebound headaches. Perhaps a more informative warning label on this and other over-the-counter medications used for headaches would be helpful for consumers. (Chapter 3)

Case 9

Although this was the first headache of this type for the patient, the headache seemed consistent with a migraine triggered by her menses. She had headache with syncope at 8 and 18 years of age that were probably of the migraine type. I advised the patient and her husband that this was probably a migraine but could not exclude other causes, such as SAH, meningitis, and sinusitis, without testing, such as a scan of the brain and possibly a lumbar puncture, which they declined. The headache returned that evening and was described as a right hemicranial and generalized pain with nausea and light sensitivity. A MRI scan of the brain demonstrated a hemorrhagic pituitary macroadenoma for which she underwent transphenoidal removal 1 month later.

Pituitary hemorrhage can result in pituitary apoplexy with headache and visual findings, be clinically silent, or, as this case demonstrates, present as a migrainelike headache without associated signs. Pituitary hemorrhage even in a macroadenoma can be overlooked and underimaged on a routine CT scan of the head for acute headache using 10-mm cuts. A MRI scan even without pituitary views will routinely identify the pathology. Sphenoid sinusitis, which can also cause a similar headache, is also well visualized on routine MRI scans of the brain but not necessarily on a routine CT scan of the head. (Chapter 12)

Case 10

There was a history of tension-type headaches every 2 weeks for a few years and perimenstrual migraine aura without headache for 2 years. She presented with a new type of headache for 4 days consistent with migraine, but there was no history of at least five similar attacks. A MRI scan of the brain was normal. The headache was gone the next day. The patient and mother declined a lumbar puncture. This was probably a first-time migraine headache of this type. It is possible that the oral contraceptive started 4 months previously was responsible for the new type of migraine.

Migraine often has different presentations in the same person. Seventy percent of patients with migraine with aura also have migraine without aura. Those with migraine aura without headache often have migraine headache with and without aura. Patients who usually have hemicranial migraines can also have occasional generalized headaches. Headaches can also be on one side or can move from one side to the other during an attack. The presence of associated symptoms, such as nausea, vomiting, and noise sensitivity, can vary from attack to attack. Those with typical migraine headaches without aura can develop transient migrainous accompaniments such as scintillating scotoma, numbness, dysarthria, and weakness for the first time after 45 years of age. (Chapter 9)

Case 11

This is a typical history of cluster headaches. The patient was started on verapamil sustained release 240 mg daily for prevention and a tapering course of prednisone. Use of 100% oxygen with a nonrebreathing mask for 15 minutes relieved the headaches. The headaches were gone within 2 weeks, at least until the next cluster attack. (Chapter 4)

Case 12

A MRI scan of the brain, a lumbar puncture and CSF examination, and blood studies were all normal. This presentation is consistent with new-onset daily persistent headaches. Medication rebound, always a concern in patients with frequent headaches, was not a factor here. About 5% of women and 3% of men have chronic daily headaches, with headaches occurring more than 15 days per month. Chronic daily headaches can begin after a prior history of episodic tension and/or migraine headaches or develop de novo. (Chapter 3)

Case 13

This patient also seemed to have new-onset daily persistent headaches with a muscle contraction component and left greater occipital neuralgia. The recent stress in her life could be the precipitant. I performed a left greater occipital nerve block and placed her on Naprosyn. We discussed obtaining a scan of the brain but she felt the headaches were due to stress and wanted to try treatment first. She called back 2 days later and the headaches were no better. She agreed to a MRI scan of the brain, which revealed a left cerebellar hemangioblastoma with mass effect. She underwent cerebellar hemispherectomy with a cure of the benign neoplasm that would have resulted in herniation and death in a short time without surgery. There was no family history or other lesions of the retina, spinal cord, kidneys, or pancreas to suggest Von Hippel-Lindau disease. Postoperatively, she had no neurologic deficit. Two months later, she unhappily moved out of state but had no headaches.

Statistically, the odds were high that she had a benign headache type. However, there is about a 2% chance that a patient with chronic headaches and a normal neurologic exam will have pathology such as a brain tumor. She was one of the 2%. When you obtain numerous normal scans on patients with headaches, it is easy to become frustrated and think that you are wasting time and money. When you detect a case such as this, for a while you become paranoid about the possible presence of brain tumors in everyone with benign headaches that you see.

In addition, it is easy to attribute all kinds of physical symptoms to stress. Although psychosomatic illness is common, everyone seems to have some stressors if you ask enough questions. The presence of stress is not diagnostic of a functional disorder, which is still a diagnosis of exclusion. (The use of the term *functional* is interesting. Although it seems to refer to a disorder of function, the term is used in neurology and psychiatry to indicate a nonorganic problem. This use dates to the nineteenth century. In his 1893 textbook of neurology, William Gowers divided neurologic disorders into organic and functional disease. As another aside, he also described "Gowers test," pulling on the pubic hair, for the detection of hysterical paraplegia. Disorders once believed to be functional, such as migraine, Tourette's syndrome, and dystonia, are now believed to have an organic basis.) (Chapters 1 and 12)

Case 14

This could be a case of transformed migraine or migraine status and new-onset daily persistent headaches. However, these are diagnoses of exclusion. A MRI scan of the brain demonstrated a pilocytic astrocytoma of the right cerebellar hemisphere with severe mass effect and hydrocephalus due to obstruction of the aqueduct of Sylvius. She was started on Decadron and underwent a ventriculoperitoneal shunt. Two days later, she underwent a craniotomy and resection of the neoplasm with clean margins. At 36 weeks, she underwent elective C-section with delivery of healthy twins. Two months postpartum, a follow-up MRI showed tumor recurrence. She had additional surgery and then radiotherapy. Six years later, she is doing well.

As in case 13, a normal neurologic examination is not the same as the absence of pathology. Papilledema is present in only 40% of patients with brain tumors. Even in patients with mass effect such as these two, papilledema can be absent and the examination may be normal. Although neuroimaging should not be obtained without appropriate indications, when the indications are present, imaging should be performed. MRI scans during pregnancy have not been associated with any type of birth defects. (Chapters 8 and 12)

Case 15

This is a case of ice cream headache, also known as "brain freeze" or "slurpy headache." Ice cream headache, first reported in 1850 as a hazard of eating ice cream, is more common in migraineurs. This case description is my own and I also have migraines with and without aura.

The point of the case is that pain is more easily tolerated when it is brief and the cause, especially when benign, is known. (Imagine working in the emergency room when a patient comes in and says, "Doc, I was eating some Haagen-

Daz frozen yogurt and I got this terrible pain in my head.")
Some patients may come to see you with an obvious migraine
or even mild tension-type headaches. If you dismiss them
without directly addressing their concerns about possible
underlying pathology, then they may still be quite anxious and
may even obtain another opinion. It is important to find out if
there is a hidden agenda or hidden concerns. They may think
they have a brain tumor because their aunt had one, an
aneurysm because their cousin had one, or sinus headaches
because of all the television commercials they have seen. All
you have to do is ask what they think may be causing the
headache or if they have any other questions or concerns. I
sometimes have a hard time convincing patients and/or their
families that their headaches are actually of the migraine type
and not due to something else. In some cases, they demand a
scan of the brain even when they have a typical definite
migraine history. (Chapters 1 and 13)

Case 16

We discussed obtaining a MRI scan of the brain, which would
have a low yield, and she declined. The headaches every 3 to 4
months are consistent with migraine without aura and with aura,
when she occasionally would see spots before the headache.
Imitrex 50 mg orally reduced the headache to a mild level. Other
medications that might completely relieve the migraine include
Imitrex 20 mg nasal spray, Imitrex 6 mg subcutaneously, Amerge
2.5 mg, Zomig 2.5 mg, Maxalt 10 mg, and Migranal nasal spray.

The daily headaches are best explained by medication rebound.
Vanquish contains acetaminophen 194 mg, aspirin 227 mg, and
caffeine 33 mg. I recommended that she taper off Vanquish,
Tylenol, and caffeinated coffee and try Aleve for the mild headaches. She was also started on amitriptyline 25 mg at bedtime for
headache prevention.

She was seen in follow-up 4 weeks later. She had had no headaches in the prior week, one mild headache in the previous week
relieved by Aleve, and no migraines. She was having no side
effects of amitriptyline, which I advised her to continue at the
same dose. (Chapters 2 and 3)

Case 17

Pseudotumor cerebri, which occurs 90% of the time in obese
women, was the most likely consideration. First, however, other
causes need to be excluded, including tumor cerebri, cerebral
venous thrombosis, and chronic meningitis. A MRI scan of the
brain was normal. A lumbar puncture revealed an opening pressure of 36 cm, and the CSF analysis was normal. Examination
by an ophthalmologist revealed enlarged blind spots. She was
placed on Diamox 500 mg po BID and advised to lose weight.
Serial follow-up visits with the ophthalmologist and visual field
testing are essential to detect the evidence of visual loss requiring more aggressive treatment, such as shunting or optic nerve
sheath fenestration. A MRI scan of the brain is the preferred
study rather than CT scan for the evaluation of this disorder
because the MRI especially with MRV can detect the occasional

case of cerebral venous thrombosis which can be a fatal disease. (Chapters 11 and 12)

Case 18

A MRI of the brain was normal. An electroencephalogram was normal. Three and one-half years later, she has had no further episodes. I do not know the cause of these episodes, which can be termed *short-lasting unilateral vibrating exertional headache* (SUV). Although the headaches were triggered by exertion, the features are different from benign exertional headaches, which are typically throbbing at the onset, are bilateral, and last 5 minutes to 24 hours. (Chapter 13)

Occasionally, you may see a new type of headache which is unfamiliar to you. First, check with a neurologist (or another neurologist if you are one) and the literature to see if you can label the headache. Rarely, you might identify a new type of headache. In fact, many neurologic disorders remain unrecognized, waiting for a first description by an astute physician.

Case 19

A MRI of the brain was normal. Magnetic resonance angiography (MRA) showed dissection of the upper left cervical internal carotid artery (ICA) but was otherwise normal. An arteriogram confirmed the left cervical ICA dissection but also demonstrated dissections of both distal vertebrals. She underwent extensive testing with no evidence of any underlying disorder as the cause of the spontaneous dissections. She was placed on Coumadin for more than 6 months, during which time serial MRA studies revealed resolution of the dissections.

Four years later, she developed right jaw pain. An arteriogram demonstrated a small short-segment dissection of the right ICA just superior to the carotid bulb. She was again placed on Coumadin.

Her initial presentation of anterior neck and facial pain raised concern about the possibility of an ICA dissection despite the absence of a Horner's syndrome or carotid bruit. Although the MRA demonstrated the ICA dissection, the vertebral dissection was only seen on the arteriogram. The occurrence of jaw pain 4 years later with this history raised concern about a recurrent dissection. Fortunately, she has never had any cerebral ischemic events from the dissections. The cause of her recurrent spontaneous dissections is unknown but may be due to cystic medial necrosis.

Head, face, orbital, or neck pain, usually ipsilateral to the site of the dissection, is the initial manifestation in about 80% of patients with extracranial ICA dissection. Focal cerebral ischemic symptoms occur in about 60% of patients and may follow the headache by up to 4 weeks or precede it. The presence of deficits is as follows: neurologically normal, 50%; mild deficits only, 21%; moderate to severe deficits, 25%; and death, 4%. An incomplete ipsilateral Horner's syndrome with ptosis and miosis but not anhidrosis is present in about 50% of cases due to damage of the sympathetic fibers. Either subjective or objective bruits or both are present in about 45% of patients. (Chapter 11)

Case 20

The headaches are probably of the migraine and tension type. Daily use of ibuprofen can cause medication rebound in some people. We discussed obtaining a MRI scan of the brain, but the mother declined. She was started on nortriptyline 10 mg at bedtime for three nights, increasing to 20 mg at bedtime, and was advised to stop ibuprofen for a week.

She was seen again 4 months later. She had not had any recent migraines but continued to have daily mild headaches. The girl had stopped taking nortriptyline after a week because her mother was concerned about the possibility of side effects, even though she had had none. She reported increased stress at school. We again discussed obtaining a MRI scan of the brain, which the mother declined. After a discussion of the possible side effects, they agreed to trying the nortriptyline again.

I also recommended evaluation by a psychologist and a trial of biofeedback. (Chapters 1, 2, and 7)

Case 21

The patient had a history of migraine without aura when she was younger. Status migrainosus, a possibility, is a diagnosis of exclusion. Other considerations included SAH, a subdural hematoma, neoplasm, and aseptic meningitis. Her complaint of low back pain raised concern of meningeal irritation due to SAH. I obtained a MRI of the brain with MRA on the day of the consultation because this study was available. A CT scan of the brain, and if negative, a lumbar puncture would have been appropriate alternative tests. (The probability that the CT scan would have shown evidence of SAH 11 days after the ictus is about 40%. The CSF would still be xanthochromic.) The MR studies showed a saccular aneurysm, which was confirmed on cerebral arteriography the next morning to be a 10-mm right supraclinoid internal carotid artery posterior wall aneurysm. The neck of the aneurysm was too wide for endovascular coil embolization. The next day, she underwent craniotomy. As the neurosurgeon approached the aneurysm, it ruptured but the clip was successfully placed. She has no postoperative neurologic deficit. (Chapter 5)

Case 22

Although this could be a case of benign weightlifter's headache, 50% of the headaches associated with Chiari I malformation are of this type. The CT scan, although normal, does not exclude Chiari malformation, which can be easily visualized on a routine MRI scan of the brain. (A CT scan with thin slices through the cervicomedullary region following injection of subarachnoid contrast, a myelogram, can detect this malformation.) The MRI of the brain was normal except for extension of the cerebellar tonsils through the foramen magnum to the level of the inferior surface of C2. MRI of the cervical and thoracic spine was otherwise negative with no evidence of syrinx. He underwent suboccipital craniectomy and C1 and C2 laminectomy followed by dural patch grafting. Postoperatively, the headaches were no longer present. (Chapter 13)

Case 23

I advised the mother that this was probably a migraine triggered by the minor head injury ("footballer's migraine" originally described in adolescent boys with minor head injuries playing soccer but made world famous by Terrell Davis in the 1998 Superbowl), although there was a small chance of a more serious problem (subdural or epidural hematoma). He was seen by a pediatric resident who found a normal neurologic exam. The symptoms cleared completely within 2 hours. The resident did not recommend a scan of the brain. When I saw the mother and the boy a few weeks later, he was doing fine and had experienced no further headaches. If I had seen the child during the acute attack, I would have ordered a CT scan. (Chapters 6 and 7)

Case 24

This was a 15-year history of migraine without aura. The persistent aching headache present on the day of consultation was probably a muscle contraction type with occipital neuralgia triggered by the migraine. A right greater occipital nerve block completely relieved the headache within minutes. The patient was placed on amitriptyline 25 mg at bedtime, which reduced the frequency of the headaches to about twice monthly. Midrin at the onset decreased the headache. One year later, she was seen again with a similar history of a right-sided headache for 4 days with nausea and vomiting for the first 2 days. A greater occipital nerve block again promptly relieved the headache. (Chapters 1 and 6)

Case 25

The blood pressure in both arms was 200/100 mm Hg. There was no history of hypertension. Prior blood pressures taken in the office were about 100/70 mm Hg. The patient was started on lisinopril. An MRI of the brain was normal. An extensive workup by a cardiologist for secondary causes of hypertension, including pheochromocytoma, was negative. With control of the hypertension, the new-onset daily headaches resolved. The blood pressure should be routinely taken in adults presenting with headaches. Although hypertension is much less common, do not forget also to check the blood pressure of children presenting with headaches. (Chapter 11)

Case 26

On admission, the patient's temperature was 99.4 degrees Fahrenheit. On the second hospital day, when I saw her initially, she had developed a fever of 101 degrees with the same symptoms. Her neck was supple. Although the headache was very similar to her migraines, the light and noise sensitivity were new symptoms. Now with the development of fever, meningitis and SAH had to be excluded. A CT scan of the brain was normal. A lumbar puncture revealed an opening pressure of 24 cm and the following: glucose, 56; protein, 74; white blood cell count (WBC), 1,317, with 87% lymphocytes and 13% polymorphonuclear cells; and red blood cell count, 56. Gram stain, cryptococcal antigen, and meningitis latex screen were negative. She was placed on Rocephin, which was discontinued after 2 days with normal cultures and discharged with a milder headache. The headache resolved a few days following discharge.

The diagnosis was viral meningitis, probably due to an enterovirus. Diagnostic confusion can occur when viral meningitis causes a headache similar to migraine with low-grade fever or without fever. (Chapter 13)

Case 27

The diagnosis is trigeminal neuralgia. An MRI of the brain, obtained to exclude the occasional neoplasm, was normal. The patient was started on Tegretol XL 200 mg for 1 day, then one every 12 hours. The pain resolved within 1 day of starting Tegretol. (Chapter 10)

Case 28

What the patient described as "sinus headaches" was consistent with perimenstrual migraine. I wondered if this acute different type of headache was due to status migrainosus. However, a worse headache supine did not fit. An MRI scan of the brain revealed acute sphenoid sinusitis (complete opacification of the right and partial opacification of the left) that in retrospect was also present but not reported on the CT scan. She was seen that day by an ENT physician and was started on antibiotics and decongestants with resolution of the headache and sinusitis. In summary, a patient with a history of perimenstrual migraines which she thought were sinus headaches presented with a severe headache similar to migraine but due to acute sphenoid sinusitis.

Sphenoid sinusitis can mimic migraine, SAH, and meningitis. In patients presenting with "first or worst" headaches, sphenoid sinusitis should be specifically excluded. Nasal discharge is present in only about 30% of patients, and fever is present in more than 50%. Acute sphenoid sinusitis is an important diagnosis to make because complications include bacterial meningitis, cavernous sinus thrombosis, subdural abscess, cortical vein thrombosis, ophthalmoplegia, and pituitary insufficiency. Plain sinus x-rays may not detect sphenoid sinusitis in about 25% of cases. (Chapter 12)

Case 29

A new-onset headache in someone more than 50 years of age raises concern about such conditions as temporal arteritis and brain tumors. However, benign types of headaches can also occur. I suspected that this headache was associated with neck muscle tightness and greater occipital neuralgia and performed a greater occipital nerve block with 3 ml of 1% lidocaine and placed her on Soma. The headache resolved. She returned 2 years later with an identical headache. I again performed an occipital nerve block and superior trapezius trigger point injection that decreased the headache. When the headache was still present 3 days later, she returned and the injections were repeated. The headache and neck discomfort resolved.

I saw another woman, 68 years old, with a similar headache that also resolved with an occipital nerve block. An ESR was 18. This patient returned a year later with a more intense hemicranial headache. The ESR was 40, a minimal elevation from the range of normal ([the woman's age + 10]/2 = 39) but significantly elevated from the year before. A superficial temporal artery biopsy was positive and the headache promptly resolved when she was started on prednisone. (Chapters 6 and 9)

Case 30

The occasional severe headaches since the patient was a teenager are consistent with migraine without aura. The mild headaches of increasing frequency are probably tension type and medication rebound with the daily use of Tylenol ES and caffeinated beverages. The new headache with the 30-minute prodrome is a thunderclap headache. Although this could be due to "crash migraine," other causes of thunderclap headache should be excluded, including SAH and carotid dissection. Although the CT scan of the head in the emergency room was normal, she should have also had a lumbar puncture.

I obtained a MRI scan of the brain with intracranial and neck MRA with normal findings. Because an MRA has about about a 90% sensitivity for intracranial aneurysms, I recommended a lumbar puncture to check for xanthochromia, which would still be present if a SAH had occurred. The patient declined. I also discussed with her the possibility of obtaining a cerebral arteriogram, which she also declined.

As treatment for the daily headaches, I advised her to stop the Tylenol ES and taper off the caffeinated beverages. For prevention, she was placed on amitriptyline 25 mg at bedtime. (Chapters 1, 3, and 5)

Case 31

The headaches occurring several times per year are consistent with migraine without aura. The acute headache, her worst ever, could be a migraine because migraines frequently are triggered by falling estrogen levels in the first week post partum. When patients with migraine develop a new type of severe headache, this can certainly be migraine. Unfortunately, a history of migraine is not protective against other diseases that can cause severe headaches.

Complications of the epidural anesthetic should be considered. Although post–lumbar puncture-type headaches occur after about 20% of epidurals due to inadvertent puncture of the dura and although post–lumbar puncture headaches can be delayed for as long as 14 days, her headaches were not consistent with the diagnosis because they were not better supine. A lumbar epidural abscess causing meningitis and a headache is also a consideration but she had a supple neck and no fever or back pain, which argue against that diagnosis. Pregnancy-induced hypertension can cause postpartum headaches, but her blood pressure was normal. Because up to 20% of aneurysmal ruptures occur during pregnancy or in the early postpartum period, SAH should also be ruled out. Cerebral venous thrombosis should also be considered because 90% of cases occur during the puerperium, most commonly in the second or third weeks post partum.

An MRI of the brain, MRA, and MRV were normal. The lumbar puncture revealed a normal opening pressure and normal

CSF. The headache resolved after two injections of Demerol and Phenergan 4 hours apart. The diagnosis is migraine. She was prescribed Vicodin if she were to have further migraines while pregnant. Triptans are relatively contraindicated while breast-feeding. (Chapter 8)

Case 32

This new headache in an elderly person warranted investigation even though the intensity was mild. A CT scan of the brain revealed a right frontal hemorrhagic infarction. I told the patient that he should get a "stroke handicap" for his round that morning.

Headaches commonly accompany stroke. In one study, headache occurred in 29% with bland infarcts, 57% with parenchymal hemorrhage, 36% with transient ischemic attacks, and 17% with lacunar infarcts. The headache began before the event in 60% and at its onset in 25%. The headaches are equally likely to be abrupt or gradual in onset. The headache is usually unilateral and focal of mild to moderate severity, although up to 46% of patients may have an incapacitating headache. The headache may be throbbing or nonthrobbing and may rarely be stabbing. The headache is more often ipsilateral than contralateral to the side of the cerebral ischemia. Headache is more common in ischemia of the posterior than the anterior circulation and is more common in cortical than in subcortical events. The duration of the headache is longest in cardioembolic infarcts and thrombotic infarcts, of medium duration in lacunar infarction, and shortest in transient ischemic attacks. Associated symptoms in one study include nausea in 44%, vomiting in 23%, and light and noise sensitivity in 25%. Bending, straining, and jarring the head usually increase the intensity. (Chapter 11)

Case 33

Pseudotumor cerebri is a consideration but is less much less common in males than in females. Infectious causes of headache should be excluded. A lumbar puncture revealed an opening pressure of 35 cm. CSF analysis included a glucose of 30, protein of 65, and WBC of 350 (90% lymphocytes). CSF cryptococcal antigen was positive. The patient was HIV negative and otherwise healthy. A chest x-ray was negative. This patient was successfully treated with amphotericin B. Flucytosine is another treatment option.

Cryptococcal meningitis is rare in patients without AIDS. About 50% of these patients have an underlying association, such as lymphoma, diabetes mellitus, or chronic steroid therapy. Cryptococcal meningitis occurs in perhaps 5% of HIV-infected individuals. The CSF often shows minimal changes in AIDS patients, but in non-AIDS patients it typically shows a lymphocytic pleocytosis, low glucose, and elevated protein. CSF cryptococcal antigen is positive in 90% of patients without AIDS and in 90% to 100% of those with AIDS. Neuroimaging reveals nonspecific findings in about 30% of cases, including meningeal enhancement, hydrocephalus, cerebral edema, and mass lesions (cryptococcomas or cryptococcal abscesses). (Chapter 13)

Case 34

Because this is a new-onset daily headache in a patient more than 50 years of age, there should be a strong suspicion of a secondary headache type. A lumbar puncture was indicated to rule out infection or meningeal carcinomatosis as the cause of the headaches. An MRI scan of the brain could have been done before the lumbar puncture to further exclude the presence of neoplastic disease. A lumbar puncture revealed a normal opening pressure. The CSF evaluation showed the following: glucose, 15 mg/dl; protein, 60 mg/dl; and WBC 10. CSF cytology was positive for carcinoma. The patient was diagnosed with meningeal carcinomatosis and underwent whole-brain radiotherapy.

Breast cancer accounts for 39% of solid-tumor non–central nervous system primaries causing meningeal carcinomatosis. Headache, which is present in 33% to 62% of patients, is usually not severe. A CT scan of the brain is usually normal in meningeal carcinomatosis, although meningeal enhancement with contrast administration or hydrocephalus is sometimes present. An MRI scan with contrast often demonstrates meningeal enhancement. Initial CSF examination demonstrates elevated WBCs in 51%, elevated protein in 73%, and hypoglycorrhachia or decreased CSF glucose in 28%. CSF cytology is positive in 54% on the first lumbar puncture, is positive in an additional 30% after the second, and is positive in 1% more after the third. Sending a relatively large volume of 5 to 10 ml of CSF for cytology may increase the yield. (Chapter 12)

Case 35

An MRI scan of the brain showed a small area of high signal intensity in the left parietal periventricular area. A cerebral arteriogram was normal. Blood work for vasculitis and an echocardiogram were normal. CSF examination was normal. Oligoclonal bands were absent. A visual evoked response study showed a prolonged P wave latency on the right. Visual fields demonstrated bilateral prechiasmal defects. The patient has been subsequently followed for 13 years with relapsing/remitting multiple sclerosis.

Although there was no history of migraine, the initial differential diagnosis included complicated migraine and the many other causes of cerebrovascular disease. This case is an example of an occasional acute stroke–like presentation of multiple sclerosis. Although headache can herald strokes, tension- and migraine-like headaches can occur with a first or subsequent attack of multiple sclerosis in 1.4% to 7% of cases. (Chapters 11 and 13)

Case 36

A CT scan of the brain was normal. A benign ipsilateral frontotemporal intense headache may follow endarterectomy with a latency of 36 to 72 hours. The headache may recur intermittently for up to 6 months. Headache can also develop postoperatively because of intracerebral hemorrhage, which is a complication of 0.75% of operations. The hemorrhage occurs at a median of 3 days after surgery with a range of 0 to 18 days. Although the latency of this patient's headache was shorter than the cases in the literature, a benign postcarotid endarterectomy headache is the best explanation. Although the cause is unknown, the headache could be due to afferent impulses from the carotid arterial wall or restoration of normal cerebral perfusion pressure. (Chapter 11)

Case 37

A lumbar puncture was performed revealing WBC 10, RBC 650, glucose 47, and protein 112. The opening pressure was not measured. Cryptococcal antigen and venereal disease research laboratory (VDRL) titers were negative. HIV was negative. A meningeal biopsy showed acute and chronic inflammation. A repeat lumbar puncture showed an opening pressure too low to be recorded. The CSF showed 63 WBCs (61% lymphocytes), glucose 58, and protein 88. Starting the day after admission, the patient became progressively encephalopathic. Two weeks after admission, he was comatose. Oculocephalics were intact. He withdrew all extremities to painful stimuli. Plantars were extensor bilaterally. A repeat MRI scan of the brain showed subdural accumulations of fluid, low cerebellar tonsils, and decreased fluid around the suprasellar cistern and the chiasmatic cisterns. An MRI scan of the cervical, thoracic, and lumbar spine showed no evidence of a CSF leak.

The patient underwent a lumbar epidural blood patch with injection of 50 ml of autologous blood. Within 1 day, the patient awoke and was confused. An MRI scan of the brain 3 days after the blood patch demonstrated some restoration of CSF in the chiasmatic and suprasellar cisterns and elevation of the brain stem. Two weeks later, he was alert and oriented. He had no recollection of the prior month. Neurologic exam was otherwise normal except for a right-pupil-sparing third nerve palsy.

This is a case of spontaneous intracranial hypotension resulting in coma. Only one similar case has been reported.[1] These two cases expand the clinical spectrum of low-CSF-pressure headache extending from headache alone, which may or may not have orthostatic features,[2] to coma. The cause of spontaneous CSF leaks is unknown but may be due to meningeal diverticula or dural tears.

Dural enhancement can be caused by dural metastates (lymphoma, leukemia, adenocarcinoma, and melanoma), infection (tuberculosis, syphilis, Lyme disease, etc), inflammatory disease (sarcoid, vasculitis, nonsteroidal antiinflammatory drugs, sagittal sinus thrombosis), or intracranial hypotension. Infectious meningitis usually presents as leptomeningeal (the arachnoid and pia) enhancement and carcinomatous meningitis as dural enhancement. (Chapter 12)

Case 38

The patient went to physical therapy with a report of mild benefit. When I saw him on referral from the orthopedist, the neck was nontender with a decreased range of motion. The speech was slightly slurred and the tongue deviated to the right. An MRI scan of the brain revealed a skull base tumor on the right that was found to be a chordoma at the time of surgery.

This is a difficult presentation to diagnose without cranial nerve findings because skull base tumors can be associated with significant complaints of neck pain which may be more prominent than the headache. The tumor would have been detected with a cervical spine MRI. (Chapter 12)

Case 39

The patient had a history of migraine headaches without aura occurring around her menses for many years. She also reported a 5-year history of frequent left-sided headaches that could be of the tension type or related to medication rebound. The acute headache, the worst of her life, could have been a new type of migraine for her, but secondary causes could not be excluded without testing. I gave her a Demerol and Phenergan injection. She wanted to have testing done for the headaches. An MRI scan of the brain with intracranial MRA was normal. A lumbar puncture produced clear CSF, which had normal constituents. She was then given an injection of Imitrex 6 mg subcutaneously that reduced the headache intensity from a 10/10 to a 2/10 within 20 minutes. I advised her to discontinue the Tylenol, Fiorecet, and Prozac and placed her on nortriptyline 25 mg at bedtime for headache prevention. When she was seen 2 weeks later, she had had no mild headaches and only one migraine. Thus she had episodic migraine, tension-type headaches with medication rebound, and the worst headache of her life due to a different presentation of migraine than previously. This case was similar to cases 10, 30, and 31 with an acute presentation of a "first or worst" migraine. (Chapters 1 and 3)

CONCLUSION

I hope you enjoyed playing, "What's my headache?" The cases were selected to demonstrate the spectrum of primary and secondary headaches. If you are in primary care, most of your patients will have primary and benign headaches that can be easily diagnosed and successfully treated. However, you should be aware of the many secondary causes of headaches. If you are a neurologist, you can collect your own interesting series from the wide world of headaches.

REFERENCES

1. Pleasure SJ, Abosch A, Friedman J, et al. Spontaneous intracranial hypotension resulting in stupor caused by diencephalic compression. *Neurology* 1998;50:1854–1857.
2. Schievink WI, Smith KA. Nonpositional headache caused by spontaneous intracranial hypotension. *Neurology* 1998;51:1768–1769.

The Headache Quiz

Randolph W. Evans

Review books based upon questions and answers are becoming increasingly popular. Some of us learn better when it seems as though we are taking a test.

This chapter reviews many of the topics previously covered through questions and answers that are provided in outline form. If you do not like this style of questions, you can make up your own multiple-choice questions for extra credit. If you want to read more about the topic, please refer back to the chapter that is cited.

1. What are the features of tension-type headaches? (Chapter 3)

Often bilateral, pressure or tight feeling

Prevalence, 90%; chronic type, 3%

Average age of onset between 25 and 30 years

Female/male ratio, 5/4

Seventy-five percent of those with chronic tension headaches are females

Prevalence in children through 11 years of age, 35%

2. How do you diagnose tension-type headaches? (Chapters 1 and 3)

Usually on clinical criteria

Early in course or if increased frequency, magnetic resonance imaging (MRI)or computed tomography (CT) scan

In those with chronic headaches and a normal neuro exam, yield on MRI or CT scan is about 2%

EEG not helpful

3. What is the epidemiology of migraine? (Chapter 2)

Prevalence, 18% for women and 6% for men

Prevalence for boys and girls before puberty, 4%

First migraine usually occurs before 40 years of age and 2% of the time after 50 years of age

Sixty percent of migraineurs do not know they have migraine—often "sinus headache"

4. How do you diagnose migraine without aura? (Chapters 1 and 2)

IHS criteria

Simpler criteria for migraine without aura: presence of two out of four

    Unilateral site

    Throbbing quality

    Nausea

    Photophobia or phonophobia

Do not diagnose based on first attack

There should be no evidence of other causes

5. What are migraine triggers? (Chapters 1 and 2)

Present in 85%; median of three triggers/migraineur

Stress, 49%, or let-down headache

Certain foods, 45%

Alcoholic beverages, 52%

Menses for 48% of females

Missing a meal, 40%

Bright sunlight, 38%

Environmental factors: flickering lights, loud noise, high altitude, heat and humidity, smoky rooms, and strong odors

Lack of sleep or oversleeping

Medications such as NTG (nitroglycerin) or OCPs (oral contraceptive pills)

Mild head trauma

6. What are the features of migraine? (Chapter 2)

Typically last 4 to 72 hours in adults without treatment and can last less than 2 hours in children

Unilateral in 60% and bilateral in 40%

Pulsating or throbbing in 50%

Nausea, 90%; vomiting, 30%; light and noise sensitivity, 80%

Migraine without aura, 80%

7. What are the features of migraine with aura? (Chapter 2)

Twenty percent of migraines are migraine with aura

Seventy percent of those with migraine with aura also have headaches without aura

Headache may be unilateral or contralateral to symptoms

Visual auras: photopsias (flashes of light), scotoma (partial loss of vision), teichopsia (fortification spectrum: scotoma that spreads outward with a scintillating edge of zigzag, flashing or occasionally colored)

Unilateral paresthesias and/or numbness often in ipsilateral hand, arm, and side of the face, especially involving the tongue and lips

8. What features of childhood migraine are different from those of adults? (Chapter 7)

Sixty-five percent bilateral (often bifrontal or bitemporal), 35% unilateral

Headache duration often less than 2 hours

9. What are the other types of migraines? (Chapters 7 and 11)

Acephalgic migraine

Ophthalmoplegic

Basilar

Retinal

Complicated with neurologic deficit lasting more than 1 day

Migrainous infarction: deficit lasting more than 7 days

10. What are the results of neuroimaging in migraine? (Chapter 1)

Yield on CT or MRI studies low: about 1%

White matter abnormalities (foci of hyperintensity on both proton density and T2-weighted images in the deep and periventricular white matter due to either interstitial edema or perivascular demyelination) reported in 12% to 46% of migraineurs but also common in controls

11. What are the effects of the menses, menopause, and pregnancy on migraines? (Chapter 8)

Menses: strictly perimenstrual migraine in 7%, trigger for 48%

Menopause: two-thirds improve

Pregnancy: improves or disappears, 60% (often during the second and third trimesters); no change, 20%; more frequent, 20%

12. What are the features of cluster headaches? (Chapter 4)

Percentage of all headache, 0.5%

Male/female ratio, 5:1

Unilateral severe stabbing pain usually in an orbital, retroorbital, or frontotemporal location

Usually accompanied by ipsilateral conjunctival injection, eyelid edema, tearing of the eye, and ipsilateral nasal congestion or clear drainage

Horner (miosis and ptosis) present in 30%

Attacks last 15 to 180 minutes and can occur one to eight times daily

Attacks often at the same time of day or night

Episodic: attacks for weeks to months

Twenty percent have chronic cluster with period exceeding 1 year without spontaneous remission or remissions for less than 2 weeks

Triggers: alcohol and NTG

Diagnosis usually by history

Secondary causes of clusterlike headaches: pituitary tumors, parasellar and upper cervical meningiomas, internal carotid artery and anterior communications artery aneurysms, and arteriovenous malformations

13. What are the features of greater occipital neuralgia? (Chapter 6)

Common and underdiagnosed

Aching, pressure, or throbbing nuchal-occipital and/or parietal, temporal, frontal, peri- or retroorbital distribution

Occasionally true neuralgia with shooting pain

Headache that can last minutes to hours to days

Headache that can occur after head and neck trauma or without trauma

Headache due to entrapment of nerve, myofascial trigger points, C2–3 facet joint, upper cervical spine, or posterior fossa pathology

14. What are the features of sinus headaches? (Chapter 12)

Acute frontal and maxillary sinusitis: frontal or maxillary pain with fever, yellowish-green nasal drainage, and tenderness to palpation

Headache worse with shaking the head or bending head forward

Sphenoid or ethmoid sinusitis: pain may be behind and between the eyes and over the vertex. Can mimic migraine or meningitis

15. What are the features of trigeminal neuralgia? (Chapters 1 and 10)

Severe, sudden, intense, stabbing, or electrical burst of pain lasting less than 30 seconds
Unilateral pain, usually involving V2 or V3; less often, V1
Bilateral pain in about 3%
Trigger zones present
Talking, swallowing, chewing, brushing of teeth, or shaving may trigger
Can have multiple daily paroxysms
Typical onset after 40 years of age
Ratio of women to men, 1.6:1; incidence, 4.3:100,000
Three percent have multiple sclerosis, often with onset before 40 years of age
Eighty percent have vascular compression of the nerve at the root entry zone, usually by branch of superior cerebellar artery
Occasionally, tumors (schwannomas, meningiomas, lymphomas, lipomas, epidermoid, and metastatic and primaries of skull base) are cause

16. What are the features of medication rebound headaches? (Chapter 3)

Can occur in susceptible people taking over-the-counter or prescription medication for more than three doses daily for 3 or more days per week on a regular basis
Medications: ergotamine, butalbital, narcotics, Xanax, ativan, acetaminophen, aspirin, triptans, and less often, nonsteroidal antiinflammatory drugs (NSAIDs)
Caffeine as little as 2 cups per day can cause withdrawal headaches

17. What is the epidemiology of brain tumors? (Chapters 7 and 12)

About 24,000 primaries per year in the United States
> Gliomas, 58%; high-grade astrocytomas, 45% (about 20% present with headaches); meningiomas, 20%; pituitary adenomas, 14%; acoustic neuromas, 8%; and primary central nervous system lymphoma, 2%

About 170,000 new cases of metastatic brain tumors per year in the United States
> Eighty percent occur after diagnosis of primary
> Seventy percent have multiple cerebral metastases
> Primaries in adults
>> Lung, 64%; breast, 14%; unknown, 8%; melanoma, 4%; colorectal, 3%, hypernephroma, 2%; other, 5%
> Primaries in children
>> Most often from sarcomas and germ cell tumors

18. What are the features of headaches due to brain tumors? (Chapter 12)

Of those with brain tumors, 31% to 71% complain of headache
There is no specific brain tumor headache
Headache usually like tension type but occasionally like migraine
"Classic" brain tumor headache only in a minority

Headache can be unilateral or bilateral and in any location

Most headaches intermittent with moderate to severe intensity but can be mild and relieved by over-the-counter medications

Headache often associated with focal findings, seizures, confusion, prolonged nausea

19. What are the features of pseudotumor cerebri? (Chapter 12)

Ninety percent are women and 90% are obese

Mean age of onset, 30 years

Headache present in 94%

Headache usually generalized, severe, pulsatile, and daily

Other symptoms

> Transient visual obscurations, 68%; pulsatile intracranial noises, 58%; photopsia, 54%; and retrobulbar pain, 44%

Signs

> Papilledema in 95%
>
> Sixth cranial nerve palsy in up to 20%
>
> Enlarged blind spots and other field defects in 20%

Secondary causes

> Venous sinus thrombosis, Addison's, hypoparathyroidism, steroid withdrawal, isotretinoin and vitamin A toxicity, anabolic steroids, and lupus

Evaluation

> Normal MRI or CT scan. Empty sella or small ventricular system may be present
>
> Normal CSF except for decreased protein concentration in some cases
>
> On LP, opening pressure >20 cm in nonobese and >25 in obese

20. What are the features of post–lumbar puncture headache? (Chapter 12)

Usually starts within 24 hours and resolves within 7 days

Occurs in up to 40%

Decreased frequency with smaller Quincke needle and atraumatic needle such as Sprotte

Headache usually bilateral, better supine

Neck stiffness, low back pain, nausea, and occasionally blurred vision and tinnitus may be present

Rarely, meningitis or subdural hematoma can occur following lumbar puncture

21. What are the features of first or worst headaches? (Chapter 5)

Chief complaint of 1% of emergency room visits

Differential diagnosis

> Subarachnoid hemorrhage, brain hemorrhage, pituitary apoplexy, acute subdural or epidural hematoma, acute severe hypertension, acute glaucoma, internal carotid dissection, acute ventricular obstruction, benign exertion or orgasmic headache, acute intoxications, acute noncephalic febrile illness, acute mountain sickness

More often subacute onset

Encephalitis, meningitis, sinusitis, periorbital cellulitis, cerebral vein thrombosis, optic neuritis, migraine, stroke, and cerebral vasculitis

Evaluation

CT or MRI scan first and if negative lumbar puncture unless acute meningitis suspected

22. What are the features of subarachnoid hemorrhage? (Chapter 5)

Eighty percent with nontraumatic SAH due to saccular aneurysm rupture that occurs in more than 30,000 people yearly in the United States with 18,000 deaths

General incidence of saccular aneurysms about 2%

Thirty-three percent of SAH during lifting, straining, or sex

Headache typically acute, severe, continuous, and generalized, often with nausea, vomiting, meningismus, focal neuro signs, and loss of consciousness

Eight percent have mild, gradually increasing headache

Headache may be unilateral

Neck or back pain may be present; 8% have no headache at onset

Stiff neck is absent in 36%

23. What are sentinel or warning leak headaches? (Chapter 5)

A sentinel or warning leak headache occurs up to 50% of time before major rupture

Headache usually lasts for several hours or days and can be associated with nausea, vomiting, and syncope

Neuro exam may be normal

Major SAH occurs in days or weeks after sentinel headache in up to 50%

Can easily be misdiagnosed as due to migraine, sinusitis, flu, hypertension, or cervical myositis

24. What does diagnostic testing reveal in subarachnoid hemorrhage? (Chapter 5)

CT scan without contrast

Day 0, 95%; day 3, 74%; 1 week, 50%; 2 weeks, 30%; 3 weeks, 0

Lumbar puncture should be performed if scan is negative

Xanthochromia due to breakdown of red blood cells with release of oxyhemoglobin and then bilirubin by third to fourth day

Xanthochromia present from 2 to 12 hours following bleed and 100% at 1 week, 100% at 2 weeks, 70% at 3 weeks, 40% at 4 weeks

Xanthochromia can be due to jaundice (total bilirubin 10 to 15)

CSF protein greater than 150 mg, dietary hypercarotenemia, malignant melanomatosis, and oral rifampin

Four-vessel cerebral angiogram necessary

Twenty percent have multiple aneurysms

Sixteen percent of initial angios may be false negative; should often be repeated after 2 weeks

MRA up to 88% sensitive in detecting aneurysms ≥5 mm

25. What is a thunderclap headache? (Chapter 5)

A severe headache of sudden maximal onset with a normal CT or MRI scan and normal lumbar puncture

A very small percentage have an unruptured saccular aneurysm or cerebral vasospasm

Expansion, thrombosis, or intramural hemorrhage of aneurysm can cause headache without SAH

26. What types of headaches are associated with sex? (Chapter 13)

Various causes

   Abstinence (according to some people)

   Viagra in about 10% of patients

   Tension type

   Five percent of subarachnoid hemorrhages

Benign orgasmic cephalalgia

   Severe headache with an explosive onset felt in the occipital region, behind the eyes or generalized

   Occurs just before or at orgasm

   Lifetime prevalence about 1%

   Men more than women

   More frequent with orgasms after the first during an encounter

   Testing may be indicated, especially with the first one

Other exertional headaches

   Can occur with running, swimming, weight lifting

27. What are the features of headaches following mild head injury? (Chapter 6)

Headaches occur in 30% to 90% of those symptomatic after mild head injury

Headaches may occur more often and with longer duration with mild than with more severe trauma

Tension type often with greater occipital neuralgia in 85%

Cervicogenic: myofascial injury, cervical disc disease, cervical spondylosis,

C2–3 facet joint injury (third occipital headache)

Footballer's migraine

   Described in young soccer players after mild head injury

   World famous as cause of Terrell Davis' 1998 Superbowl migraine

Migraine with and without aura can be triggered de novo or an increased frequency of preexisting migraine can occur

Other causes

   Supra- and infraorbital neuralgia, dysesthesias over scalp lacerations, hematomas, cluster, carotid and vertebral dissections

28. What are the features of subdural and epidural hematomas? (Chapter 6)

After mild head injury, the incidence for subdurals is about 1% and that for epidurals, less than 1%

Subdural hematomas

   Nonspecific headache

Mild to severe, paroxysmal to constant

When unilateral, usually on same side as subdural

Epidural hematomas

Acute: lucid interval, then coma within 12 hours (talks, then dies)

Chronic in up to 30%

May follow trivial head injury without loss of consciousness in child or young adult

Persistent headache develops, often with nausea, vomiting, and memory impairment, then focal findings

MRI more sensitive than CT scan, which can miss isodense hematoma

CT scan usually preferred in acute setting

29. What are the features of headaches occurring in those past 50 years of age? (Chapter 9)

New-onset tension type rather common but migraine and cluster uncommon

Hypnic headaches

Onset past 45 years of age

Diffuse, throbbing pain but can be unilateral

Awakens patients from sleep same time every night, lasts 15 to 60 minutes

Secondary headaches

Mass lesions, temporal arteritis (TA), medication related, trigeminal neuralgia, postherpetic neuralgia, systemic disease (e.g., infections, acute hypertension, hypoxia or hypercarbia, hypercalcemia, severe anemia, cervicogenic headache, glaucoma, sinusitis, stroke)

30. What are the features of temporal arteritis and headaches? (Chapter 9)

Fifty percent of those with TA have polymyalgia rheumatica (PMR)

15% with PMR have TA

Onset past 50 years of age, with mean age of onset 70 years

Prevalence in population past 50 years of age is 0.13%

Headaches present in 60% to 90%

Can be throbbing, sharp, dull, burning, or lancinating

Intermittent or continuous, more often severe than moderate or mild

May have sensitivity of scalp and face (lying on pillow, combing hair)

Fifty percent have tenderness of the superficial temporal arteries on exam

Location of headache is variable

Only the temple, 25%; temple exclusively or inclusively, 54%; not the temple, 29%; generalized, 8%

Intermittent jaw claudication in 38%

31. How do you diagnose temporal arteritis? (Chapter 9)

American College of Rheumatology 1990 criteria

Presence of three out of five gives sensitivity of 93.5% and specificity of 91%

Age ≥ 50 years
New onset of localized headache
Temporal artery tenderness or decreased pulse
Sed rate at least 50
Positive histology

Sed rate
Increases with age: upper limit of normal (divide man's age by 2; add 10 to woman's age and divide by 2)
TA can be present with normal erythrocyte sedimentation rate (ESR) in up to 36%
When abnormal, average 70 to 80; can be 130

TA biopsy
Demonstrates necrotizing arteritis
False-negative rate, 5% to 44%
Biopsy of contralateral artery increases yield up to 15%
Pathology persists for at least 4 to 5 days after starting steroids

32. What drugs can trigger headaches? (Chapter 3)

Numerous drugs, some examples are provided
Cardiovascular: nitroglycerin, beta-blockers, calcium channel blockers, angiotensin converting enzyme inhibitors, and methyldopa
Nonsteroidal antiinflammatory medications, especially indomethacin
NSAIDs, especially ibuprofen, can cause aseptic meningitis
Sex hormones: oral contraceptives, estrogen replacement therapy, tamoxifen
Amino acids: monosodium glutamate, aspartame (the sweetener)
Histamine receptor antagonists: cimetidine, ranitidine
Antibiotics: amphotericin, griseofulvin, tetracycline, sulfonamides

33. What headaches occur during sleep? (Chapter 13)

Secondary causes of nocturnal headaches: drug withdrawal, temporal arteritis, sleep apnea, oxygen desaturation, pheochromocytomas, primary and secondary neoplasms, communicating hydrocephalus, subdural hematomas, subacute angle-closure glaucoma, and vascular lesions
Primary headaches: migraine, cluster, hypnic, and chronic paroxysmal hemicrania

34. What is the association of headaches and multiple sclerosis? (Chapter 13)

Headaches can be associated with first or subsequent attacks in up to 7%, occasionally simulating migraine with aura
One percent of patients with multiple sclerosis have trigeminal neuralgia and 2% of those with trigeminal neuralgia have multiple sclerosis
Migraine is twice as common in multiple sclerosis patients as in controls

Patient Resources, Educational Materials, and Alternative Treatments

Randolph W. Evans

HEADACHE RESOURCES

American Council for Headache Education

American Council for Headache Education (ACHE) is a nonprofit patient-health professional partnership dedicated to advancing the treatment and management of headache. ACHE's goal is to help headache sufferers gain more control over all aspects of their lives—medical, social, and economic. ACHE offers contact with others, alliance for change, help finding help and education about headache.

19 Mantua Road
Mt. Royal, NJ 08061
Phone: 609-423-0258
Fax: 609-423-0082
Email: achehg@ache.smarthub.com
Web site: http://www.achenet.org

Educational materials that are available include brochures, video tapes, books, and a quarterly newsletter.

National Headache Foundation

The National Headache Foundation (NHF) disseminates free information on headache causes and treatments, funds research, and sponsors public and professional education seminars nationwide. In addition to functioning as a clearinghouse for information, NHF has audio and video tapes, books, brochures, and other helpful materials available for purchase. A nationwide network of local support groups has been organized.

428 W. St. James Place, 2nd Floor
Chicago, IL 60614-2750
Toll free: 800-843-2256
Phone: 773-388-6399
Fax: 773-525-7357
Web site: http://www.headaches.org

Internet Web Sites

There are numerous additional internet Web sites with headache information. Here are a few with migraine information:

The Journal of the American Medical Association Migraine Information Center: http://www.ama-assn.org/special/migraine
Glaxo Wellcome Migraine Resource Center: http://www.migrainehelp.com

Excedrin Headache Resource Center: http://www.excedrin.com
MAGNUM (Migraine Awareness Group: A National Under-
  standing for Migraineurs): http://www.migraines.org
Merck Migraine site: http://www.merck.com/disease/migraines

CAFFEINE CONTENT OF SELECTED BEVERAGES, FOODS, OVER-THE-COUNTER AND PRESCRIPTION MEDICATIONS*

Daily use of caffeine in susceptible persons can cause frequent
headaches, caffeine rebound headaches. People often recognize
this headache as due to coffee. In fact, as few as 2 cups of coffee
per day can be responsible. However, you may not be aware that
caffeine is also present in a variety of other beverages, foods,
over-the-counter, and prescription medications (see later). The
headache typically is present in the morning and goes away after
consuming caffeine. If you have this type of headache, slowly
tapering off of caffeine can eliminate the headaches.

Coffee

Brewed, 8 oz	135 mg
Instant, 8 oz	95 mg
Starbucks espresso, 1 oz	89 mg
Decaffeinated, 8 oz	5 mg

Soft drinks

Coca-Cola, 12 oz	45 mg
Diet Coke, 12 oz	47 mg
Dr. Pepper, 12 oz	41 mg
Pepsi-Cola, 12 oz	37 mg
Sunkist Orange Soda, 12 oz	40 mg
Mountain Dew, 12 oz	55 mg
Jolt, 12 oz	71 mg
Josta, 12 oz	58 mg
7-UP, 12 oz	0
Sprite, 12 oz	0

Tea

Lipton tea, 8 oz	35–40 mg
Snapple iced tea, all varieties, 16 oz	48 mg
Celestial Seasonings herbal tea, all varieties, 8 oz	0
Lipton Natural Brew Iced Tea Mix, decaffeinated, 8 oz	Less than 5 mg

Caffeinated waters

Java Water, 16.9 oz	125 mg
Krank20, 16.9 oz	100 mg
Aqua Blast, 16.9 oz	90 mg
Water Joe, 16.9 oz	60–70 mg
Aqua Java, 16.9 oz	50–60 mg

Chocolate

Hershey's Special Dark Chocolate Bar, 1.5 oz	31 mg

*Source: The Center for Science in the Public Interest, product labels, and the
Physicians' Desk Reference.

Hershey Bar, 10 mg.	10 mg
Hot chocolate, 8 oz	5 mg

Yogurt and Ice Cream

Ben & Jerry's No Fat Coffee Fudge Frozen Yogurt, 1 cup	85 mg
Starbucks Coffee Ice Cream, 1 cup	40–60 mg
Haagen-Dazs Coffee Fudge Ice Cream, 1 cup	30 mg
Dannon Coffee Yogurt, 8 oz	45 mg
Stonyfield Farm Cappucino Yogurt, 8 oz	0

Over-the-Counter Medications

NoDoz maximum strength, 1 tablet	200 mg
NoDoz regular strength, 1 tablet	100 mg
Excedrin, Extra-Strength, 2 tablets	130 mg
Excedrin Migraine, 2 tablets	130 mg
Anacin, 2 tablets	64 mg
Advil, Nuprin	0
Aleve	0

Prescription Medications

Fiorinal	40 mg
Esgic	40 mg
Cafergot	100 mg
Darvon Compound-65	32.4 mg

AN EXPLANATION OF HYPERVENTILATION SYNDROME*

Hyperventilation (overbreathing) attacks are the commonest cause of dizziness and are often associated with headache. They can be overcome by recognizing the cause and following a few simple rules.

What are the symptoms?

A person may have one or any number of the following symptoms:

Light-headedness, dizziness, faintness, giddiness
Tightness or pain in the chest
Shortness of breath or difficulty getting a good breath
Dry mouth
Faster heartbeat
Blurring of vision
Sweating
Trembling of hands and legs
Weakness ("jelly legs")
Pins and needles in hands, feet, and around the mouth
Headache
Anxiety, fear, or panic
Sensation of being unable to breathe
Spasms of hands and feet
A feeling of having a heart attack, passing out, losing control, or being about to die

*From Lance JW, Goadsby PJ. *Mechanism and management of headache*, 6th ed. Oxford: Butterworth-Heinemann, 1998; modified, with permission.

When you overbreathe you may swallow air, causing:

Distension of the stomach
Burping
Passing gas

What do we mean by overbreathing?

Deep, sighing breaths
Yawning often
Rapid shallow breathing
Deep breathing
There are two types of hyperventilation: acute, which affects 1%, and chronic, which affects 99% of patients
Acute hyperventilation is obvious when someone is breathing way too fast
Chronic hyperventilation is not obvious: You can breathe a little too fast and a little too deeply and cause hyperventilation, but neither you nor your doctor can tell just by looking at you during a spell

When is this most likely to happen?

When you are tense, bored, or depressed
In crowds, at a party, or out shopping

How does this cause symptoms?

Normally, nature takes care of the rate and depth of breathing. The carbon dioxide in your blood makes you breathe enough to eliminate it and get sufficient oxygen. If you override nature and breathe too much, you wash out too much carbon dioxide. This reduces the blood flow to your brain and makes you feel dizzy. It also reduces the available calcium in the blood, which can cause "pins and needles," numbness and tingling, and cause spasms of the hands and feet. Adrenaline increases in the bloodstream, causing a feeling of anxiety, sweating, and trembling, and makes the heart beat faster.
Contraction of muscles causes pain and tightness in the chest and headache.

How can you stop it?

Look for the first signs of sighing or yawning
Do not:
Open the windows.
Run outside.
Take deep breaths.
Instead:
Sit down.
Hold your breath and count to 10.
Breathe out slowly and say "relax" to yourself.
Then breathe in and out slowly every 6 seconds (10 breaths per minute).
If you wish, you may instead breathe into a lunch bag placed over your nose and mouth for a minute or so.
As soon as possible, forget about your breathing and let nature do it for you.

General principles

Take it easy. It is not a disaster if you forget someone's name, burn the dinner, or don't have time to mow the lawn. Talk more slowly. Walk more slowly. You have plenty of time.

Think positively. You can handle a problem as well as the next person.

Everyone else has problems, too. Spread out your workload through the day.

Give yourself enough time for each task.

Remain calm.

Don't bottle up your feelings—discuss any worries or things that make you angry or upset.

Eat regular meals and don't hurry them.

Limit caffeine in soft drinks, coffee, or tea.

Learn to recognize any tendency to overbreathe.

Learn to relax your muscles—no frowning or jaw-clenching.

Exercise regularly.

Take time out for social activities and holidays.

You can control your attacks completely by following these rules.

A HEADACHE DIARY

For patients with frequent headaches, a headache diary is very useful to document the frequency, possible triggers, and response to treatment. Headache diaries can range from just a piece of paper to a formal headache diary. See pages 298 and 299 for an example of a key for a headache diary, as well as a headache diary in chart form.

A BRIEF DESCRIPTION OF ALTERNATIVE AND COMPLEMENTARY TREATMENTS USED FOR HEADACHES: ALTERNATIVE TREATMENTS FROM A-Y

In the United States, 42% of the adult population used alternative therapy in 1997.[1] Thirteen percent used alternative treatments for headaches, including 42% who saw a medical doctor and used alternative therapy and 20% who saw a medical doctor and an alternative practitioner for headaches. According to a patient survey in the United States, alternative medicine users find these approaches to be more congruent with their own values, beliefs, and philosophical orientations toward health and life.[2]

Despite advances, physicians and patients need all the help they can get in treating headaches. Consider the pharmacotherapy of migraine. Individual preventive medications have an efficacy of only about 60%, with a number of possible side effects. Triptans reduce or relieve migraine for 70% to 80%, depending upon the route of administration, but what about the unaided 20% to 30%? In addition, transformed migraine and medication rebound are significant concerns.

Informed physicians can do their patients a service by providing unbiased information and suggesting and reading reference sources such as the books by Cassileth,[3] Mauskop and Brill,[4] and Jonas and Levin.[5] As Jonas states, "Alternative medicine is here to stay. It is no longer an option to ignore it or treat it as something outside the normal processes of science and medicine."[6]

KEYS FOR HEADACHE DIARY

1. INTENSITY

1=Mild   2=Moderate   3=Severe

2. HEADACHE INTENSITY AFTER MEDICATION

0=None   1=Mild   2=Moderate   3=Severe

3. EMOTIONAL STRESS TRIGGERS

1—Family or friends
2—Work
3—Social life
4—Financial difficulties
5—Relaxation after stress
6—Other

4. PHYSICAL TRIGGERS

1—Fatigue
2—Lack of sleep
3—Oversleeping
4—Bright/flashing lights
5—Sun or glare
6—Loud noise
7—Strong smells
8—Heat/high humidity
9—Menstruation
10—Exercise or labor
11—High altitude
12—Travel
13—Vacation
14—Weekend
15—Other

5. FOOD AND DRINK TRIGGERS

1—Missing a meal
2—Chocolate
3—Cheese
4—Citrus fruit
5—MSG
6—Hot dogs or cured meat
7—Alcohol or beer
8—Wine
9—Other

HEADACHE DIARY

Patient's name _____

Date started _____

Date of Headache	Time Started	Time Stopped	1 Intensity	Medication taken	2 Intensity after medication	3 Emotional stress triggers	4 Physical triggers	5 Food and drink triggers

Although many alternative medicine treatments may have merit, others may be no better than expensive placebos. As Angell and Kassirer insist, "Alternative treatments should be subjected to scientific testing no less rigorous than that required for conventional treatments."[7] In a sense, there is no alternative medicine; there is only medicine that works and medicine that does not work.

Numerous alternative and complementary treatments are used for headaches. There are varying amounts of scientific evidence for effectiveness.[8a] A brief description of some of the treatments from A to Y follows.

Acupuncture

Acupuncture is a medical therapy developed in China more than 2,000 years ago. Hua Tuo, a third-century A.D. Chinese surgeon, is credited with being the first to use acupuncture for headache. Acupuncture was introduced to physicians in the United States by William Osler in the late nineteenth century.

Very thin, disposable needles of varying length are placed into the skin at specific points along meridians or channels. There are 12 main meridians that are believed to be connected to a specific organ system of the body. By needling acupoints of a particular meridian, a problem in a distant area of the body can be treated. Needles are usually kept in place for less than 30 minutes. Twirling or other motion of the needles is believed to enhance the effect. Acupuncture may be effective in reducing a variety of headaches,[8a] including migraine,[9] tension,[10] and posttraumatic.

Aromatherapy

Practitioners believe that when essential oils from plants are inhaled or absorbed through the skin, they can alleviate headaches, including migraines and tension-type headaches.[11] Aromatherapy may help reduce stress. Some people can have allergic reactions to the oils.

Biofeedback

Biofeedback is a Western approach to meditation (see later) with the goal of producing beneficial physiologic changes. Monitoring equipment provides visual or audible signs of muscle and autonomic activity. The most common types of biofeedback are electromyography (surface electrodes are used to monitor muscle activity), thermal (measurement of skin temperature), electrodermal activity (measures changes in perspiration), finger pulse (measures pulse rate and the amount of blood in each pulse), and respiration feedback (measures the rate, volume, and rhythm of the patient's breathing).

EMG and thermal biofeedback are used for treatment of headaches. The therapist teaches relaxation techniques to use in conjunction with biofeeback. Biofeedback has been demonstrated to be effective in treating pediatric migraine[12] and tension headaches[13] and adult migraine and tension headaches.[14,15]

Chiropractic

Chiropractic (from the Greek for "done by hand") was founded in the 1890s in Davenport, Iowa, by D. D. Palmer. There are now some 50,000 chiropractors in the United States who saw 11% of the adult population in 1997. Misaligned vertebrae or subluxations are believed to interfere with the transmission of nerve impulses. "Straight" chiropractors focus almost exclusively on manual manipulation, whereas "mixers" use other treatments, such as nutritional counseling and exercise with manipulation. The hand is used to manipulate the spine with high-velocity, low-force recoiling thrusts or rotational thrusts with the hands or elbows. Some patients with headaches may benefit from chiropractic treatment.[16] Recent studies have found benefit for cervicogenic headaches[17] but no benefit for treatment of episodic tension-type headache.[18] Uncontrolled studies have reported benefit for migraine.[19]

Herbal medicine

There are numerous herbs (plants or plant parts) with purported medicinal value. The use of herbal medicine has been documented as far back as Neanderthal man 60,000 years ago. More than one-fourth of conventional pharmaceuticals come from herbs. Feverfew may be effective in reducing migraines.[20]

Hypnosis

The induction of hypnotic states has existed at least since early recorded history. The Viennese physician Franz Mesmer popularized medical hypnosis in the late 1700s to treat imbalances of animal magnetism ("mesmerize"). Freud used hypnosis in conjunction with psychoanalysis in the early 1900s.

Hypnosis (from the Greek word for "sleep") is a state of focused attention or altered consciousness that makes the participant highly receptive to suggestion and allows a person to concentrate intently on a particular subject, memory, sensation, or problem. Patients can go to a hypnotherapist or learn self-hypnosis. Hypnosis can be effective in treating pediatric[21] and adult migraine.[22]

Massage

Therapeutic touch can reduce headaches such as chronic tension type.[23] The history of massage goes back 4,000 to 5,000 years. Hippocrates described massage as an effective treatment for sports and war injuries. There are numerous types of massage.

Swedish massage (devised by the nineteenth-century Swedish physician Per Henrik Ling) uses a system of long strokes, kneading, and friction techniques on superficial muscles and active and passive movements of joints. There are five types of strokes: effleurage (long, gliding stroke performed with the whole hand or thumb), petrissage (kneading and compression movements), friction (deep circular movements made with the thumb pads or fingertips), vibration (a fine, rapid, shaking movement), and tapotement (use of the hands to alternatively strike or tap the muscles).

Deep-muscle and connective-tissue massage uses deep finger pressure and slow strokes on contracted areas. Trigger-point therapy uses concentrated finger pressure on trigger points.

Shiatsu (Japanese for "finger pressure") and acupressure use finger pressure massage on special points along acupuncture meridiens to unblock and balance qi, the body's hypothesized flow of energy.

Reflexology uses digital pressure on target points on the feet, which refer, or "reflex," to all areas of the body to help heal distant areas. Reflexology was started by an ENT physician, William Fitzgerald, in the early twentieth century.

Rolfing, or structural integration, was devised by Ida Rolf, who had a doctorate in physiology, in the 1950s. The therapist uses fingertips, knuckles, elbows, and sometimes knees to knead muscle and tissue layers.

Meditation

Medicine and *meditation* have the same Latin root meaning "to cure" and "to measure" (in the sense of bringing the mind and body to its right inward measure). Most meditation techniques derive from Eastern religious practices and involve intense concentration on a breath, word, sound, prayer, or phrase while excluding all outside thoughts. Meditation can be practiced while sitting (Transcendental meditation), standing or lying down (e.g., qigong—the willful manipulation of the vital life force, or *qi*), or moving (tai chi chu'an—Buddhist mindfulness meditation). Meditation and other relaxation techniques may be effective in treating migraines, tension, and other headaches.

There are some Western approaches to meditation. The German physician Schultz developed *autogenic training*, which means "coming from the self." This is a simple exercise that combines verbal, visual, and sensory imagery to relax different parts of the body. In the late 1960s, the cardiologist Herbert Benson studied the beneficial physiologic effects of meditation, which he termed the *relaxation response*. This response can be induced by a variety of techniques, including meditation, prayer, progressive muscle relaxation, hypnosis, and yoga.

Osteopathy

Andrew Taylor Still founded the first medical school for osteopathy (literally, "disease from the bones") in Missouri in 1874. Today medical school for osteopaths is similar to that for medical doctors with the addition of training in osteopathic medical manipulations or manual therapy, including soft-tissue technique, myofascial release, cranial osteopathy, lymphatic technique, thrust technique, muscle energy technique, counterstrain, and visceral techniques. Osteopaths can specialize in medical and surgical specialties or primary care.

Cranial osteopathy involves pressure and massage of the muscles and fascia surrounding the skull to take pressure off the nerves of the skull, improve blood flow, and improve the flow of cerebrospinal fluid within the head. Craniosacral therapy is also practiced by chiropractors.

Progressive Relaxation

Progressive relaxation, developed by Edmund Jacobsen in the 1920s, is a series of steps or exercises to relax the muscles that may be effective for tension- and migraine-type headaches.[24,25] Relaxation techniques are often used in combination with biofeedback. An example of progressive relaxation exercises is provided in the next section.

Yoga

Yoga (from the Sanskrit word for "union") is an ancient Eastern philosophy and exercise of health and well-being that combines movements and simple poses with deep breathing and meditation to unite the soul with a universal spirit. A life energy, Prana, is believed to flow through and vitalize the body. Yoga may be beneficial for headaches, including migraines.[26]

A SIMPLE MEDITATION EXERCISE*

This simple meditation exercise can be practiced by anyone.

1. Find a comfortable position—lying down or sitting either on the floor or in a straight-backed chair. If sitting, keep your back straight without being rigid and let your hands rest in your lap. If your feet don't reach the floor, place a stool or books beneath them so that they rest on a firm surface.
2. Scan your body for tension from head to toe and relax your muscles. Unknit your eyebrows and unclench your jaw. Release your shoulders, arms, and belly. Let your spine lengthen, without becoming rigid, and your chin pull gently inward. Let your pelvis sink into the chair or ground.
3. Be aware of the sensation of your body touching the earth (or firm surface).
4. Close your eyes if you feel it's more comfortable.
5. Focus your mind on your breath as you inhale naturally. Breathe through your nose if you can. Feel the breath fill your chest and then your belly. Keep focused on the breath as you exhale, feeling it leave your belly and your chest. Alternatively, you can focus on the sensation of breath entering and leaving your nostrils.
6. Keep your eyes directed toward the end of your nose.
7. Keep your mind focused on your breath.
8. When thoughts cross your mind, gently note them, let them pass, and return to your breathing. Each time this happens, simply return to the breath.
9. Continue for fifteen minutes. It's okay to check the clock every so often.
10. Sit quietly for a few minutes.

You can use the breath as a focus, or select a word. Any simple, positive word or name will suffice.

A PROGRESSIVE RELAXATION EXERCISE†

1. Get comfortable. Wear loose clothing, remove your shoes. Make sure you are neither too warm nor too cold. Find a quiet room where you won't be distracted for fifteen minutes.
2. Sit in a comfortable chair, or lie down on the ground on your back, using an exercise mat or soft carpet.
3. Take a few deep, easy breaths.
4. Tense all of the muscles in your body, from head to toe. Hold the tension for several seconds. Let your mind feel the sensation of this tension.
5. Holding on to the tension, inhale deeply and hold your breath for several seconds. Let your mind and body register the sensation of this tension.

*From Mauskop A, Brill MA. *The headache alternative: a neurologist's guide to drug-free relief.* New York: Dell, 1997:276–277, with permission.
†From Mauskop A, Brill MA. *The headache alternative: a neurologist's guide to drug-free relief.* New York: Dell, 1997:264–265, with permission.

6. Exhale slowly as you let the tension go by. Let your mind and body register the sensation of this relaxation.

Now, work on individual muscle groups. As you tense the following muscles, try to keep the rest of your muscles as relaxed as possible. Repeat each of the following exercises three times.

1. Tighten your fists. Feel the tension radiating up your arms. Inhale deeply and hold the tension for several seconds. Exhale and let your hands relax.
2. Press your arms against the ground or chair. Inhale and hold the tension for several seconds, concentrating on the sensation. Exhale and let your arms relax.
3. Shrug your shoulders up to your eyes. Experience the tension in your neck and shoulders. Inhale and hold. Exhale and let your shoulders drop.
4. Frown and raise your eyebrows. Study the tightness in your face. Inhale and hold the tension. Exhale and release.
5. Press your eyelids closed as tightly as possible. Inhale and hold. Exhale and open your eyes gently.
6. Open your mouth as wide as possible. Inhale and hold. Exhale and release your jaw.
7. Clench your jaw, biting down with your teeth. Feel the tension spread across your skull. Inhale and hold. Exhale and release.
8. Inhale deeply into your belly, letting your chest expand. Hold the chest tension. Exhale and let your breath return to normal.
9. Tighten your abdominal muscles. Hold, then relax.
10. Arch your back, chest up and hips down. Inhale and hold. Exhale and release your back gently.
11. Tighten your hips and buttocks. Inhale and hold. Exhale and relax.
12. Tense your left leg, from thigh to heel. Inhale and hold. Exhale and relax.
13. Tense your right leg, from thigh to heel. Inhale and hold. Exhale and relax.
14. Curl your toes under. Inhale and hold. Exhale and relax.
15. Remaining still, scan your body. Experience the relaxation over your entire body. If you need to, return to areas of tension and repeat the exercise for that muscle group. Breathe naturally and deeply for several moments, experiencing the relaxed state. Gently and slowly stand up.

REFERENCES

1. Eisenberg DM, Davis RB, Ettner SL, et al. Trends in alternative medicine use in the United States, 1990–1997: results of a follow-up national survey. *JAMA* 1998;280:1569–1575.
2. Astin J. Why patients use alternative medicine: results of a national study. *JAMA* 1998;279:1548–1553.
3. Cassileth BR. *The alternative medicine handbook: the complete reference guide to alternative and complementary therapies.* New York: WW Norton, 1998.
4. Mauskop A, Brill MA. *The headache alternative: a neurologist's guide to drug-free relief.* New York: Dell, 1997.
5. Jonas WB, Levin JS. *Essentials of complementary and alternative medicine.* Philadelphia: Lippincott-Williams & Wilkins, 1999.

6. Jonas WB. Alternative medicine: learning from the past, examining the present, advancing to the future. *JAMA* 1998;280: 1616–1618.

7. Angell M, Kassirer JP. Alternative medicine: the risks of untested and unregulated remedies. *N Engl J Med* 1998;339:839–841.

8. Henninger MI, Holroyd KA, Lipchik GI. Acupuncture and chiropractic treatments for headache. *Headache* 1999;39:357.

8a. Melchart D, Linde K, Fischer P, et al. Acupuncture for recurrent headaches: a systematic review of randomized controlled trials. *Cephalagia* 1999;19:779–786.

9. Baischer W. Acupuncture in migraine: long-term outcome and predicting factors. *Headache* 1995;35:472–474.

10. Vincent CA. The treatment of tension headache by acupuncture: a controlled single case design with time series analysis. *J Psychosom Res* 1990;34:553–561.

11. Schattner P, Randerson D. Tiger balm as a treatment of tension headache. *Austral Family Physician* 1996;25:216–222.

12. Hermann C, Blanchard EB, Flor H. Biofeedback treatment for pediatric migraine: prediction of treatment outcome. *J Consult Clin Psychol* 1997;65:611–616.

13. Grazzi L, Leone M, Fediani F, Bussone G. A therapeutic alternative for tension headache in children: treatment and one-year follow-up results. *Biofeedback Self Regul* 1990;15:1–6.

14. Arena JG, Bruno GM, Hannah SL, Meador KJ. A comparison of frontal electromyographic biofeedback training, trapezius electromyographic biofeedback training, and progressive muscle relaxation therapy in the treatment of tension headache. *Headache* 1995;35:411–419.

15. Grazzi L, Bussone G. Effect of biofeedback treatment on sympathetic function in common migraine and tension-type headache. *Cephalalgia* 1993;13:197–200.

16. Shekelle PG, Coulter I. Cervical spine manipulation: summary report of a systematic review of the literature and a multidisciplinary expert panel. *J Spinal Disorders* 1997;10:223–228.

17. Nilsson N, Christensen HW, Hartvigsen J. The effect of spinal manipulation in the treatment of cervicogenic headache. *J Manipulative Physiol Ther* 1997;20:326–330.

18. Bove G, Nilsson N. Spinal manipulation in the treatment of episodic tension-type headache: a randomized controlled trial. *JAMA* 1998;280:1576–1579.

19. Chapman-Smith D. Chiropractic management of headache. *Chiropractic Rep* 1991;5:1–6.

20. Murphy JJ, Heptinstall S, Mitchell JRA. Randomized double-blind placebo-controlled trial of feverfew in migraine prevention. *Lancet* 1988;2:189–192.

21. Olness K, MacDonald JT, Uden DL. Comparison of self-hypnosis and propranolol in the treatment of juvenile classic migraine. *Pediatrics* 1987;79:593–597.

22. Reich BA. Non-invasive treatment of vascular and muscle contraction headache: a comparative longitudinal clinical study. *Headache* 1989;29:34–41.

23. Puustjarvi K, Airaksinen O, Pontinen PJ. The effects of massage in patients with chronic tension headache. *Acupunct Electrother Res* 1990;15:159–162.

24. Holroyd KA, Penzien DB. Pharmacological versus non-pharma-

cological prophylaxis of recurrent migraine headache: a meta-analytic review of clinical trials. *Pain* 1990;42:1–13.
25. Engel JM, Rapoff MA, Pressman AR. Long-term follow-up of relaxation training for pediatric headache disorders. *Headache* 1992;32:152–156.
26. Monro R, Ghosh AK, Kalish D. *Yoga research bibliography, scientific studies on yoga and meditation.* Cambridge, England: Yoga Biomedical Trust, 1989.

Subject Index

Subject Index

Range-of-motion exercise, 134
Ranitidine-related migraine, 29t
Rational copharmacy
  for chronic daily headache,
    80
  in migraine prophylaxis,
    54–55
Rebound headache. *See also*
    Analgesic rebound
    headache; Medication
    rebound headache
  case presentation of, 266
  definition of, 70
Recurrence, definition of, 70
Recurrent headache, 264
Red blood cells, 113
Red ear syndrome, 231
Red eye, 223t
Reflexology, 301
Relaxation response, 302
Relaxation therapy, 302
  for childhood migraine, 145
  for episodic tension-type
    headache, 77
  exercise for, 303–304
Relieving factors, 9
Relpax (eletriptan), 41, 56t
  dosage and preparations of,
    40t
REM rebound, 72
REM sleep, 88
Reserpine-related migraine, 29t
Resource organizations,
    293–294
Respiratory alkalosis, 250
Retinal migraine, 195–196
Retroorbital pain, 265–266
Rhinosinusitis, 224
Rhizotomy, radiofrequency
    trigeminal
  for intractable cluster
    headache, 101–102
  observations on, 102
Riboflavin, 45t, 53
Rifampin, 241
Rizatriptan (Maxalt)
  cautions and
    contraindications to
    combination therapy
    with, 56t
  clinical use of, 42
  dosage and preparations of,
    40t
  efficacy rate of, 41

  for migraine, 37, 274
  pharmacokinetics of, 39t
Rocephin, 278
Rolfing, 301

S
Sarcoidosis, nervous system,
    246
Scalp lacerations, 122
Scintigraphic imaging, 204
Scleritis, 223
Scotoma, migraine, 28f
Second-impact syndrome, 124
Seizure disorder, posttraumatic,
    124
Seizures
  headaches and, 253–254
  versus migraine, 172
  migraine and, 253
  partial
    in basilar migraine, 143
    in vertigo, 143–144
Selective serotonin receptor
    agonists, 1
Selective serotonin reuptake
    inhibitors
  in combination therapy for
    migraine, 55
  efficacy and side effects of,
    49t
  for migraine prophylaxis, 45t,
    50
  withdrawal of, 46
Sensory root section, 191
Sentinel headache
  definition of, 289
  in subarachnoid hemorrhage,
    197
Serotonin
  in migraine, 36
  mobilization of precipitating
    migraine, 44–45
  in pain modulation, 74–75
  receptors for, 36
Serum Lyme antibody testing,
    246
Serzone (nefazodone), 50
Sex hormones, triggering
    headache, 292
Sexual headache
  benign explosive type, 270
  case presentation of, 259–260
  clinical manifestations of,
    236–237